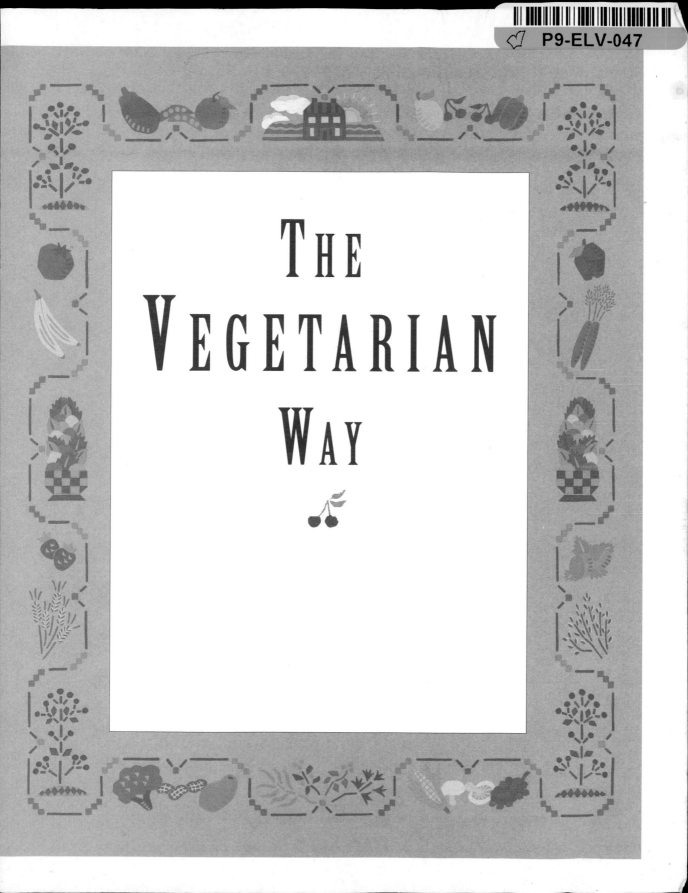

THE VEGETARIAN WAY

THE VEGETARIAN WAY

Total Health for You and Your Family

VIRGINIA MESSINA, MPH, RD
AND
MARK MESSINA, PHD

Crown Trade Paperbacks • New York

To Noah, Sarah, Christen, Christopher, B.J., Lenore, and Miss Juliet—
may the world you inherit be one where people are healthy, kind to animals,
and respectful of the environment.

Copyright © 1996 by Virginia Messina and Mark Messina
Published by Crown Trade Paperbacks, 201 East 50th Street, New York, New York 10022.
Member of the Crown Publishing Group.
Random House, Inc. New York, Toronto, London, Sydney, Auckland
CROWN TRADE PAPERBACKS and colophon are trademarks of Crown Publishers, Inc.
Printed in the U.S.A.
Design by Blond on Pond
Library of Congress Cataloging-in-Publication Data
Messina, Virginia.
   The vegetarian way: total health for you and your family / Virginia and Mark Messina. — 1st ed.
   Includes index.
   1. Vegetarianism.   2. Vegetarian cookery.   I. Messina, Mark.   II. Title.
RM236.M444 1996
613.2'62—dc20   95-34599
ISBN 0-517-88275-2
10 9 8 7 6 5 4 3

ACKNOWLEDGMENTS

Joseph Campbell said, "Follow your heart and the world rushes to help." When we first told friends and colleagues about our plan to write this book, and how much this project meant to us, the response was always the same: "What a great idea! How can I help?" And, over the two years during which this project evolved from an outline to a book, many, many people did help—sometimes in ways that probably weren't even apparent to them.

First and always, our thanks to Patti Breitman, our talented agent whose enthusiasm for this book matched our own from the very start and never waned for a second. We were lucky to work with two excellent editors at Harmony Books. Valerie Kuscenko cheerfully and skillfully dealt with two stubborn authors and helped us to sort and shift and refine and rewrite. Sherri Rifkin picked up our book right in the middle of the project and with amazing aplomb saw it through its final stages. We also were fortunate to have the world's best copy editor, Susan Betz, work on this manuscript.

We are fortunate to count among our friends dietitians who are some of the most knowledgeable experts on vegetarian nutrition. Our wonderful friend Mary Clifford, R.D., spent hours in the library tracking down obscure dietary details for us, read drafts, reviewed guidelines, and contributed recipes—and, as if that wasn't enough, she helped to move us and a bevy of neurotic cats 3,500 miles across the country right smack in the middle of this project. Reed Mangels, Ph.D., R.D., took time to review all of our chapters on vegetarian diets for children and pregnant women. Reed's generous help and her extensive knowledge on these topics were indispensable to us in writing this book. Suzanne Havala, M.S., R.D., also gave us helpful comments about our meal planning guidelines for vegetarians, helped us to formulate the best recommendations for meatless meal planning, and was always there to commiserate about or share in the joys of book-writing.

Sally Clinton, publisher of the teen vegetarian magazine *How On Earth!* and a tireless advocate for the vegetarian diet, took time out of a very busy schedule to perform laborious nutritional analyses on the menus in this book. We're grateful for her friendship, her work on this book, and all the wonderful things she does to teach young people about vegetarian diet. Chy Lin, a *How on Earth!* volunteer, made numerous runs to the library for us to track down answers to our questions about environmental and farm animal issues.

It's easy to write a book when you have friends who are talented geniuses. Our computer gurus made our lives infinitely easier. Brad Scott, of the Vegetarian Resource Group, can solve any computer problem in the world and can even do so long distance. His computer savvy is matched only by his unending patience. Kevin Cook set our computers up so that we could actually find things on them. Bobbi Pasternak knows every vegetarian resource on the Internet and is tireless in her efforts to educate vegetarians via that resource. We're grateful to her for helping us to get plugged into vegetarianism on the Net.

And we would never have *been* plugged in if not for our wonderful friends Kate and Ned Schumann, who brought the Internet to Port Townsend, Washington, and brought *us* to this paradise as well. A special thank-you to Kate for her helpful comments on chapter drafts, for encouraging Ginny to take a few stress breaks now and then, for great coffee and conversation, and for all those wonderful flowers.

We spent much time tracking down the "real story" on vitamin B_{12} and are grateful to two true vegetarian pioneers for taking the time to talk with us about this complex issue. Thanks to Dr. Agatha Thrash of the Yucchi Pines Institute for warmly and generously sharing her time with us and for being so enthusiastic about this book. And our gratitude to long-time vegetarian nutrition researcher Dr. Mervyn Hardinge, who came out of retirement for a few minutes to give us the real scoop on vitamin B_{12}.

In order to have a few "strangers" review portions of this book, we sent out a plea for help to the vegan-1 mailing list on the Internet and were completely overwhelmed with responses. We thank the more than sixty people from that list who responded and wish we could have used the services of every one of them. A special thanks to those who did read portions of the book—Larry Kaiser, Jeanne Kaiser, Jim Ferraiolo, and Judy Ferraiolo—and especially to Elyse Abraham, who put her expertise as a psycholinguist to use in reviewing chapters and to Mary Daly for bringing the almost-vegetarian perspective to her review.

Good friends make anything possible. Thanks to Ginny's friends from way, way back—Joan Petrokofsky and Lynn Myhal—for testing recipes and reading drafts, for cheery phone calls and silly e-mail. To our wonderful vegetarian friends, especially those from PCRM, Louise Holton, Chrissie and Dale Bartlett, and Melissa Goldman, for all those great vegetarian dinners in D.C. and the never-ending alley cat escapades. A very special thanks to Mark's friend David Snyder, the world's biggest veggie burger fan.

There would be no interest in a book of this type if not for the fact that many, many people have worked so hard to educate Americans about vegetarianism and to promote interest in this way of eating. We're honored to know and work with some of these people. Most importantly, we thank Charles Stahler and Debra Wasserman of the Vegetarian Resource Group, two people who have done more to educate consumers about vegetarianism than anyone else we can think of. Warm thanks to Dr. Neal Barnard, president of the Physicians Committee for Responsible Medicine and indefatigable vegetarian advocate, for his important work and for letting us play some small role in that work. Our thanks also to Bill Shurtleff of the Soyfoods Center for sharing his incredible knowledge of soyfoods and vegetarian history, and to Jennie

Collura of the North American Vegetarian Society for letting us participate in her efforts toward vegetarian education.

Finally and most importantly, we thank our families for their love and support. Our greatest thanks and love go to our parents Bill and Willie Kisch and Carmen and Eileen Messina for always believing in us and for always having some vegetarian food on the table. To Bill and Irma and Steve and Agnes for putting up with meatless lasagna and tofu cream pie (and for admitting that they taste good!), and to John and Pat for being terrific vegetarian role models.

CONTENTS

INTRODUCTION

It always amuses us when someone describes a vegetarian diet as "alternative." Well, it may seem alternative compared with the style of eating that most of us were raised on, but in the bigger scheme of things, a diet based on plant foods is actually the most ordinary way of eating in the world. What's more, a diet centered on grains, beans, vegetables, and fruits is the natural diet of humans and the one that best supports our optimal health.

Vegetarianism isn't a radical departure from "normal" eating patterns. Rather, it takes us back to where we belong. It is the diet best suited to human nutrition and health needs. It is the diet most compatible with the earth's resources. It is the diet that best addresses world food needs and world hunger.

But despite that, a vegetarian diet is likely to raise questions and concerns for many people. These run the whole gamut. Not just "where do you get your protein" but "where do you shop, how do you get kids to eat vegetables, and what happens when you have dinner at the boss's house and she serves filet mignon." We wrote this book in order to answer those questions and deal with such concerns. Our goal is to give you a complete overview of what you need to know about vegetarian diets—from raising vegetarian children, to losing weight on a meatless diet, to figuring out what to do with tofu.

We expect that our readers will approach this book from varied perspectives. Perhaps you are a new vegetarian or are contemplating the plunge, but you have questions about meeting nutrient needs and planning meals. Maybe you and your spouse have been carefree, healthy vegetarians for years, but the imminent arrival of a new baby has raised all kinds of questions. Or maybe you had absolutely no interest in a vegetarian diet until last week when your sixteen-year-old daughter arrived home for dinner—the very night you made her favorite spaghetti with meat sauce—and announced that she had gone meatless. Finally, you may be looking to cut down your meat intake, exploring meatless meals for fun and as a way to improve your health.

Whatever motivates you to learn more about a vegetarian diet, your knowledge can only make your life better. Confirmed vegetarians may learn nutrition tips here that will make their diets even healthier. We hope that new vegetarians will feel more relaxed about vegetarian nutrition and that prospective vegetarians will gain enough confidence to change their diets.

We also hope to convey some of our own enthusiasm for vegetarian eating. We bring a dual perspective to this subject. First, we are professional nutritionists—a registered dietitian and a Ph.D. in nutrition—who have chosen to make vegetarian diet our area of expertise. Not surprisingly, we're also vegetarians. In fact, between the two of us, we have more than thirty years of experience in meatless eating.

Our own experience as vegetarians has been a true evolution. We've explored all the reasons for eating this way—health, concern for animals and the environment, spiritual and world-hunger issues. We've evolved from semivegetarians to lacto-ovo (including dairy and eggs in our diet) to total veganism (no animal products whatsoever).

For us, a vegetarian diet is more than a responsible way of eating. It's a way of living the good life. Many friends and family members have tried tempting us with a juicy steak, afraid that we were missing out on something. But we know that they are the ones who are *really* missing out on something special. For one thing, vegetarian food is wonderful. It's fun and it's delicious. It includes exotic Indian curries, pasta tossed with fresh spring vegetables, tender marinated vegetables grilled to perfection and served on crusty rolls, and spicy Caribbean bean dishes. It can also be familiar, comforting foods, like tacos, potpies, and warm, savory soups. We started eating the best food of our lives when we went vegetarian. What a wonderful bonus that this food is also the healthiest there is.

But if people should be eating vegetarian meals, how did most Americans and northern Europeans end up eating such a meaty diet? It's purely an accident of prosperity. Throughout most of the world, people can't afford to eat much meat. It's just too costly to produce, requiring much land, water, and animal feed. But in the United States, many kinds of food are relatively abundant and cheap, so we can afford to eat anything we want. Most people elsewhere do not have the same food choices that we enjoy, and their diets are more closely linked to local products.

When people do eat a less expensive diet of grains, beans, vegetables, and fruits—all locally produced—they are actually much better off. Those of us who eat everything we please pay the price for it in a big way. Not just in terms of medical bills but also in the cost of dwindling environmental resources.

There is good evidence that this trend is reversing. Many people are reducing their intake of meat—mostly for health reasons. But even more dramatic are the numbers of people embracing a vegetarian diet— twelve million of us, according to a recent Gallup poll. We used to be the counterculture. Now all of a sudden we're trendsetters. And the decided opinion of the media, the nutrition profession, and the food industry is that we are important consumers and that we are here to stay. Just look at what has happened in the past few years.

In a 1991 Gallup poll, 20 percent of all people who eat in restaurants said that they patronize *only* those establishments that offer vegetarian entrées. While these people aren't all vegetarians, they care enough about having the choice to limit the restaurants they go to. The National Restaurant Association took this poll seriously and recommends that all its member restaurants add vegetarian entrées to their menus.

The grocery business has taken note of its vegetarian customers as well. Veggie burgers, once the domain of the health-food store, are showing up in the freezer case of supermarkets and are being produced by some of the world's largest food manufacturers. In the past ten years alone, more than two thousand new soy-based meat and dairy substitutes have appeared in food markets. And one national grocery chain that offers regular coupons for free meat to its customers recently amended the offer to include meat substitutes for vegetarian customers.

Nowhere is vegetarianism more popular than in the media. Vegetarian cookbooks are appearing on best-seller lists, and a number of magazines aimed exclusively at vegetarians are appearing on newsstands.

But despite all the growing interest in meatless eating, there is no single, comprehensive guide for vegetarians of all ages and types—from the parents of a new vegan baby to the vegetarian senior citizen. Our goal in writing this book is to address the full spectrum of vegetarian issues, including nutrition basics, meatless cooking, socializing, and special situations like diabetes and weight control.

In exploring the nutrition issues surrounding vegetarianism, we looked at as many scientific studies as we could find and examined every perspective. We tried to be objective, honest, and balanced in our assessment of the health effects and nutritional adequacy of a meatless diet. In examining other, nonhealth reasons for choosing a vegetarian diet, we studied agricultural publications and research on the effects of animal agriculture on the environment. As a result, we believe we are giving you the most reliable, up-to-date information that is available.

As we wrote this book, our goal was to be informative; we weren't necessarily aiming to write an inspirational text on the virtues of vegetarianism. But as you learn more about this way of eating, it is difficult not to be inspired. There is a perfect and comforting symmetry here. What is good for your body turns out to be good for the planet. When we eat in a way that is respectful and kind to our bodies, it is also respectful and kind toward the rest of the world—humans and animals as well.

Vegetarians no longer must defend and explain their diet. Vegetarianism is gradually being recognized for the smart, healthy, caring, and responsible choice that it is. We hope that this book makes some small contribution to this more accurate view of dietary choices.

It makes sense to choose a vegetarian diet. Even if there were no health advantages to eating this way, meatless eating has profoundly positive effects on the environment and on animal welfare. We feel that these factors are reason enough to opt for vegetarianism.

However, as nutritionists, we've chosen to focus on health in this book. And we are happy to conclude that not only are vegetarian diets perfectly safe and nutritious choices, they are also superior to meat-based diets. Vegetarians are healthier than omnivores. It isn't possible to conclude otherwise when you review the hundreds of scientific studies on vegetarians and health.

But as you read this book, you'll find that not every study we examine supports this viewpoint. And, in some instances, we acknowledge that for a particular issue the picture is a bit murky, and we are hesitant to draw any firm conclusions. We've tried to bring an objective perspective to the subject of vegetarianism, and we expect that some readers may find this somewhat disconcerting. For those who feel strongly about the virtues of vegetarianism, it is natural to want to read about only the most positive findings on the subject. However, we think it is in the best interests of vegetarianism when we invite you to explore *all* of the information about this way of eating. For one thing, it will help you to be a healthier vegetarian. For another, we think you'll feel more confident than ever that vegetarianism is the best choice.

The fact is that the overwhelming preponderance of scientific findings supports a vegetarian diet as the healthiest pattern of eating. However, sometimes supporters of meatless diets have been eager to draw favorable conclusions even when evidence is weak or have ignored evidence that may be less than favorable. As a result, there are concepts about vegetarian diets that have been repeated over and over again and have been embraced as fact. Some of these ideas are shaky at best; others are just plain wrong.

Our goal is to present you with information about a vegetarian diet in the most objective and comprehensive manner possible. In doing so, we have examined all of the studies—including those that at face value don't support vegetarianism. And we don't hesitate to admit that we don't have every answer. It would be easy—and tempting—to simply ignore the findings that don't support our position or to overstate the findings that do. But there is nothing to be gained by doing so. In fact, we believe that an objective view of a vegetarian diet does the most to promote it. Opponents of vegetarianism—those who would like to see vegetarian diets debunked—can easily expose the weaknesses in a pro-vegetarian argument if that argument is based on inaccurate or incomplete information. It is best to explore an issue completely and to know exactly where science stands on a particular matter. Only then is it possible to argue confidently and effectively in favor of a vegetarian diet. Because, in the final analysis, after all the data are in, vegetarianism wins hands down over meat-based diets.

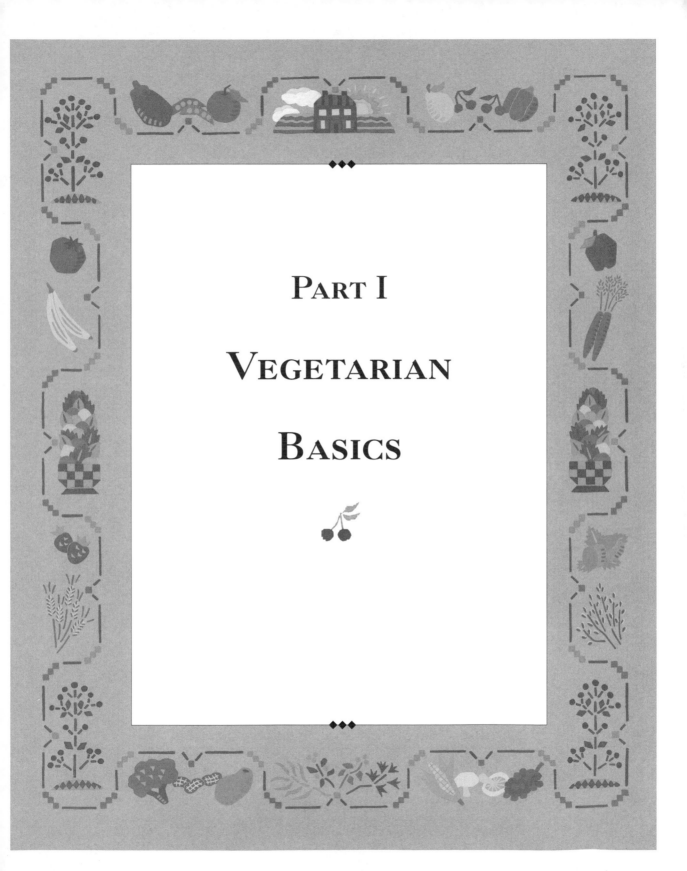

PART I

VEGETARIAN

BASICS

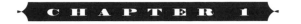

CHAPTER 1

VEGETARIANISM THROUGH THE AGES

◆◆◆

I have no doubt that it is part of the destiny of the human race in its gradual improvement to leave off eating animals.

—HENRY DAVID THOREAU, *Walden*, 1854

◆

Who were the first vegetarians? Well, the answer depends upon whom you ask. A biblical account says the first vegetarians were the first humans—Adam and Eve. God's commandment to the Garden of Eden dwellers to eat a strictly vegetarian diet was quite clear: "And God said, 'Behold, I have given you every plant yielding seed which is upon the face of all the earth, and every tree with seed in its fruit; you shall have them for food.'"[1]

Anthropology tells a somewhat different story. Fossil records show that throughout our evolution, humans and their ancestors definitely ate meat. How much meat we ate varied quite a bit. During the Ice Age, for example, when vegetation was sparse, the human diet relied more on meat. At other times, especially after the development of agriculture, the diet was much more likely to be plant based.[2]

Some accepted ideas about our historical relationship to meat are pure myths. "Early man, the mighty hunter" is one of them. Our earliest ancestors probably didn't hunt animals. Rather, they scavenged, eating the meager leftovers at the kill site after other animals

had feasted and left. Prehumans used tools to cut food from the bones of animals, but marks left by those tools show that they cut bones in places where there was likely to be very little meat.[3] Some anthropologists have suggested that our ancestors may have broken the bones apart to get to the nutrient-rich marrow and may not have eaten much of the meat at all.

One thing is for certain: our earliest ancestors did not eat from the four basic food groups. Many of those foods simply weren't available in earlier times. Diets were centered on vegetables, fruits, nuts, seeds, and meat. Animals had not been domesticated, and early humans were unable to digest milk, so dairy foods were never on the prehistoric menu. Despite that, our early ancestors may have had a higher intake of calcium than today's average milk drinker, since the wild greens that made up so much of their diet were abundant in this mineral.[4] Both Neanderthals and Cro-Magnons had massive bones, an indication that they consumed adequate amounts of calcium.[5]

Early ideas about humans as hunters may have come from some confusion over the fact that fossils of early man have been discovered in reverse order. That is, the most recent fossils were discovered first. The idea that our early ancestors were mighty hunters was a hypothesis firmly established by Charles Darwin. But by the time Darwin died, the only human bones that had

◆◆◆

been unearthed were those of Neanderthal man, who lived just thirty-five thousand to fifty thousand years ago. Neanderthal man was a big meat eater. He had to be, since he lived during the Ice Age, when other types of food were more scarce.[6]

In general, even before the birth of agriculture ten thousand to twelve thousand years ago, plants were most likely the staples of the diet throughout much of our history, though meat played a varying role. With the advent of agriculture, plant foods probably made up close to 90 percent of the human diet.[7] And for those who believe that meat is a natural part of our diet because that's what our ancestors ate, it is worth noting that they also ate human flesh.[8]

THE EARLY GREEKS AND ROMANS

Although the word "vegetarian" wasn't coined until the mid-1800s, the concept was alive and well in much earlier times. In ancient Greece and Rome, vegetarianism was linked to religious and moral beliefs. In the sixth century B.C. philosopher Pythagoras believed that a vegetarian diet was the most natural and healthiest way of eating. He taught that for the attainment of spiritual and physical health it was necessary to adhere to a prescribed lifestyle that included simple clothing, an ordered daily regimen, and a vegetarian diet of fresh foods.[9] Other philosophers probably weren't vegetarians themselves, but Socrates, Plato, Horace, Ovid, and Virgil definitely favored the idea of meatless diets.

The Pythagorean diet had a resurgence in popularity in Europe in the 1700s. According to those who repopularized this way of eating, the diet included the "free and universal use of everything that is vegetable, tender and fresh . . . and which requires little

BILL OF FARE FROM THE FIFTH ANNUAL MEETING OF THE AMERICAN VEGETARIAN SOCIETY, AUGUST 30, 1854

FIRST COURSE	SECOND COURSE
Potato pie	
Green corn	Vegetarian mince pie
Savory omelette	Coconut custard
Graham bread	Cheese cake
Baked sweet potatoes	Peach pie
White bread	Apple custard
Fried eggplant	Moulded rice
Lima beans	Fruit pudding
Pickled beets	Washington cream sauce
Tomatoes	Sweet cakes
Pickled martenoes	Apples, peaches, watermelon, cantaloupe
Ice water	

or no preparation to make it fit to eat, such as roots, leaves, fruits, and seeds."[10]

THE FIRST VEGETARIAN MOVEMENT

Down through the centuries adherents of certain religions and philosophies have followed a vegetarian diet. Political and religious leaders as well as celebrities embraced vegetarianism. One of the best known was Benjamin Franklin, whose vegetarian diet fit in well with his simple-living credo. Methodist-church founder John Wesley was also a vegetarian for at least part of his life. As long ago as 1641, English physician George Cheyne was advocating a vegetarian diet for his patients. But it wasn't until the nineteenth century that anything akin to an actual vegetarian movement developed. And although there were vegetarians throughout the world—and in many areas of the world, vegetarianism was a much stronger force than in the West—what we can describe as the first vegetarian movement was largely the product of "diet reformers" in the United Kingdom and the United States.

One of the earliest experiments in vegetarian living in the United States was Fruitlands, a vegan community founded in Harvard, Massachusetts, in 1843. It was established by the English educational reformer Charles Lane and by Amos Bronson Alcott, father of writer Louisa May Alcott. Fruitlands put into practice the Utopian principles that both men embraced. The Fruitlands diet consisted of fruit, grains, beans, and peas. Meat, fish, butter, cheese, eggs, and milk were denounced as causing corruption. Tea, coffee, rice, molasses, and sugar were prohibited in the community because they were produced by slave labor. Alcott himself wore only linen clothes, since all other clothes either came from animals or were produced by slaves.[11]

The goals of Fruitlands were lofty ones, but it wasn't a particularly productive community. Alcott, Lane, and their friends spent much of their time sitting and discussing philosophy—a luxury afforded them by Mrs. Alcott's laboring in the vegetable garden to feed the members. Daughter Louisa remembered her parents' roles this way: "While Mother . . . tried to help everybody . . . Father talked."[12] In fact, Amos Alcott's lifelong advocacy of the social reform that would include a vegetarian diet made it difficult for him to support his family. Louisa May Alcott's prolific writing was in part due to her role as family breadwinner. An inside look at life

in the Fruitlands Community can be found in her satire *Transcendental Wild Oats*.

The impact of Fruitlands may have been somewhat limited—the experiment in communal living lasted only seven months. But other influences on vegetarianism were cropping up in nineteenth-century America. The two with the largest impact came from—surprisingly—the Christian church.

The Bible Christians

In 1800 the Reverend William Cowherd, a minister of the Church of England, broke with that church to establish a congregation with Bible literalism as its foundation. One reason for the rift was that Cowherd believed that meat eating was prohibited by the Bible. Cowherd's church members, called Bible Christians, avoided all meat, and many did not eat dairy products or eggs. They also believed that Scripture forbade the use of coffee, tea, alcohol, and tobacco.

In 1817, William Metcalf, another Bible Christian minister, left England with forty-one church members and came to America. Although his new Philadelphia-based church never exceeded one hundred members, it had a considerable influence on the promotion of a vegetarian lifestyle.[13] One of Metcalf's converts was Sylvester Graham, a Presbyterian minister who toured the country giving lectures on the evils of certain foods and other factors that were "stimulating" and therefore both physically and morally harmful. According to Graham, stimulating hazards included white bread, meat, alcohol, coffee, extramarital sex, and tight pants.[14] Graham became a great advocate of a meatless diet, but his real legacy was in promoting the use of whole grain flour. In fact, it eventually became known as graham flour (as in graham

FAMOUS VEGETARIANS IN HISTORY

Louisa May Alcott

Clara Barton

Charles Darwin

Leonardo da Vinci

Isadora Duncan

Thomas Edison

Albert Einstein

Mahatma Gandhi

Sylvester Graham

John Harvey Kellogg

John Milton

Sir Isaac Newton

Pythagoras

Albert Schweitzer

George Bernard Shaw

Mary Wollstonecraft Shelley

Percy Bysshe Shelley

Upton Sinclair

Isaac Bashevis Singer

Henry David Thoreau

Leo Tolstoy

John Wesley

FAMOUS VEGETARIANS TODAY

Henry (Hank) Aaron, Major League baseball player

Bryan Adams, rock musician

Maxine Andrews, singer with the Andrews Sisters

Bob Barker, TV personality

Kim Basinger, actress

Jeff Beck, rock guitarist

Cindy Blum, opera singer

Surya Bonaly, Olympic figure skater

David Bowie, rock musician

Boy George, rock singer

Berke Breathed, cartoonist

Christie Brinkley, model

Roger Brown, professional football player

Ellen Burstyn, actress

Andreas Cahling, champion bodybuilder

Chris Campbell, Olympic medalist in wrestling

Skeeter Davis, country singer

Peter Falk, actor

Sara Gilbert, actress

Elliot Gould, actor

Richie Havens, rock musician

Henry Heimlich, physician and inventor of the Heimlich maneuver

Doug Henning, magician

Dustin Hoffman, actor

Desmond Howard, professional football player and Heisman-trophy winner

Chrissie Hynde, rock musician

Andrew Jacobs Jr., Indiana U.S. congressman

Mick Jagger, rock musician

Elton John, rock musician

Casey Kasem, radio personality

Billie Jean King, tennis champion

k. d. lang, country singer

Tony La Russa, manager of the Oakland Athletics

Cloris Leachman, actress

Annie Lennox, rock singer

Marv Levy, head coach of the Buffalo Bills

Carl Lewis, Olympic runner

Madonna, rock singer

Catherine Malfitano, opera singer

Bill Manetti, power-lifting champion

Steve Martin, comedian and actor

Paul and Linda McCartney, rock musicians

Michael Medved, film critic

Edwin Moses, Olympic gold medalist in track

Martina Navratilova, tennis champion

Kevin Nealon, comedian

Olivia Newton-John, rock singer

Stevie Nicks, rock singer

Paavo Nurmi, long-distance runner with twenty world records

Dean Ornish, physician and author of *Dr. Dean Ornish's Program for Reversing Heart Disease*

Bill Pearl, four-time Mr. Universe

Martha Plimpton, actress

Bonnie Raitt, rock singer

Phylicia Rashad, actress

Tony Robbins, motivational speaker

Fred Rogers, TV's Mr. Rogers

Todd Rundgren, rock musician

Dave Scott, six-time Ironman triathalon winner

Grace Slick, rock musician

Leigh Taylor-Young, actress

John Tesh, TV personality

Tina Turner, rock singer

Cicely Tyson, actress

Lindsay Wagner, actress

Lesley Ann Warren, actress

Dennis Weaver, actor

---

crackers). Graham's work made him one of the nineteenth century's greatest diet reformers.

In 1847, members of the Bible Christian church who had remained in England established the Vegetarian Society of Great Britain. In response, Metcalf invited U.S. diet reformers to establish the American Vegetarian Society. The society met for the first time in 1850. Its publication, the *American Vegetarian and Health Journal*, presented arguments against meat eating that focused on ethical, environmental, and health issues. The Reverend Metcalf spent fifty-two years in the Bible Christian ministry and can be largely credited with initiating and organizing the first true vegetarian movement in the United States.[15]

Seventh-day Adventist Church

The Seventh-day Adventist (SDA) church has been one of the most important influences on vegetarianism in the United States since the middle of the nineteenth century. It was founded in the 1840s by Ellen White, who produced copious teachings on the relationship of physical health to religious life. Mrs. White noted that the diet prescribed by God is spelled out for us in Genesis and that eating a healthy diet "for the glory of God" is truly a spiritual responsibility. In 1890 she wrote, "Every faculty with which the Creator has endowed us should be cultivated to the highest degree of perfection, that we may be able to do the greatest amount of good of which we are capable. Hence, that time is spent to good account which is used in the establishment and preservation of physical and mental health."[16] To that end, the Seventh-day Adventists focused on spiritual health, diet, and exercise.

The Seventh-day Adventist church continues to be a major influence on the vegetarian scene. Its members are among the most authoritative and active forces in the world promoting a vegetarian diet. Fifty percent of church members are vegetarians (close to 100 percent of Seventh-day Adventist clergy are vegetarians).

Since its earliest days, the church has given rise to community outreach programs in the areas of diet and health. Seventh-day Adventist–run food companies and restaurants offer vegetarian foods, and church-associated universities are centers of scientific research on vegetarian diet.

John Harvey Kellogg

The man who was eventually to give the world cornflakes was closely associated with the SDA church. John Harvey Kellogg worked for Ellen White and her husband, James, as a printer for their health-centered publication, the *Review and Herald Press*. The couple sponsored him through medical school and then hired him as physician in chief for the Adventist-run Western Health Reform Institute in Battle Creek, Michigan. Kellogg promptly renamed it the Battle Creek Sanitarium and set out to produce an appealing vegetarian menu. Kellogg and his wife set up a research kitchen in 1877 to develop the recipes. Here they invented the first meat analogue, called nuttose, which was made from peanuts and flour and was seasoned to taste like meat. Many such products would come out of the Kelloggs' test kitchen.[17]

Although he performed more than twenty-two thousand operations in his lifetime, Kellogg's interest was in preventive medicine. He called the system that he made famous at the Battle Creek Sanitarium "biologic living." It included a vegetarian diet with total abstinence from meat, alcohol, tea, coffee, sugar, chocolate, and strong spices. The program also emphasized exercise, hydrotherapy, fresh air, sunshine, good posture, simple dress, and good mental health.

Kellogg was greatly concerned with the effects of meat on the colon. He believed this to be the source of "nine-tenths of all the chronic ills from which civilized human beings suffer." He blamed poor diet and colon problems for the country's "national inefficiency and physical unpreparedness."[18] Kellogg noted that the bowel problems related to meat eating were so horrible that "the marvel is not that human life is so short and so full of miseries, . . . but that civilized human beings are able to live at all."[19]

Kellogg's work had far-reaching and positive effects. His sanitarium was a mecca for the rich and famous and especially for forward-thinking inventors, businesspeople, and artists. His guests included such notables as William Howard Taft, William Jennings Bryan, John D. Rockefeller, Alfred Dupont, J. C. Penney, Montgomery Ward, Thomas Edison, Henry Ford, George Bernard Shaw, and Admiral Richard Byrd.

In addition to meat analogues Kellogg also produced foods that have become staples in most American diets. In 1892 he invented peanut butter. And the cereals that made his name a household word began in 1877 with the invention of one many Americans mistakenly believe was created in the 1960s—granola. In 1898 he developed cornflakes with his brother W. K. Kellogg, who later added sugar to the cereal and founded the Kellogg's cereal company. A rival company was founded by C. W. Post, who developed an interest in these foods when he was a patient at the sanitarium.

Kellogg himself was an excellent advertisement for the healthy lifestyle he advocated. He slept only four to five hours a night, cycled or jogged daily into his eighties, dictated twenty-five to fifty letters a day, adopted and raised forty-two children, wrote nearly fifty books, edited a magazine, and gave nearly all of his money to charitable organizations. He lived in good health until the age of ninety-one, performing the last of his operations at the age of eighty-eight.[20]

One anecdote reveals Kellogg's charisma in promoting the lifestyle he so believed in. In the early part of the century, the U.S. Department of Agriculture (USDA) displayed posters in post offices depicting the nutritional virtues of meat. Kellogg printed up an almost identical poster; it differed only in that it listed the problems associated with meat consumption. This enraged meat packers, who filed a complaint with the Federal Trade Commission, which immediately dispatched an attorney to Battle Creek to investigate. After the attorney left the sanitarium the investigation was dropped. Some time later, the attorney saw Dr. Kellogg again and confessed to him, "You know, Doctor, I haven't tasted meat since I saw you in Battle Creek."[21]

Other Early Influences on Vegetarianism
In the United States, interest in vegetarianism was at its peak in the mid-nineteenth century through the early part of the twentieth century. The Battle Creek Sanitarium was one of several vegetarian sanitariums that opened across the country. Vegetarian restaurants opened in several large cities. One of New York City's popular eateries of the time was the Physical Culture and Strength Food Restaurant. Although Philadelphia was the undisputed center of vegetarian activity (where the Bible Christians had opened their first church), there were vegetarian societies in Kansas City, St. Louis, Minneapolis, Boston, Pittsburgh, Chicago, and Washington, D.C. Vegetarian move-

ments also sprang up in most European countries.[22]

Interest in diet and diet reform ebbed toward the middle of the twentieth century. Around this time, government organizations began to produce food guides for Americans, all of which placed a heavy emphasis on meat and dairy products. But even though vegetarianism was hardly a hot issue in the middle part of this century, results of a 1943 Gallup poll, reported in the *Washington Post* on October 2 of that year, revealed that there were between 2.5 and 3 million vegetarians living in the United States, or about 2 percent of the total population.[23] In 1944, in Great Britain, the term "vegan" was used for the first time to define a vegetarian who didn't consume dairy products or eggs, and the Vegan Society—which just celebrated its fiftieth anniversary—was formed in Great Britain that same year.[24]

THE SECOND VEGETARIAN MOVEMENT

Vegetarianism enjoyed a resurgence in popularity in the 1960s and 1970s, when it seemed a natural dietary choice for the new health-conscious counterculture. One important influence was the introduction of macrobiotic teachings by Michio Kushi in the 1960s. But vegetarianism was viewed then as a nuts-and-berries regimen. Although it was popular with young people, it didn't have much mainstream appeal.

But all of that changed a decade and a half ago, largely due to two influences. The first was the 1971 publication of Frances Moore Lappé's book *Diet for a Small Planet*. This book offered a stunning revelation of the effects of food production on the environment. It became an important influence on the way Americans thought

TABLE 1.1 VEGETARIAN DIET—THE NATURAL DIET OF MAN?

One popular argument in favor of a vegetarian diet is based on the idea that the anatomy and physiology of humans is best suited to a plant-based diet. Here, we've compared some key anatomical features of humans with those of animals who are carnivores (a meat diet only), herbivores (plant foods only), and omnivores (both plant and animal foods).

Feature	Carnivore	Herbivore	Omnivore	Human
Teeth Incisors	Short and pointed	Broad, flattened, and spade-shaped	Short and pointed	Broad, flattened, and spade-shaped
Canines	Long, sharp, and curved	Dull and short or long or none	Long, sharp, and curved	Short and blunted
Molars	Sharp, jagged, and blade-shaped	Flattened with cusps vs. complex surface	Sharp blades and/or flattened	Flattened with nodular cusps
Colon	Simple and short	Long and complex	Simple and short	Long and complex
Nails	Sharp claws	Flattened nails or blunt hooves	Sharp claws	Flattened
Length of small intestine	3–6 times body length	10–12+ times body length	4–6 times body length	10–11 times body length
Saliva	No digestive enzymes	Carbohydrate-digesting enzymes	No digestive enzymes	Carbohydrate-digesting enzymes

about diet, and it made a strong case for a vegetarian diet based on environmental concerns.

A second influence was the birth of the animal rights movement, largely due to the publication of the book *Animal Liberation*, by Peter Singer, in 1975, and the formation of the nonprofit People for the Ethical Treatment of Animals (PETA) in 1980. Both made a case for a vegetarian diet based on humane concerns.

The vegetarian movement of the 1980s and 1990s is clearly of greater impact than the first movement of the nineteenth century. Today, there is a stronger case for a vegetarian diet than ever before. First, diet-related illnesses, like heart disease and cancer, are much bigger problems today than they were 150 years ago, and the relationship between diet and these diseases is more firmly established. Second, concerns about the environment are more pressing. Finally, animal agriculture has become more intensive, and the inhumane aspects of that industry are better publicized. All of these factors make a vegetarian diet more attractive to a growing number of people from many different walks of life.

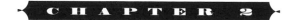
DEFINING VEGETARIANISM

◆◆◆

Vegetarianism, of course, like any other cultural phenomenon is very diverse.

—JULIA TWIGG, *The Sociology of Food and Eating,* 1983

◆

Vegetarianism is changing its image. Twenty years ago vegetarians were viewed as food faddists, members of the counterculture, people who held a particular set of political and personal beliefs. Today, the average vegetarian is as likely to show up at a PTA meeting as at a peace rally—or to be the CEO of a major corporation just as easily as the cashier at your local health-food store.

A vegetarian diet is becoming downright mainstream as people abandon meat at an ever-growing rate. More than 12 million American adults—or about 6.5 percent of the population—call themselves vegetarians.[1] That's about a 100 percent increase since 1985.

For most vegetarians, meatless eating is more than a passing fancy. According to a 1992 poll, close to half of all vegetarians have been eating a meatless diet for more than ten years; about one-quarter have been vegetarian for more than twenty years.[2]

VEGETARIAN DIETS

It is no simple matter to define a common vegetarian diet. At its broadest, a vegetarian diet is one that excludes meat, fish, and poultry. Beyond that, there are many variations on the theme.

Lacto-Ovo Vegetarianism

This is the most popular type of vegetarian diet. Lacto-ovo vegetarians avoid all meat, fish, and poultry but do consume milk, cheese, yogurt, other dairy products, and eggs. Subdivisions exist within this group. Vegetarians who eat dairy products but avoid eggs technically are referred to as lacto vegetarians. A smaller percentage who eat eggs but no dairy are known as ovo vegetarians.

A lacto-ovo-vegetarian diet plan will almost certainly meet a person's nutritional needs. If there is any cause for concern it lies in the fact that some lacto-ovo vegetarians overemphasize dairy and eggs in their diet so they end up eating too much fat and cholesterol. New vegetarians in particular may be likely to eat a lot of cheese during the transition to a plant-based diet.

Lacto-ovo vegetarians can guard against excessive fat in their diet by using only non-fat or very low-fat dairy foods. Since even low-fat dairy foods can replace healthier,

◆◆◆

fiber-rich plant foods, milk, cheese, and other animal products shouldn't play too large a role in the diet. You'll see throughout this book, and in the chapter on meal planning in particular, that we encourage lacto-ovo vegetarians to be moderate in their use of dairy foods and eggs and to explore plant sources of calcium and other nutrients.

Vegan

A growing number of vegetarians are embracing a vegan diet. Vegans avoid all animal products in their meals. They do not eat meat, fish, poultry, eggs, or dairy products. Vegan diets are based on grains, legumes, vegetables, fruits, nuts, and seeds. These diets tend to be moderate in fat and protein and high in fiber.

A vegan diet may seem more complex than a lacto-ovo-vegetarian diet. Many seemingly innocent foods actually contain animal ingredients. For example, commercially baked breads may contain eggs or dairy. Even products that boast nondairy on the label, such as nondairy whipped toppings, are likely to contain casein, a protein derived from milk. In fact, many newer vegetarian products are not suitable for vegans. Vegetarian burgers often contain eggs as a binder. Soy cheese, which might sound like a great choice for vegans, frequently contains milk protein to give it better "meltability."

But most vegans quickly become savvy about their diets. A few weeks of label reading in the grocery store help a new vegan to be comfortable with certain brands of foods and to know which ones to avoid.

Well-planned vegan diets are always an excellent choice for health reasons. They are more likely to be low in fat and high in fiber than either omnivorous patterns of eating or lacto-ovo-vegetarian menus. There is some evidence that vegans have an even lower risk of chronic disease than lacto-ovo vegetarians.[3] However, those who are new to a vegan diet need to be aware that in traditional Western diets the foods that are most likely to supply calcium, zinc, vitamin D, and vitamin B_{12} are animal foods. It isn't at all difficult to get these nutrients in a vegan diet, but new vegans should expect to explore new foods in order to meet their nutrient needs. In fact, that's half the fun of a vegan diet.

Many vegans are also motivated by ethical reasons. (Some of the ethical concerns associated with the production of dairy products and eggs are addressed in chapter 4.) Vegans who adopt their diet for ethical reasons often avoid all animal products—not just those in the diet. So a vegan might not wear leather or wool and is likely to avoid cosmetics and household products that contain animal by-products or are tested on animals.

Macrobiotics

Macrobiotics represents a particular dietary philosophy. Because it emphasizes consuming seasonal foods that are locally produced, the diet will vary according to region. However, people living in temperate zones, including most of North America, Europe, most of Asia, parts of Latin America, and parts of Australia, will eat more or less the same diet. Meals are predominantly based on whole grains, which make up about 50 to

TABLE 2.1 WHO ARE VEGETARIANS?

	Vegetarians (%)	General Population (%)
GENDER		
Female	68	52
Male	32	48
EDUCATION		
College graduate	30	25
High school graduate	45	56
No high school degree	21	18
MARITAL STATUS		
Married	48	59
Single	24	22
Widowed	14	8
Divorced/separated	11	11
HAVE CHILDREN UNDER 18		
Yes	37	24
No	60	75
INCOME		
Less than $35,000	56	55
More than $35,000	44	45
OCCUPATION		
White collar	37	35
Not white collar	60	62
AGE		
Under 40	42	49
Over 40	55	50

Source: Survey of adult Americans conducted by Yankelovich Clancy Shulman for *Time* magazine and CNN in April 1992

60 percent of the diet, and locally grown vegetables, which make up about 25 percent of the diet. The rest of the diet includes soups, beans, and limited amounts of fruits, nuts, and seeds. Some macrobiotic traditions allow seafood. However, for macrobiotics who don't eat fish, the diet is vegan, since meat, poultry, dairy products, and eggs are not included in macrobiotic meals. Other foods that are *not* consumed are vegetables of the nightshade botanical family (potatoes, eggplant, peppers), tropical fruits, and processed sweeteners.[4]

Macrobiotics is loosely related to Bud-

TABLE 2.2 TYPES OF VEGETARIANS AND THEIR DIETS

Types of Vegetarians	Foods Consumed	Comments	Typical Meal Patterns
Lacto-ovo	Grains, legumes, fruits, vegetables, nuts, seeds, dairy, eggs	Total and saturated fat can be high if full-fat dairy products and eggs are used.	**BREAKFAST** 1 cup bran flakes, with 1 cup skim milk Sliced banana 6 ounces orange juice **LUNCH** Missing-egg-salad sandwich, with 2 slices whole wheat bread Raw carrot Peach **SNACK** 1 cup low-fat vanilla yogurt ½ cup strawberries **DINNER** 1 slice lentil-walnut loaf 1 cup quinoa mixed with corn ½ cup steamed spinach
Vegan	Grains, legumes, vegetables, fruits, nuts, seeds (no dairy or eggs)	Some vegans avoid honey, white sugar, beer, and other foods that involve animal products in their processing.	**BREAKFAST** 1 cup Raisin Bran, with ½ cup soymilk Sliced banana 2 slices whole wheat toast, with jam **LUNCH** Broiled tofu burger, with 1 whole wheat hamburger roll Avocado slices, tomato slices, carrot sticks 2 oatmeal cookies Orange **SNACK** 2 rice cakes, with 2 tablespoons almond butter **DINNER** 1 cup Caribbean black beans 1 cup brown rice 1½ cups sautéed mixed vegetables (broccoli, bok choy, mushrooms, snow peas) **SNACK** Strawberry soymilk shake

TABLE 2.2 TYPES OF VEGETARIANS AND THEIR DIETS (cont.)

Types of Vegetarians	Foods Consumed	Comments	Typical Meal Patterns
Macrobiotic	Grains, legumes, vegetables, fruits and nuts to a lesser extent; grains heavily emphasized; sea vegetables, soy products, and Asian condiments frequent parts of the diet (dairy, eggs, and some vegetables avoided)	Some macrobiotics consume fish. Guidelines for this diet need to be adjusted to make it appropriate for children	BREAKFAST 1 cup oatmeal, with 1 tablespoon sesame seeds Grain coffee LUNCH 1 cup barley–shiitake mushroom soup, with miso broth ½ cup steamed tofu 1 cup steamed broccoli 1 cup brown rice SNACK ¼ cup roasted sunflower seeds DINNER 1 cup chickpea soup, with onions, carrots, and wakame (a sea vegetable) 1 cup steamed collards ¼ cup daikon 2 cups mixed brown rice and bulgur ½ cup cantaloupe cubes
Fruitarian	Fruits, vegetables that are botanically fruits (tomatoes, eggplant, avocado, zucchini), nuts, and seeds	Planning nutritionally adequate diets on a true fruitarian plan is difficult. *This diet is not recommended for children.*	Modified plan with some grains. BREAKFAST Granola, with raisins, almonds Sliced banana Fresh pineaple-orange juice LUNCH Steamed eggplant and zucchini in tomato sauce Fruit salad (bananas, figs, apples, Brazil nuts) Almond milk DINNER Eggplant, stuffed with sprouted barley, raisins, and walnuts with tahini sauce Apples, spread with almond butter Sliced mango Fresh figs

TABLE 2.2 TYPES OF VEGETARIANS AND THEIR DIETS (cont.)

Types of Vegetarians	Foods Consumed	Comments	Typical Meal Patterns
Raw-foods diet	Vegetables, fruits, nuts, seeds, sprouted grains, and sprouted beans, eaten in the raw state	Percentage of raw foods in the diet varies considerably among followers of this plan. *A completely raw-foods diet is not recommended for children.*	**BREAKFAST** Granola, with almond milk Fresh fruit **LUNCH** Gazpacho soup Salad (baby kale, endive, escarole, spinach, tahini dressing) Almond-fig-oat bars **DINNER** Sprouted wheat berries and lentils, raw vegetables, with olive oil, fresh lemon juice, and herbs Apple-cherry juice Celery and carrots, spread with almond butter
Natural-hygiene diet	Emphasis on raw vegetables and fruits, with whole grains, legumes, nuts, and sprouted grains, seeds, legumes	The emphasis is placed on eating or avoiding certain combinations of foods. Meat is included in some plans. *Some natural-hygiene menus are not recommended for children.*	**BREAKFAST** 2 cups fresh pineapple-orange juice **MIDMORNING** Papaya 1 cup cantaloupe **LUNCH** 1 cup carrot juice Salad (3 cups lettuce, 2 cups raw vegetables, 1/2 cup chickpeas), with olive oil and lemon juice dressing **DINNER** 1 cup vegetable juice cocktail Cream of broccoli soup Baked potato Salad (1 cup lettuce, 1 cup raw vegetables) **EVENING** 1 cup watermelon

dhism and linked to the ancient Chinese principles of yin and yang. Foods typically used in macrobiotic cooking reflect these Asian influences. For example, macrobiotic diets make considerable use of sea vegetables such as kelp, nori, and arame, root vegetables like daikon and lotus, miso soup, and pickled vegetables. Macrobiotics is actually more than a diet. It is a lifestyle and philosophy based on principles of balance and harmony with nature and the universe. Macrobiotic adherents often choose this diet as a part of a larger set of beliefs.

However, many people choose macrobiotics because they consider it the healthiest way to eat. Others believe that it can cure or slow the process of some diseases, such as cancer. Although there is little scientific proof for this, some researchers have noted that cancer patients following macrobiotic diets live longer.[5]

Among traditional nutritionists, macrobiotics has long and erroneously been considered a dangerous and nutritionally unsound practice. However, it can actually be a healthy dietary choice that provides nutritious, well-balanced meals. In fact, with its emphasis on whole grains and vegetables, including mineral-rich sea vegetables, and its deemphasis on fats and processed foods, it is certainly a healthier diet than that consumed by the average American. Although the founder of macrobiotics, George Ohsawa, claims that a diet of only brown rice cured him of a fatal disease, modern macrobiotics eat a varied menu of nutrient-rich foods. There *are* some lingering concerns about the safety of macrobiotic diets for children, however. In the 1970s, studies of macrobiotic children in the United States and the Netherlands showed severe nutrient deficiencies.[6] Although the modern macrobiotic diet is likely to be more liberal than that consumed in the 1970s, some current macrobiotic recommendations are unsound. In the popular book *Macrobiotic Diet,* water in which brown rice has been cooked is recommended as one possible milk substitute for infants.[7] However, homemade brown-rice formula does not offer adequate nutrition for an infant or a toddler.

Also, because the macrobiotic diet is especially low in fat and limits the use of foods like nuts and seeds, the diet can be too low in calories for some children. The emphasis on various foods should be slightly different for macrobiotic children than for adults. That is, children need fewer whole grains and more nuts, seeds, legumes, and soy products than do macrobiotic adults. Michio Kushi, who is considered the leading authority and teacher on the macrobiotic diet, has recently revised some of his recommendations for macrobiotic children, based on the findings of nutrition researchers.[8] Unfortunately, these newer recommendations encourage the use of dairy foods and fish in the diet. Actually, macrobiotic children can meet nutrient needs without the use of animal foods. Parents of macrobiotic children can use the guidelines for meal planning for infants and children described in chapters 12 and 13 of this book. All of these recommendations can be met with foods that are acceptable on a macrobiotic diet.

In terms of nutritional profile, macrobiotics is similar to a vegan eating pattern. Throughout this book, whatever we recommend for vegans applies to macrobiotics as well.

Other Vegetarian Patterns

There are a few other vegetarian patterns that deserve mention. A fruitarian diet has relatively few followers and is a rather specific version of vegetarianism. People are attracted to this eating pattern usually for either health or spiritual reasons. It is based on fruits (including some foods that we often think of as vegetables but that are botanically fruits, such as squash, tomatoes, eggplant, peppers, and avocados), nuts, and seeds.

It is certainly possible to meet nutrient needs with a fruitarian diet. However, of all the vegetarian choices, this one is probably the trickiest menu to plan. Also, the extremely high amount of bulk in the diet would make it difficult for children to eat enough food to meet their needs.

A natural-hygiene diet is traditionally based on vegetables, fruits, nuts, and sprouts (including sprouted grains and beans), all eaten in raw form. However, natural-hygiene proponents follow considerable variations of this diet. Some include cooked whole grains and legumes in their meals. Some versions of the diet are not completely vegetarian but make very limited use of animal products.

The purpose of the natural-hygiene regimen is to continuously cleanse the body of waste material. At the heart of this philosophy is a set of beliefs regarding food combining. That is, foods must be eaten in certain combinations and other combina-

tions must be avoided to allow for efficient digestion. For example, natural hygienists do not eat starchy foods and high-protein foods at the same time, believing that the body's enzymes can't digest these foods together. Also, fruits are always eaten alone.

The rules regarding food combining are largely unfounded, since the human body is perfectly capable of digesting a wide variety of foods at the same time. Also, some natural-hygiene menu plans that we've seen have not been nutritionally adequate for either adults or children. However, there is a fair amount of flexibility in the natural-hygiene diet; if a good variety of plant foods is used, this diet can certainly be planned to meet nutrient needs.

A raw-foods diet is similar to a natural-hygiene diet except that the emphasis is on consuming only uncooked foods. Raw-foods advocates eat vegetables, fruits, nuts, seeds, and sprouted grains and beans, all in their raw state. One underlying belief is that this is the natural diet of humans, since it is certainly our original diet, consumed for many thousands of years before fire was discovered. Of course, the earliest raw foodists also ate raw meat, which is not part of today's raw-foods diet. Another principle of raw-foods diets is that enzymes in foods can be destroyed with cooking. However, since enzymes are proteins, they are destroyed upon digestion anyway, so there is little advantage to consuming them in their natural state.

Many raw-foods advocates don't necessarily recommend a diet that is 100 percent raw, but rather they adhere to one that includes between 50 and 80 percent raw foods. As is true with the other vegetarian patterns, there is quite a bit of variation in both philosophy and practices among people following raw-foods diets.

There is certainly some merit to raw foods, since cooking does destroy nutrients. However, heating foods also makes them more easily digested and destroys antinutritional factors. Also, a completely raw-foods diet would not be appropriate for babies and very young children. Early humans breastfed children for much longer than people do now, providing them with one very digestible source of nutrition. It is also likely that before cooking was available mothers prechewed food for babies and children to make it more digestible.

A raw-foods diet can meet the nutrient needs of adults with some planning, but we don't recommend it for children.

SEMI- OR NEAR VEGETARIAN

With an interest in choosing healthier diets, a growing number of people call themselves semivegetarian or near vegetarian. Many of these people are actually in a transition stage approaching true vegetarianism. The dietary patterns of this group vary widely. While some do eat a near-vegetarian diet by consuming animal flesh infrequently, many people who consider themselves semi-vegetarians actually consume fairly large amounts of fish and poultry. In fact, the myth persists that a diet free of red meat is a vegetarian menu and that it will offer the same health benefits as a total-vegetarian diet. But replacing red meat in the diet with liberal amounts of chicken and fish does little to improve overall diet and will not produce the health benefits of vegetarianism.

People who limit their meat intake to one or two small portions per week or who use only tiny amounts of meat to flavor foods may enjoy some of the benefits associated with a vegetarian diet. But meat intake is certainly linked to some health risks, and we really don't know how much meat is too much.

One survey shows that of the 12 million people in the United States who call themselves lacto-ovo vegetarians, about half eat meat occasionally. Does that make them semi-vegetarians? In fact, a 1994 Roper poll commissioned by the Vegetarian Resource Group revealed that only 1 percent or less of the population can truly say that they *never* eat meat.[9]

Does this mean that most vegetarians are actually semivegetarians? Is a person who eats meat once or twice a year a semivegetarian? Admittedly, the definitions get a little murky here. We can't establish any precise definition, but there does seem to be a fine distinction. We would say that *semivegetarians* eat limited amounts of meat regularly. For *true vegetarians*, meat might represent a very occasional departure from their normally meat-free diet.

NONVEGETARIANS

A word that you will see used frequently throughout this book is "omnivore," which comes from two Latin roots: *omni*, meaning "all," and *vorare*, meaning "to devour." For our purposes, an omnivore is a person who consumes animal flesh, other animal foods, and plant foods. An omnivore usually eats red meat, fish, poultry, dairy products, eggs, vegetables, fruits, legumes, grains, nuts, and seeds. A semivegetarian is actually an omnivore who limits his or her meat intake—perhaps to a daily intake of just one or two ounces or larger amounts of meat just one or two times a week.

WHICH DIET TO CHOOSE

This book and the meal-planning guidelines in chapter 10 focus primarily on lacto-ovo and vegan diets, since these are the two most common types of vegetarian diet and the ones we recommend. We don't particularly aim to discourage adherents to other vegetarian patterns, but we also see no reason to rec-

ommend them. While there are hundreds of studies pointing to the health advantage of eating a vegetarian diet, there is no evidence that natural-hygiene, raw-foods, or fruitarian diets produce any additional benefits. Evidence for the superiority of macrobiotic diets is fairly limited at this time.

We also have some concerns about the advisability of fruitarian and raw-foods patterns for children. A macrobiotic and a more flexible natural-hygiene diet are likely to meet nutrient needs of all age groups if they are well planned. Macrobiotics can easily use the food guides in this book by choosing foods that are compatible with their diet.

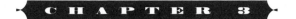

CHAPTER 3

THE WORLD'S HEALTHIEST DIET

Although we think we are one and we act as if we are one, human beings are not natural carnivores. When we kill animals to eat them, they end up killing us because their flesh, which contains cholesterol and saturated fat, was never intended for human beings, who are natural herbivores.

—WILLIAM CLIFFORD ROBERTS, M.D., EDITOR IN CHIEF, *American Journal of Cardiology,* 1991

◆

If you step back and look at the data, the optimum amount of red meat you should eat is zero.

— WALTER WILLETT, PH.D., HARVARD UNIVERSITY SCHOOL OF PUBLIC HEALTH, 1990

◆

There is no disease, bodily or mental, which adoption of vegetable diet and pure water has not infallibly mitigated, wherever the experiment has been fairly tried. Debility is gradually converted into strength, disease into healthfulness . . . the unaccountable irrationalities of ill temper, that make hell of domestic life, into a calm and considerable evenness of temper.

—PERCY BYSSHE SHELLEY, *A Vindication of Natural Diet,* 1813

◆

Thanks be to God, since the time I gave up the use of flesh meat and wine, I have been delivered from all physical ills.

— JOHN WESLEY, LETTER TO THE BISHOP OF LONDON, 1747

◆

Men dig their graves with their own teeth and die more by those fatal instruments than the weapons of their enemies.

—THOMAS MOFFETT, *"Health's Improvement,"* 1600

◆

THE POWER OF A VEGETARIAN DIET

A vegetarian diet is a powerful way to protect health. Vegetarians have lower rates of cancer, particularly colon and lung cancer, less heart disease, lower blood pressure, less diabetes, fewer gallstones, less kidney disease, and less colon disease. Vegetarian diets have been shown to prevent the onset of these diseases; in some cases they are also useful treatments for these diseases. Vegan diets appear to be even healthier than lacto-ovo-vegetarian diets.

We can point to many aspects of plant-based diets that help to explain the good health of vegetarians. For example, vegetar-

Vegetarians Have Lower Rates Of

Cancer	Hypertension
Heart disease	Gallstones
Diabetes	Kidney stones
Obesity	

Protective Factors in Vegetarian Diets

• Vegetarians eat less fat. High-fat diets are linked to a risk for diabetes, heart disease, obesity, and cancer. American omnivores eat a diet that is 36 to 40 percent fat; lacto-ovo vegetarians eat a 33 to 35 percent fat diet; vegans eat a 30 percent fat diet.

• Vegetarians eat less cholesterol. Cholesterol raises the risk for heart disease and possibly for cancer. American omnivores consume about five hundred milligrams of cholesterol per day; lacto-ovo vegetarians eat two hundred milligrams of cholesterol a day; vegans eat no cholesterol.

• Vegetarians eat more fiber. Dietary fiber appears to lower the risk for cancer and heart disease, and helps to control diabetes. Typical Americans eat only about twelve grams of fiber each day. Vegetarians eat about two to four times this much.

• Vegetarians consume more antioxidants. Antioxidants reduce the risk for cancer, heart disease, cataracts, and other diseases. They include vitamin E, vitamin C, and beta-carotene, as well as many phytochemicals.

• Vegetarians consume adequate protein, but less total protein and less animal protein. Omnivores consume a diet that is 15 to 17 percent protein, lacto-ovos eat 13 to 15 percent protein, while vegans get only about 11 percent of their calories from protein. Excess protein, especially animal protein, is linked to higher risk for osteoporosis, kidney stone formation, and kidney disease. Animal protein may raise blood cholesterol levels and may increase cancer risk.

• Vegetarians consume phytochemicals. These biologically active nonnutritive plant components are associated with reduced risk for a wide range of diseases. There may be literally thousands of phytochemicals in plant foods that provide health benefits.

ian diets are generally lower in fat, higher in fiber, and higher in key vitamins and phytochemicals, or plant chemicals, that are protective. Also, plant protein may have some important health benefits over animal proteins. But it really seems to be the whole package that matters, and in some cases there are pieces that we haven't yet fit into the puzzle. Meat eaters can reap some of the benefits of vegetarian diets by lowering their fat intake and by increasing their intake of whole grains, beans, fruits, and vegetables. But it is doubtful that they can fully match the health of vegetarians. Most of the evidence points to this: the less meat and other animal products you eat, the better. A vegetarian diet seems to be the best choice for protecting health.

NUTRITION PRIMER

Nutrients are the substances in foods that we need for the maintenance, repair, and growth of body tissues. They fall into six categories—carbohydrates, protein, fat, vitamins, minerals, and water, and we need them all in order to stay alive. The superior health of vegetarians is often because their nutrient intake is in balance with the body's needs—not too much and not too little. So before we look at the health of vegetarians, let's review the substances that foods contain and their importance.

Carbohydrates

Carbohydrates provide energy to the body. There are two kinds of carbohydrates: complex and simple. Complex carbohydrates include starch and fiber. Starches are found in grains, beans, and some vegetables. Fiber is found in grains, beans, vegetables, fruits, nuts, and seeds. No animal foods contain any fiber. Simple carbohydrates are sugars, which occur naturally in fruits in high amounts and in lesser amounts in other plant foods and in milk.

The healthiest populations in the world build their diets around foods that are rich in complex carbohydrates, which are found only in plant foods. In healthy diets, carbohydrates should provide at least 65 percent of calories, mostly as starch. Vegetarians eat diets that are much higher in complex carbohydrates than nonvegetarians, and they especially have much higher intakes of fiber, typically two to four times as much.

Protein

Protein is needed for the structural parts of the body—such as the bones and muscles—and it is also needed to produce the enzymes and many hormones that are necessary for the processes that support life. Protein is found in all foods except fats. Healthy populations tend to eat diets that are moderate in protein and that include mostly plant protein. Americans typically eat about twice the RDA of protein. High-protein diets, especially diets high in animal protein, may raise the risk for a number of chronic diseases.

Optimal diets include between 10 and 15 percent of calories from protein. Vegetarians eat diets that are moderate in protein and low in animal protein (or, in the case of vegans, that contain no animal protein at all).

Fats

Fats are high in calories. A gram of fat has more than twice as many calories as a gram of either carbohydrates or protein. There are three types of fat: saturated fat, polyunsaturated fat, and monounsaturated fat. Most foods that contain fat contain all three, though the amounts of each vary in different foods. Saturated fat is mostly found in meats, poultry, dairy foods, eggs, and a few vegetable oils, like palm oil and coconut oil. Polyunsaturated fats are found in most vegetable oils, nuts, seeds, soyfoods, and in smaller amounts in grains, beans, and vegetables. Monounsaturated fats are found in olive oil, olives, canola oil, avocados, and nuts.

The optimal diet should get no more than 15 to 20 percent of its calories from fat, and most of that should be either polyunsaturated or monounsaturated fat. Evidence from Mediterranean countries, however, suggests that higher fat intakes can be healthy when most of the fat is monounsaturated. Vegetarians eat less total fat and less saturated fat than meat eaters, although the fat intake of Western lacto-ovo vegetarians, and even of vegans, is still too high.

Our actual fat requirement is very small. There are two polyunsaturated fatty acids that are essential in the diet and we need very small amounts of these. One of these, linoleic acid, is known as an *omega-6 fatty acid*. About 1 to 2 percent of our calories should come from linoleic acid, which is the predominant fat in many vegetable oils. For a person consuming 2,000 calories per day, ½ tablespoon of corn oil would provide enough linoleic acid. But you don't have to consume oils to meet the need for this nutri-

ent since it is also found in whole grains, vegetables, nuts, seeds, and legumes in small amounts. Eating a mixed diet of whole plant foods will provide enough linoleic acid. However, it is possible that higher intakes of linoleic acid are beneficial to health, especially for people who have high intakes of saturated fat. The amount of polyunsaturated acid relative to the amount of saturated fat in the diet plays a role in determining blood cholesterol levels.

The second essential fatty acid is linolenic acid, which is an *omega-3 fatty acid*. Omega-3 fatty acids may help to reduce heart disease and cancer risk. As little as one-third of a gram of linolenic acid is probably enough to meet our nutritional needs. Although fish oil has the highest content of omega-3 fatty acids, vegetarians can get this nutrient in soybeans and foods made from them (like soy oil, tofu, and soymilk), flax seed, canola oil, walnuts, and wheat germ. For example, one-half cup of tofu provides almost one-half gram of linolenic acid, or more than enough to meet nutritional needs.

The balance of these two essential fatty acids in the diet is an important issue. They are involved in the production of hormones with competing effects, so the ratio of the two fatty acids affects our ability to produce optimal levels of these hormones. The exact ratio isn't known, but scientists suggest that for every ten grams of linoleic acid consumed we need between one and three grams of linolenic acid.

Although most of the fat in vegetarian diets is unsaturated, they can still be high in *trans* fatty acids. Produced when vegetable oils are hydrogenated to make them more solid, trans fatty acids are found in processed foods, especially baked goods, and margarine, and they may increase the risk for heart disease. However, if the overall diet is low in fat, small amounts of trans fatty acids will probably be fine.

Vitamins

We need vitamins in very tiny amounts, but deficiencies of these nutrients have extensive, harmful effects on the body. They have a wide variety of functions and are involved in every aspect of the growth and maintenance of cells. This group includes the water-soluble vitamins—vitamin C, thiamin (B_1), riboflavin (B_2), niacin, B_6 (pyridoxine), B_{12} (cobalamin), folic acid, pantothenic acid, and biotin—and the fat-soluble vitamins, A, D, E, and K.

Minerals

Minerals are indestructible elements in foods that we need for a variety of reactions in the body and for the structures of body cells. An adult male's body has about six pounds of minerals. Although our bodies contain more than sixty different minerals, only seventeen of them are needed in the diet. The minerals we need are calcium, phosphorus, magnesium, sodium, potassium, chlorine, sulfur, iron, iodine, zinc, copper, chromium, fluorine, silicon, selenium, manganese, and molybdenum.

Water

Water is the most abundant substance found in the body. In fact, about two-thirds of your body weight is water. Without this essential nutrient, we can die in as few as three days. About half of the water in the diet actually comes from food, since food is mostly water.

Other Components in Foods

The following are not considered nutrients but do have effects on health.

Cholesterol. Although it is essential to health, the body makes all of the cholesterol it needs. The diets of healthy populations are low in cholesterol. Because cholesterol is found only in animal foods, lacto-ovo vegetarians have low-cholesterol diets and vegans have cholesterol-free diets. The average nonvegetarian consumes about five hundred milligrams of cholesterol a day.

Alcohol. Like carbohydrates, protein, and fats, alcohol provides calories to the body, but it is not a nutrient. Studies of Mediterranean populations indicate that moderate consumption of red wine lowers the risk for cardiovascular disease.

Phytochemicals. A vast array of active compounds in plant foods, phytochemicals don't function as nutrients, but they do affect health. Phytochemicals in all plants, but particularly in fruits and vegetables, may be powerful disease deterrents. Vegetarians have higher levels of these compounds in their diet.

HEART DISEASE

In 1925, British physician Sir John McNee described to his colleagues two cases of atherosclerosis, a "rare disease" that he had observed in the United States.[1] Today, just seventy years later, this disease kills more than one hundred people each

Figure 3.1 Average Serum Cholesterol Levels in Vegetarians and Omnivores

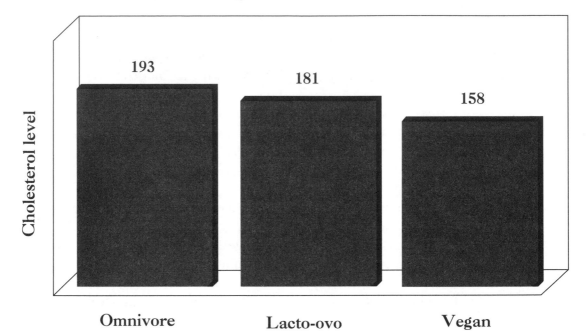

Thorogood M, Carter R, Benfield L, McPherson K, Mann JI. Plasma lipids and lipoprotein cholesterol concentrations in people with different diets in Britain. Br Med J 295:351–353, 1992.

hour in this country.[2] It is the leading cause of American deaths. Elevated blood cholesterol levels greatly increase the risk for atherosclerosis, which is the underlying cause of heart disease and heart attacks. Approximately 50 million Americans have blood cholesterol levels that are too high.

But cholesterol levels and the risk of heart disease vary considerably throughout the world. It's well established that lifestyle and diet play a big role. It is also very clear that vegetarians are much less likely to die from heart disease than meat eaters—about 50 percent less likely according to studies of vegetarians in the United States, Great Britain, the Netherlands, Norway, Germany, and Japan.[3]

Defining Heart Disease

Atherosclerosis is a hardening and narrowing of the arteries resulting from the buildup of fatty plaques. When blood flow becomes impeded or blocked, organs that depend on that blood supply for oxygen and nutrients will suffer. Atherosclerosis can therefore affect the health of the kidneys, the brain, the heart, and the reproductive organs. A blockage of blood flow to the heart may result in a heart attack.

Several factors raise the risk for developing atherosclerosis or having a heart attack. High blood cholesterol is one, since cholesterol makes up a significant portion of the plaques in the arteries. However, the *total* amount of cholesterol in your blood is just one part of the story. Since cholesterol is a waxy, fatlike substance, it won't mix in the blood very well, so it is always transported around the body attached to protein. The whole package of cholesterol and protein is called a lipoprotein, of which there are two types. One type of lipoprotein is called low-density lipoprotein, or LDL. LDLs raise the risk for heart disease because they carry cholesterol to the arteries to be deposited there. You've probably heard this referred to as "bad cholesterol." Cholesterol that is part of high-density lipoproteins, or HDLs, protects against heart disease because they carry cholesterol away from the arteries to be broken down and excreted. In fact, low levels of HDL—called good cholesterol—are considered a significant risk factor for heart disease. So the ideal situation is low levels of total cholesterol, but relatively high levels of HDL. That is, most of the cholesterol in your blood should be carried in HDL packages.

However, populations with low-fat, carbohydrate-rich diets tend to have low levels of the desirable HDL cholesterol, but they still have a low incidence of heart disease.[4] This is because people who eat vegetarian diets have lower *total* cholesterol and have less need for the protection of HDLs. Even with their lower HDL levels, they still have a favorable ratio of HDL to total cholesterol. But where people eat a typical Western diet and have high total cholesterol, they need higher levels of HDL.

When HDLs get too low in these groups, the risk of heart disease goes up.

Dietary Fat and Cholesterol Levels

Cholesterol levels respond very readily to changes in the diet. We see this in laboratory studies and in populations. For example, in Japan, a significant increase in cholesterol levels corresponded to a threefold increase in animal-food consumption between 1960 and 1980.[5] A number of dietary factors affect blood cholesterol levels:

• Saturated fat, which is abundant in animal foods, raises cholesterol levels more than any other dietary component. Although there are some kinds of saturated fat that don't raise blood cholesterol, they are often found in foods with those types that do. For example, red meat is high in a type of saturated fat called stearic acid that has no effect or very little effect on blood cholesterol levels. But it also contains considerable amounts of another saturated fat—palmitic acid—that does affect cholesterol. The net effect is that red meat will raise blood cholesterol.

• Dietary cholesterol, which is found only in animal foods, also raises blood cholesterol levels. Even very low fat animal foods can be high in cholesterol.

• Polyunsaturated fat and monounsaturated fat can lower blood cholesterol levels when they replace saturated fat in the diet. Plant foods tend to be higher in these types of fats. Studies of people living in Mediterranean countries indicate that higher-fat diets (30 percent or so) can be healthy when most of the fat is the monounsaturated type found in olives and olive oil.[6] However, most experts recommend reducing all types of dietary fat to help prevent heart disease.

• Trans-fatty acids also raise blood cholesterol levels somewhat.[7] These are the fats formed when vegetable oil is hydrogenated to make it solid. They are in margarine and other solid vegetable fats and are abundant in commercial baked goods. However, replacing the margarine in your diet with butter isn't the solution because butter is high in saturated fat. The best approach is to reduce your use of all fats.

Many studies have shown that vegetarians have lower levels of blood cholesterol. The American Health Foundation in Valhalla, New York, found that the blood cholesterol levels of vegans were 35 percent lower than those of omnivores.[8] Lacto-ovo vegetarians have cholesterol levels that are usually at least 10 percent lower than those of omnivores and often as much as 20 percent lower.[9] Even when vegetarians are compared with people who eat just small amounts of meat, the vegetarians have lower cholesterol.[10] In fact, in a study of Seventh-day Adventists, those who ate meat just once or twice a week had higher levels of cholesterol than vegetarians.[11]

Although many lifestyle habits can affect cholesterol, diet is most likely the important factor in these studies. Putting omnivores on a vegetarian diet without any other lifestyle change results in a drop in cholesterol levels.[12]

One of the most publicized studies of heart disease was led by Dr. Dean Ornish of the University of California, San Francisco. He showed that a very low-fat vegetarian diet produced a 25 percent reduction in cholesterol levels.[13] For every 1% decrease in cholesterol, there is a 2 to 3% decrease in heart disease risk. The most exciting thing about this study was that the diet was actually able to reverse heart disease by reducing the amount of plaque in the arteries. In the past, only drugs or surgery could achieve this.

Traditional diets for lowering blood cholesterol, like the American Heart Association (AHA) diet, can sometimes slow the progression of plaque in the arteries, but they rarely stop it and never reverse it. This dietary approach doesn't go far enough in producing healthful changes. The AHA diet is 30 percent fat and allows meat, including red meat, daily. Ornish's diet was 10 percent fat and allowed no meat and only limited amounts of nonfat dairy products. Note, however, that Ornish's plan also involved exercise and stress management through daily meditation. It may be the combined effect of these factors that made the program so successful a treatment, not just diet.

Protein and Cholesterol

The traditional wisdom is that it is the lower fat content of vegetarian diets that makes them protective against heart disease. However, this may be only part of the story. A lacto-ovo-vegetarian diet was shown to lower blood cholesterol levels more than a meat-based diet even when both diets contained the exact same amounts of fat, saturated fat, and cholesterol.[14] Although this is still a controversial area, it seems that animal *protein* may raise the risk for heart disease by directly affecting blood cholesterol levels. The effects of plant protein—in particular, soy protein—are really nothing new. The first studies to show these were conducted in the 1960s.[15] Of the 38 trials conducted since that time, 34 found that soy protein effectively lowered cholesterol—on average by about 13%. But people with very high cholesterol experience a much bigger decrease.[16] In fact, the national health service of Italy actually provides soy protein free of charge to physicians for treatment of patients with high cholesterol.[17]

Other Protective Effects of Vegetarian Diets

Vegetarians also eat more fiber. One type of fiber, called soluble fiber, lowers blood cholesterol between 5 and 10 percent.[18] Legumes, oat bran, and barley are especially good sources of this type of fiber.

Antioxidants in plant foods can protect against heart disease. In order for LDL cholesterol to be taken up by the arteries and to damage the artery walls, it has to be oxidized first. This occurs when LDLs are attacked by unstable oxygen molecules called free radicals. Antioxidants, which are especially abundant in fruits and vegetables, prevent this from happening and can protect the arteries from the damaging effects of cholesterol.

Three vitamins in particular seem to be powerful antioxidants. These are vitamin C, beta-carotene (actually a previtamin), and vitamin E. All of these tend to be higher in the diets of vegetarians than of omnivores.

Vitamin E is an especially important antioxidant, and vegetarians have higher levels of this nutrient in their bloodstream.

High levels of iron in the blood may raise heart disease risk because iron plays a role in oxidation.[19] Although iron levels are generally adequate in vegetarians, they do tend to be lower than in meat eaters.[20] This is probably the optimal situation: iron levels that are on the low side of normal. Also, researchers at Harvard found that it is only the type of iron found in animal foods that raises risk for heart disease. The iron in plant foods has no effect.[21]

Finally, there are other risks for heart disease that don't necessarily have anything to do with blood cholesterol. Heart attacks are often the result of blood clots forming in the arteries and blocking the flow of blood. The more viscous the blood, the more likely a clot will form. For reasons that aren't clearly understood, vegetarians tend to have less viscous blood.[22]

Vegetarian Diets versus Other Low-Fat Diets

Some nutritionists have suggested that low-fat diets that use lean meats can have the same cholesterol-lowering effects that vegetarian diets have. Conventional wisdom has been that it isn't a vegetarian diet per se that reduces heart disease risk, but that it is low-fat, high-fiber diets (which would include vegetarianism) that are protective. But we have good reason to believe that meat eaters who take pains to reduce fat and increase fiber in their diet won't necessarily have the same benefits as vegetarians. Plant protein as well as other compounds in plants may be

Figure 3.2 Leading Causes of Cancer Death

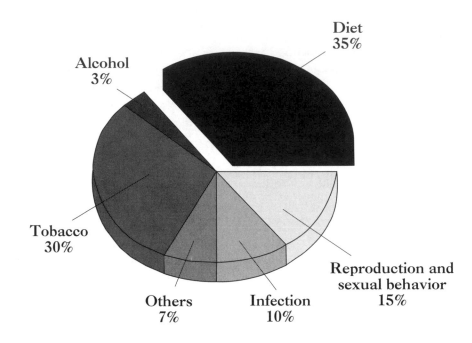

Diet
35%

Alcohol
3%

Tobacco
30%

Others
7%

Infection
10%

Reproduction and
sexual behavior
15%

protective. The iron that is abundant in lean meat may be harmful. So it's not surprising that studies have shown that even people with very small amounts of meat in their diet have higher cholesterol than vegetarians. There is good evidence that the farther you go in replacing animal foods with plant foods in your diet, the less your chance of developing heart disease. So it appears that a vegetarian diet—most likely a vegan diet—is the best choice of all.

CANCER

People who eat vegetarian or near-vegetarian diets have rates of cancer among the lowest in the world. It isn't too surprising. A vegetarian diet comes closest to the dietary guidelines for reduc-ing cancer risk set forth by the National Cancer Institute. In fact, it is estimated that Americans could reduce their cancer incidence by 50 to 90 percent if they adopted the lifestyle and diet of low-risk countries.[23] Although other lifestyle factors—and genetics, for that matter—have a lot to do with cancer risk, the National Cancer Institute estimates that one-third of all cancer deaths in this country and eight out of ten of the most common cancers are related to diet.[24] It's no wonder that among different populations, cancer rates vary by as much as a hundredfold.

Defining Cancer

The incredible destruction of cancer is thought to start with just one cell. Every time cells divide, there is the possibility one of them will become a cancer cell. Over a lifetime, each of the 100 trillion (that's 100,000,000,000,000) cells in the human body divides approximately 10 trillion times. This means that every minute of the day, about 10 million of your cells are dividing. (However, only certain types of cells, called stem cells, are thought to be converted into cancer cells.)

Under the best conditions, cells divide normally, producing new, exact copies of themselves. But sometimes the genetic material in the cell—the DNA—is altered in some way by a compound called a mutagen. Most mutagens are also carcinogens. When these attack the DNA at certain sites, the result can be a cancer cell. Carcinogens include many pesticides, environmental contaminants, and some dietary components.

A cell that is damaged by a carcinogen is *initiated*. Most initiated cells stay dormant or inactive until they are acted on by a promoter that prompts them to divide. Some dietary factors, likely among them dietary fat, are promoters. The promotion stage of cancer lasts for many years. Fortunately, it is also reversible. Dietary changes, such as reducing fat intake, made after the cancer process has begun can still be effective in stopping it.

There are also enzymes in the body that can "detoxify" carcinogens. Certain dietary components in plant foods may enhance some of these enzymes. Other dietary components like fiber—also found only in plant foods—can actually help the body to get rid of carcinogens. These are just a few of the ways that plant-based diets might lower the risk for cancer.

But there are many important questions about vegetarians and cancer risk. First, is it truly diet and not some other factor that protects vegetarians? Does a vegetarian diet protect against all types of cancer? And if it is diet, what is it about a vegetarian diet that is so protective? We'll see that the answers are actually harder to come by than you might think.

Does a Vegetarian Diet Protect against Cancer?

In trying to determine whether a vegetarian diet is protective against cancer, we run into two problems. First, vegetarians tend to differ from the rest of the population in several ways. They smoke less, drink less, and are more highly educated. All of these things probably reduce the risk for cancer, so it is difficult to determine how big a role diet plays. Second, most studies of vegetarians have looked at the effects of a lacto-ovo-vegetarian diet on cancer risk or have involved people who have followed a vegan diet for only a short period of time. Therefore, we have very little information about the cancer rates of vegetarians who consume no animal products. Nevertheless, we can see some interesting trends. Studies in Great Britain, Germany, Japan, and Sweden all show that vegetarians have lower cancer mortality rates than meat eaters.[25] One British study of six thousand vegetarians found that vegetarians were only half as likely to die from cancer as omnivores.[26] And when they were compared with a group of people who had similar lifestyles—except for diet—the vegetarians were still 40 percent less likely to die from cancer. This indicates that diet is the protective factor.

Vegetarians and Breast Cancer

Worldwide, populations that eat plant-based diets have much less breast cancer than those that eat more Western-type diets. Also, there is evidence that vegetarian diets—or diets that are largely based on plant foods—produce changes that seem to protect against breast cancer:

- Vegetarians have lower levels of blood estrogens, hormones that raise the risk for breast cancer.[27]

- Menstrual cycles of vegetarians are also different, and this might impact cancer risk. First, vegetarians begin menstruation somewhat later than average—an occurrence that lowers breast cancer risk.[28] Also, in Asian countries, where diets are more plant based, women have longer menstrual cycles; that is, there is a longer time between periods. Longer menstrual cycles mean that a woman is exposed to less estrogen over her lifetime and are also linked to a lower risk of breast cancer.[29] It's interesting to note that dietary fat shortens the menstrual cycle, while fiber increases it.[30]

- Soyfood consumption may also affect breast cancer risk. Soybeans, and many of the foods made from them, contain chemicals called isoflavones, which act against cancer in a variety of ways. They can block the activity of estrogen, which may help to explain the lower incidence of breast cancer in women in Asian coun-

tries, where soyfood consumption is high compared with that in the West.[31] Western vegetarians are also much more likely than omnivores to use soy products like tofu, soymilk, tempeh, and miso.

With these kinds of findings, it is somewhat surprising to find that *Western* vegetarian women actually have about the same rates of breast cancer as Western meat eaters. One reason might be that most of the available studies have involved Seventh-day Adventist vegetarians, most of whom are lacto-ovo vegetarians and who have diets that are fairly high in fat. So we don't know whether studies of vegetarians of other cultural groups, and particularly studies of vegans, would give us a different picture of vegetarian diet and breast cancer risk.

Vegetarians and Colon Cancer

Diet is more strongly linked to colon cancer than to any other type of cancer. Vegetarians clearly are less likely to get this disease.[32] In fact, the whole environment of the colon may be quite different in vegetarians than in meat eaters in the following ways.

Cell proliferation. The more colon cells grow and divide—or proliferate—the greater the risk for cancer. Colon cells of vegetarians tend to be much less active in this regard.[33]

Bile acids. These are compounds in the intestines that are necessary for the absorption of fat. Most bile acids—called primary bile acids—are harmless, but they can be converted into *secondary bile acids*, which are carcinogenic. Vegetarians and other people consuming mostly plant-based diets have fewer of these carcinogenic bile acids.[34]

Vegans have even lower levels than lacto-ovo vegetarians.[35]

Intestinal bacteria. Our intestines are home to more than four hundred different species of bacteria, numbering in the billions. Some studies indicate that vegetarians have somewhat different types of bacteria. They may have fewer of the bacteria that convert the harmless bile acids into the ones that are carcinogens.[36]

Fecal enzyme activity. Some studies show that vegetarians have lower levels of fecal enzymes that enhance the absorption of carcinogens.[37]

Fecal mutagens. Most studies indicate that vegetarians have lower levels of mutagens, compounds that can lead to cancer cell formation, in their feces.[38]

Other Cancers

Diet may also play a role in lung cancer, although there is much debate about this.[39] In a Japanese study of more than 122,000 people, meat intake increased lung cancer risk in people who smoked.[40] In nonsmoking women, saturated fat intake increased lung cancer risk dramatically.[41] One advantage for vegetarians might be the fact that they have higher blood levels of beta-carotene, which is thought to protect against lung cancer.[42]

We don't know whether a vegetarian diet protects against prostate cancer, but diet may play some role here. It is interesting to note that early prostate cancer is just as common in Japan as in the United States. However, something seems to delay the growth of prostate cancer in Japanese men, since their tumors are much less likely to develop into full-blown cancer.[43] Diet may be one factor. High fiber intakes decrease the risk of prostate cancer, and high fat intakes raise the risk.[44] Animal fat in particular may raise the risk. There is some evidence that varying levels of male hormones affect prostate cancer. In one study, when omnivore men were fed a vegetarian diet, levels of the hormones that may raise the risk for prostate cancer decreased.[45]

Low-fat diets have also been shown to reduce the occurrence of non-melanoma skin cancer.

What Makes a Vegetarian Diet an Anticancer Diet?

Western vegetarians are less likely to die from cancer in general; specifically, they have lower rates of colon and lung cancer, two of the most common cancers in developed countries. International comparisons show that where people eat plant-based diets, their risk for *many* kinds of cancer is lower.

There are many factors in vegetarian diets that might lower the risk for cancer. Foods that are central to vegetarian diets—whole grains, legumes, fruits, and vegetables, for example—are loaded with compounds that have anticancer activity. Also, meat, animal fat, and high-protein diets might be directly linked to a higher risk of cancer. Red meat, in particular, seems to raise the risk for colon cancer.

But, undoubtedly, it is the whole vegetarian package that counts. Avoiding meats, especially those cooked at high temperatures, limiting fat, especially animal fat, and eating more whole grains, fruits, and vegetables could help to explain why, worldwide, people who eat plant-based diets have less cancer.

Let's look at the dietary components that affect cancer risk.

Fat. While there continues to be quite a bit of controversy over the role of fat in breast cancer risk, studies indicate that a significantly lower fat intake lowers the risk for colon cancer. Studies also indicate that low-fat diets, and perhaps vegetarian diets, increase the levels of *natural killer cells*, which are part of the immune system and can kill tumor cells and viruses.[46] In Western countries, the fat intake of lacto-ovo vegetarians, although it is lower than that of meat eaters, is too high. This may be from an overreliance on cheese, eggs, and whole or 2 percent milk and yogurt. We would encourage lacto-ovo vegetarians to deemphasize these foods in their diet.

Protein. High intakes of protein in general, and especially animal protein, might raise the risk for breast, colon, prostate, renal, and endometrial cancer.[47] All types of vegetarian diets are lower in protein than omnivore diets, and vegan diets are lowest of all. It is a little bit difficult, however, to separate the effects of protein from those of fat, since these two nutrients occur together in foods much of the time.

Cholesterol. Dietary cholesterol, which is found only in animal foods, may specifically increase the risk for colon cancer.[48]

Animal foods. If vegetarians get less cancer and if diets high in protein and fat seem to pose some risk, then clearly meat raises the risk for cancer, right? Unfortunately, things aren't quite that simple. The role of both fat and protein in increasing cancer risk are unclear. Even if vegetarians get less cancer, that doesn't "prove" that meat causes cancer. The information is conflicting. Not all studies show that eating meat poses a cancer risk,[49] but a number of studies, including the following findings, do support a link between meat and cancer:

• Meat consumption increases the levels of mutagens in the colon.[50]

• Meat cooked at high temperature, especially when it has been grilled, produces potent mutagens called heterocyclic amines (HCA).[51] These might be associated with cancer of the colon, liver, lung, breast, small and large intestines, and other types of cancer.

• In one large study of Seventh-day Adventists, various animal foods had different effects on different cancers.[52] While there was no relationship between animal-product consumption and breast cancer, both meat and egg consumption raised the risk for ovarian cancer. When researchers looked at the combined effect of eating meat, eggs, milk, and cheese, the risk for getting cancer in general went up three and a half times.

• SDAs who consumed meat, fish, or poultry three times or more per week were two and a half times more likely to develop bladder cancer than those who consumed it fewer than three times per week.[53]

• A Harvard study of eighty-eight thousand nurses found that meat intake, especially red meat, raised their risk for colon cancer.[54]

• In the Health Professional Follow-Up Study researchers looked at the meat intake of fifty thousand male health professionals. Those who ate red meat (beef, pork, and lamb) more than four times per week had more than a three-fold increase in the risk of colon cancer compared with those who ate meat less than once per month.[55]

Fiber. Fiber clearly plays a big role in maintaining the health of the colon. It binds harmful substances like bile acids and potential carcinogens and ushers them out of the colon more quickly.[56] Fiber may also help to lower estrogen levels, which could offer protection against breast cancer.[57] Fiber is found only in plant foods, and vegetarians have much higher fiber intakes than meat eaters do—as much as two to four times higher.

Vitamins. Certain vitamins may lower the risk for cancer. Specifically, vitamin C may help to protect against colon cancer.[58] Beta-carotene, which is a precursor of vitamin A, might protect against lung cancer and other cancers as well.[59] Both these vitamins are found almost exclusively in plant foods.

Phytochemicals. These are compounds in plants that have no nutritional value but can have important biological effects that may lower the risk for cancer, heart disease, and other diseases. There are literally hundreds of them, and we haven't begun to test all of them. Since they are found only in plant foods, vegetarians have higher intakes of these compounds than nonvegetarians. Many plant pigments, the chemicals that give fruits and vegetables their bright colors, are phytochemicals that give protection against cancer. And the cruciferous vegetables, including broccoli, cauliflower, kale, and turnips, contain compounds that reduce colon cancer risk. Fruits and vegetables are especially rich in these compounds, but whole grains and legumes are also good sources.

The strongest dietary protection against cancer seems to come from eating fruits and vegetables. More than one hundred studies of eating habits throughout the world show that fruits and vegetables decrease cancer risk.[60]

HIGH BLOOD PRESSURE

Hypertension is a disease of epidemic proportions in the United States. In most industrialized countries, blood pressure typically gets higher as people get older. But this doesn't occur in developing countries.[61] Blood pressure goes up when people move from countries where blood pressure is not a problem to Western industrialized countries.[62]

As long ago as the early 1900s some researchers noted that meat raised blood pressure. In 1926, a study of vegetarian college students showed that their blood pressure increased within just two weeks of adding meat to their diet.[63] In 1930 a study of German monks showed that those who didn't eat meat had lower blood pressure than those who did.[64] Other early studies showed that adding meat to plant diets raised blood pressure in a relatively short time.[65]

Most of the more recent studies show the same thing. Vegetarians have lower blood

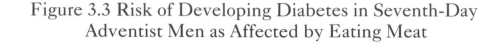

Figure 3.3 Risk of Developing Diabetes in Seventh-Day Adventist Men as Affected by Eating Meat

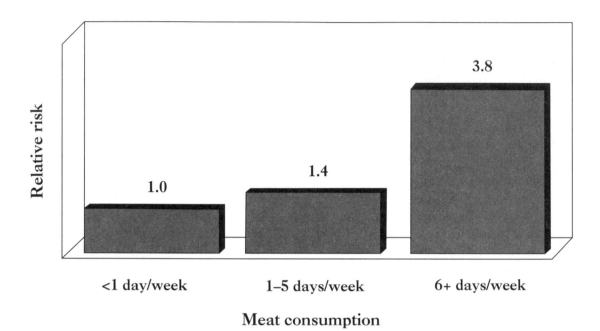

Snowdon DA, Phillips RL. Does a vegetarian diet reduce the occurrence of diabetes? Am J Publ Health 75:507–512, 1985.

pressure than meat eaters in general.[66] Vegetarians also have less hypertension. Meat eaters are also about thirteen times more likely to have very high blood pressures (defined as blood pressure above 160/95).[67] As is true for heart disease, even a little bit of meat might make a difference. Vegetarians have lower blood pressure than semivegetarians who consume meat less than once per week.[68]

People who are overweight are at much higher risk for hypertension. So we might guess that vegetarians have lower blood pressure than meat eaters because they are leaner. However, vegetarians have lower blood pressure regardless of differences in weight. The only time vegetarians don't have lower blood pressure is when they are significantly obese.[69]

In fact, researchers aren't sure what it is about vegetarian diets that protects against hypertension. Vegetarians eat about the same amount of salt as omnivores, so this wouldn't explain it.[70] The effects also don't seem to be due to the type of fat in the diet, or fiber, potassium, calcium, or magnesium, all of which have been linked to blood pressure.[71]

It may be a fairly complex set of circumstances that lowers the risk for vegetarians. But chances are, as is true for other diseases, vegetarians gain their protection through some combination of dietary factors, including, perhaps, unknown substances in plant foods that directly protect against hypertension.[72]

DIABETES

One of the most interesting things about diabetes is how varied its occurrence is throughout the world. In many parts of the world it is rare, or almost nonexistent.[73] In other areas, nearly 50 percent of the population is diabetic.[74] Although some groups are genetically susceptible to this disease, it is clear that lifestyle and diet impact the risk of diabetes. In the United States, at least 13 million people, or 5 percent of the population, are diabetic, although probably half of these people don't know it.

Again, Western diet and lifestyle raise the risk for this disease. For example, when Japanese people move from Japan to Hawaii or California, their rates of diabetes increase—probably due to changes in lifestyle, particularly diet.[75] Diabetes is also more common in people with high cholesterol levels and in people who eat more fat, animal fat, protein, animal protein, and sugar. It's less common in people who have high intakes of carbohydrates and vegetable fat.[76]

Diabetes is actually two different diseases. In Type I diabetes, people produce inadequate amounts of the hormone insulin (or, in some cases, none of it). Insulin is needed to get blood sugar, or glucose, into cells. So without insulin, glucose builds up in the bloodstream. These people must have insulin injections to live. Studies have shown that in people who are genetically susceptible to this disease, drinking cow's milk during early infancy can greatly raise the risk of eventually developing Type I diabetes.[77]

In Type II diabetes the production of insulin varies. In many cases the cells are not responsive so that, again, glucose can't move into cells. Type II diabetics may or may not use insulin injections. In most cases, this disease can be treated by diet and exercise. Most of the diabetics in this country have Type II diabetes, and most are overweight. In fact, obesity, more than any other factor, raises the risk for diabetes.[78]

Because insulin is actually involved in many processes in the body, and because high levels of blood glucose can be damaging, the effects of diabetes can be far-reaching. Diabetics are more likely to have high levels of blood cholesterol and are at very high risk for atherosclerosis.[79] Uncontrolled diabetes can lead to heart disease and can also cause nerve damage and affect reproductive organs, kidneys, eyes, and limbs.

Diet for Diabetics

Treatment of diabetes has always centered around diet. Precisely how much carbohydrate, protein, and fat diabetics should eat has been debated over the years. At one time early in this century, physicians recommended a diet that was only 20 percent carbohydrates. But it is clear that populations with the lowest rates of diabetes eat a diet that is rich in carbohydrates. Recent studies show that high-carbohydrate, low-fat diets are more effective in controlling blood glucose.

In fact, the more scientists learn about diabetes, the more their recommendations have come to resemble a vegetarian diet. Today, recommendations are for diabetics to eat a diet rich in complex carbohydrates, including plenty of fiber, to consume moderate protein, and to keep fat intake low, especially avoiding saturated fat and cholesterol.[80] The American Diabetes Association recommends a diet that is less than 30 percent fat, and there is good reason to believe that fat intake should be even lower for diabetics. It is clear that a vegetarian diet fits this prescription better than almost any other way of eating. That's why it isn't very surprising to find that vegetarian diets work well to prevent and to treat diabetes.

A very low fat vegetarian diet helped to treat symptoms of diabetic neuropathy, which is nerve damage that can cause considerable pain in diabetes.[81] In a study at the Pritikin Longevity Center in California, patients with Type II diabetes followed a diet that was just 10 percent fat and included only about three ounces of meat a week. Most of the patients were able to stop using insulin or oral medication.[82]

In fact, feeding very high fat diets to lean, healthy people can actually produce signs of mild diabetes.[83]

Diabetes in Vegetarians
We expect to see less diabetes in vegetarians, since they are leaner and they eat a diet rich in complex carbohydrates. And although there hasn't been much research in this area, the little that has been done shows that veg-

etarians are less likely to get diabetes. In a study of twenty-five thousand SDAs, non-vegetarian men were nearly twice as likely to have diabetes as vegetarian men. Non-vegetarian women were about one and a half times as likely to have diabetes as vegetarian women. In this case, the difference in the rates of diabetes seemed to have nothing to do with weight.[84]

Meat consumption seems to be directly associated with diabetes risk, although it is a more powerful factor in men than in women. Even men who ate meat just one or two times per week had a higher risk of diabetes.[85] In women, risk is higher only in those who eat meat at least six times per week.

OBESITY

Obesity isn't a disease but a condition that most people would like to avoid. And it certainly raises the risk of diseases such as atherosclerosis, hypertension, cancer, and diabetes. In the United States, about one-fourth of all adults below the age of seventy-four are overweight. Although obesity raises the risk for disease, it is important to distinguish between "apples" and "pears." People who deposit fat around their hips and thighs are referred to as "pears." This kind of fat distribution is not associated with higher risk for disease. But apples carry their weight in the belly, and this does raise risk.

Despite a multimillion-dollar dieting industry and a plethora of studies on obesity, the true cause of this condition and its cure remain unknown. Although there seems to be a strong genetic component, lifestyle—particularly diet and exercise—

has the biggest impact. A diet that is low in fat and high in carbohydrates—especially fiber—appears to be the best approach to weight control.[86]

Of course, this bodes well for vegetarians. Not surprisingly, they tend to be slimmer than omnivores.[87] And when, as in some studies, they do weigh the same, it is because they have more muscle tissue, not more body fat.[88] As we would expect, vegans tend to weigh even less than lacto-ovo vegetarians.[89]

In many studies vegetarians actually consumed more calories, and they didn't exercise any more than omnivores. Clearly there is no mysterious or unusual quality of vegetarian diets that helps to keep people slim. Vegetarian diets are lower in fat and higher in fiber. Vegetarians who eat high-fat diets are likely to gain weight just as easily as those who eat meat. (We discuss the relationship of vegetarian diets to weight loss in more detail in chapter 17.)

KIDNEY DISEASE

The kidneys are clusters of mini-filters that sift unwanted chemicals out of the bloodstream and excrete them in urine. Every day, the kidneys filter your entire volume of plasma—the liquid portion of the blood—about sixty times for a total of forty-five gallons a day. But only about 1 percent of what passes through the kidneys is actually excreted.

Anything that increases the rate at which kidneys filter blood will stress the kidneys to some degree by forcing them to work harder. One thing that boosts this filtration rate is protein. So it isn't surprising that the filtra-tion rate of vegetarians is about half that of meat eaters.[90] And vegans, whose diets are lower in protein, filter blood at an even slower rate than lacto-ovo vegetarians.[91]

The type of protein in the diet may be just as important as the amount in determining the filtration rate. In a British study, the filtration rate was about 16 percent higher after people ate a meal of animal protein than after they ate a meal of soy protein—even though total amounts of protein were the same.[92]

In people who already have kidney disease, protein restriction is generally recommended.[93] But newer recommendations for treating kidney disease may be to replace animal protein with plant protein (particularly soy) rather than decrease overall protein intake. Since the pathology of kidney disease is very similar to that of atherosclerosis, high cholesterol levels can also increase its risk. This is another reason that vegetarian diets may protect against kidney disease.

KIDNEY STONES

A separate issue related to the kidneys is the formation of kidney stones in the urinary tract. They are rarely life threatening, but can be an excruciatingly painful disorder. Although about 12 percent of Americans will develop them at some time in their life (mostly men), they are rare in other parts of the world.

Kidney stones are made up mostly of calcium and a substance called oxalate that is found in a variety of foods, including many fruits and vegetables. It is also produced in the body. Contrary to popular belief, though, dietary calcium seems to reduce the risk for kidney stones.[94] It does this by binding oxalates in the digestive tract and making them unavailable for kidney stone formation.

Lacto-ovo vegetarians have fewer kidney stones, since they often have high-calcium diets. But why do vegans, who have *lower* calcium intake than omnivores, also form fewer kidney stones? Once again, the answer seems to lie in the type of protein in their diet. We'll see in chapter 7 that animal protein increases the excretion of calcium in the urine. The more protein in the diet, the greater the risk of stone formation.[95] In one study of fifty thousand men, animal protein increased the risk of kidney stones by 30 percent. The more animal protein in the diet, the more likely the men were to have kidney stones.[96] And, British vegetarians were only half as likely to form kidney stones as the general population.[97]

Although most kidney stones are made up of calcium oxalate, some are formed of uric acid. Diets high in compounds called purines promote these kinds of stones. Protein-rich foods tend to be higher in purines.[98]

There may also be components of vegetarian diets that directly inhibit stone formation. For example, citrate, an organic acid that is abundant in vegetarian diets, interferes with kidney stone formation.[99]

GALLSTONES

Gallstones are another common problem in Western societies, affecting about 10 percent of the U.S. population. The gallbladder releases bile into the intestines, where it helps in the digestion of fat. Bile can crystallize into small stones that block the gallbladder, producing pain or jaundice. The chief ingredient of gallstones is cholesterol, which is also the chief ingredient in bile.

Meat eaters are twice as likely as vegetarians to form gallstones.[100] In contrast, rural Africans, who eat a largely vegan diet, rarely, if ever, develop gallstones.[101] Western vegetarians are also much less likely to form them. We don't know why this is, though. People who are obese are more likely to form gallstones, and people who eat meat are more likely to be fat. A higher intake of saturated fat also raises risk. Moderate alcohol consumption and high fiber intake both reduce the risk for gallstones.[102] Also, plant protein, particularly soy protein, is linked to a reduced risk for gallstones.[103]

DIVERTICULAR DISEASE

Diverticular disease involves small pouches along the lining of the large intestine. When these pouches become inflamed, the condition is called diverticulitis, which can be quite painful. This common Western ailment affects as many as 40 percent of Americans over the age of fifty.[104] It is much less common in rural populations and in people who eat plant-based diets. In some cultures, it is almost nonexistent.[105] As is true for so many other conditions, vegetarians are only half as likely to develop diverticular disease as meat eaters.[106]

It is most likely the fiber content of vegetarian diets that lowers the risk for this disease. But high fat intake may also promote diverticular disease. A diet that is low in fiber and high in fat is twice as likely to produce diverticulosis. But a diet that is specifically high in red meat and low in fiber is three times more likely to result in this disease.[107] One theory is that red meat influences some bacteria in the colon to produce toxins that weaken the colon wall and promote the formation of diverticula.[108]

OTHER CONDITIONS

Vegetarians may be less likely to suffer from a number of other conditions, although the evidence is not nearly as strong as for those diseases we discussed above.

Arthritis. Arthritis is a general term for inflammation of the joints. Rheumatoid arthritis is the most common type, and it can result in irreversible damage to the joints. It is thought to be an autoimmune disease; that is, the body's immune system attacks itself. Arthritis sufferers spend billions of dollars each year in search of relief for this painful, debilitating condition. A few studies have suggested some relief is obtained from a vegan diet that includes substantial amounts of raw foods.[109] In one study, patients began with a seven- to ten-day fast, followed by a wheat-free vegan diet for three to five months, and then a lacto-ovo-vegetarian diet for six months. There was significant reduction in pain and stiffness.[110] Unfortunately, the studies on diet and arthritis suffer from a number of problems, so we can't draw any firm conclusions about the effects of vegetarianism on this disease.

Multiple sclerosis. MS is a degenerative disease of the central nervous system that produces symptoms of numbness, impaired vision, tremors, and lack of coordination.

The speed with which the disease progresses varies quite a bit among people who have it. No studies exist on vegetarian diet and MS, but saturated fat may have an impact. Patients who consumed fewer than twenty grams of saturated fat per day had many fewer symptoms than those who ate more than twenty grams of saturated fat per day.[111] Another study found that progression of the disease was slowed in people who ate a diet higher in polyunsaturated fat, but low in total fat.[112]

Dementia. Dementia is a major economic and public-health problem. As many as 50 percent of the over-sixty-five population may have mild forms of this condition, with 5 percent suffering from severe dementia.[113] One report indicates that vegetarians may be less likely to develop dementia. Seventh-day Adventists who ate meat were more than twice as likely to develop dementia than those who didn't eat meat.[114] If they had been eating meat for many years, they were more than three times as likely to show symptoms. One theory is that cell damage from free radicals might be involved in the onset of dementia.[115] Vegetarian diets are higher in the antioxidants that protect against free-radical damage.

Constipation and hemorrhoids. The key to avoiding constipation is to consume plenty of liquids and fiber. Insoluble fiber (such as that found in wheat bran) is especially helpful. When people become constipated, they strain to pass stools, which can result in hemorrhoids, clusters of enlarged veins near the rectum. Hemorrhoids are painful and uncomfortable and sometimes require surgery. Since vegetarians consume two to four times as much fiber as meat eaters, they are less likely to suffer from either constipation or hemorrhoids.

Tooth decay. Vegetarians may have better dental health than meat eaters. Several studies of Seventh-day Adventist children show that they have fewer dental cavities, although the reasons for this aren't very clear.[116]

THE DAIRY CONNECTION

Eliminating meat from your diet can have a profound impact on your health risk. But it may be that the optimal eating pattern also limits—or eliminates—milk as well. Health risks associated with dairy foods are rather speculative at this time; the amount of research on these issues is somewhat meager for the most part. However, it is interesting and worth considering in making dietary choices.

Diabetes. Early consumption of cow's milk—whether it be regular cow's milk or infant formula based on cow's milk—can increase the risk for Type I diabetes (also called insulin-dependent diabetes, or IDDM) in genetically susceptible babies. These children may form antibodies to milk protein. It is believed that these antibodies destroy the cells on the pancreas that produce insulin. In one study of 142 children with diabetes, every one of them had high levels of this antibody to milk protein.[117] Other studies have shown the same thing.[118] In fact, recent research indicates that consuming milk throughout adolescence increases diabetes risk.

Ovarian cancer. One Harvard University study revealed that women with ovarian cancer were more likely to eat dairy prod-ucts than women without ovarian cancer.[119] In this case the culprit could be the milk sugar lactose. Enzymes in the body break lactose down to a sugar called galactose. Galactose is further metabolized by enzymes. Some people may have low levels of these enzymes. If so, dairy-product consumption can lead to a buildup of galactose, which may, in some way, damage the ovaries.[120]

Colic. Sensitivity to milk proteins can cause colic, a digestive problem in infants that produces great discomfort. Even breast-fed infants can have this problem if the nursing mother is using dairy products in her own diet. Removing milk from the mother's diet has been shown to reduce symptoms of colic.[121] Also, although it is *very* speculative, milk-protein intolerance has been suggested as one possible link to sudden infant death syndrome.[122]

Contaminants. Bacteria that can cause illness have been isolated from milk and other dairy products. In some cases, the bacteria contaminate the milk after pasteurization.[123] Soft cheeses are especially vulnerable to contamination, and the Centers for Disease Control recommends that pregnant women, older people, and those with weakened immune systems, in particular, should avoid these cheeses. Milk is also contaminated with hormones and antibiotics, and in some cases with drugs that can raise cancer risk.[124]

Milk intolerance. Many people are unable to digest the milk sugar lactose. Drinking milk can cause cramping, diarrhea, and nausea in these people. Many children are also allergic to milk protein.

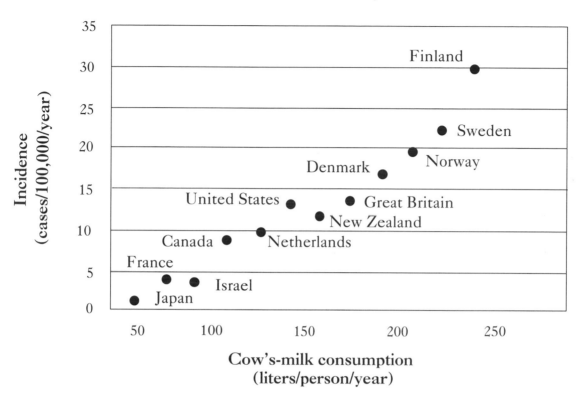

Figure 3.4 Relationship between Cow's-Milk Consumption in
Children 0–14 Years and Mean Yearly Incidence of IDDM

These values are approximate and are taken from Dahl-Jorgensen K, Joner G, Hanssen KF. Relationship between cow's-milk consumption and incidence of IDDM in childhood. Diabetes Care, 14:1081–1083, 1991.

Milk and anemia. In children, in particular, overreliance on milk can lead to anemia. This is because milk is very low in iron itself, and drinking too much of it can crowd iron-rich foods out of the diet. In young infants, protein from cow's milk can cause intestinal bleeding, which can lead to anemia. This effect isn't seen with infant formulas made from cow's milk, however. Also, the calcium in milk inhibits iron absorption.[125]

Milk and vitamin D toxicity. Milk is fortified with vitamin D. Federal regulations specify that ten micrograms of vitamin D should be added to each quart of milk. However, because such large volumes of milk are fortified at one time, the vitamin D may not be mixed properly, and some of the milk may have very high levels of this extremely toxic vitamin. In one case in which individuals were found to suffer from vitamin D toxicity, the milk they were drinking had five hundred times the amount of vitamin D that is specified by the government. (See chapter 8 for more on this issue.)

Galactose and heart disease. Heart disease risk is higher in Western countries, where people eat diets high in animal fat. In these countries, people also consume more dairy products. One theory is that galactose is directly related to heart disease risk. Galactose can attach to artery walls, which may initiate a series of reactions that can induce cholesterol to attach to the artery. This leads to plaque formation and eventually to heart disease.[126]

Galactose and cataracts. In some individuals, high blood levels of galactose cause the formation of cataracts. One condition, called galactosemia, results from a genetic deficiency of two enzymes needed to effectively process galactose. In people with this deficiency, consuming milk for just four to eight weeks can lead to cataract development.[127] Improperly metabolized galactose can lead to the formation of an alcohol called galactitol, which disrupts the structure of the lens of the eye.[128] Galactitol has been found in the lens of deceased patients who had cataracts and who had galactosemia.[129] Classic galactosemia is a rare condition, occurring in only about one out of every one hundred thousand people. More common is a situation in which people have a generally reduced ability to metabolize galactose—although they can metabolize small amounts of this sugar. As many as one out of every thousand people may have this condition.[130] In these individuals, consuming lactose—with the eventual production of galactose—greatly increases their risk of developing cataracts.[131] In India, where 39 percent of all blindness is due to cataracts, studies of patients who had cataracts and no other abnormalities revealed that nearly half had an impaired tolerance to galactose, measured by abnormal levels of galactose in the blood.[132] A recent study found that older people with impaired lactose tolerance were more likely to develop cataracts if they drank large amounts of milk.[133]

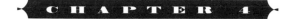
MORE REASONS TO GO MEATLESS

◆◆◆

How good it is to be well-fed, healthy and kind, all at the same time.

—DR. HENRY HEIMLICH, PHYSICIAN AND INVENTOR OF THE HEIMLICH MANEUVER

◆

Refrain at all times such foods as cannot be procured without violence and oppression. For know that all the inferior creatures, when hurt, do cry and send forth their complaints to their maker.

—THOMAS TRYON, *Wisdom's Dictates,* 1691

◆

You have just dined, and however scrupulously the slaughterhouse is concealed in the graceful distance of miles, there is complicity.

—RALPH WALDO EMERSON

◆

It is calculated that if no animal food were consumed, one-fourth of the land now used would suffice for human sustenance. And the extensive tracts of the country now appropriated to grazing, mowing, and other modes of animal provision, could be cultivated by and for intelligent and affectionate human neighbors.

—AMOS BRONSON ALCOTT AND CHARLES LANE, IN *Herald of Freedom,* SEPTEMBER 8, 1843

A VEGETARIAN DIET IS AN EARTH-FRIENDLY DIET

There are many ways to soften your impact on the environment. Using less water in your household, recycling, reducing your consumption of all material goods, driving less, and using less electricity are some of them. But it is most likely that your diet has the greatest impact. Animal agriculture has devastating effects on deforestation, water use, petroleum use, pollution, and perhaps even the ozone layer.

To a certain extent, all agriculture is destructive to the environment. But certain practices are more so than others. Organic agriculture is kinder to the earth than traditional farming methods. And the production of animal foods is much more destructive than the production of plant foods.

The 1971 publication of Frances Moore Lappé's groundbreaking work, *Diet for a Small Planet,* forever changed the way many of us look at protein and diet.[1] Through painstaking research, Lappé exposed the inefficiency of feeding a growing population with a diet based on animal foods. She dubbed beef cattle a "protein factory in reverse." That's because cattle—and other food animals—actually *consume* more protein than they *provide.* A steer consumes seven pounds of protein in the form of grain

◆◆◆

Figure 4.1 Relative Protein Production Efficiency

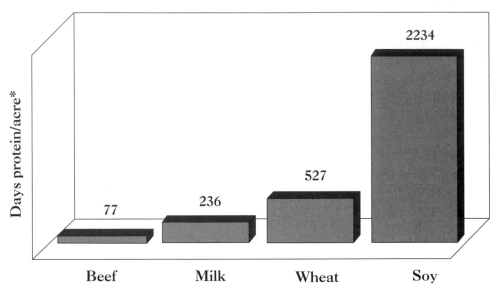

Days protein/acre*

77	236	527	2234
Beef	Milk	Wheat	Soy

*Daily protein needs met by 1 acre of land devoted to the production of various foods.

Christiansen RP. USDA Tech Bull 963, 1948.

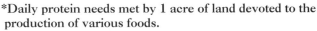

and soybeans to produce just one pound of beef protein. In the process, six pounds of high-quality protein ends up wasted.[2] It clearly would make more sense for us to eat the grain directly.

But there is much more at stake here than wasted grain. Large amounts of land, water, and fuel are used for the production of the grain that is fed to farm animals, as well as for the animals' direct use. In return, those animals give us relatively small amounts of meat and protein. This has far-reaching consequences on the environment.

Land and Forests

We have limited resources to grow food for our rapidly expanding global population, which has more than doubled since 1950, from 2.5 billion to more than 5 billion. It is expected to double again to reach more than 10 billion within fifty years.[3] It is absolutely crucial that we use land in the most efficient ways possible to produce food. Right now, we don't. When farmland is devoted to grazing animals and growing their food, the system is very inefficient. Let's assume that the average person consumes 2,500 calories per day: one acre of land will support seven people if it is used to grow grains and beans for human consumption; it will support less than one person if that same acre is given over to producing milk and meat.[4] You can see that using land for animal foods is an impractical way to feed large populations.

This inefficient use of land is directly related to forest destruction throughout the world, as it increases the demand for more farmland. The overgrazing of livestock also destroys land, turning it into desert, creating a constant need for new, arable land. One way to create new land for farming is to clear forests for grazing or for growing feed. Agriculture accounts for almost 90 percent of the nearly 30 million acres of forestland destroyed each year.[5] In Latin America, more than 50 million acres of tropical rain forest have been converted to cattle pasture.[6] Since 1960, more than one-third of the forest in Central America has been destroyed to create pastureland for cattle.[7]

The destruction of the rain forest has consequences that may be more devastating than we will ever realize. For one thing, when tropical rain forest is lost, many species of plants become extinct. At least half of all known species are native to the rain forest, and we are currently losing one hundred species per day.[8] At the present rate of rain forest destruction we can expect that 15 percent of all the earth's species will be extinct by the year 2000.[9] Although we've only identified about 1 percent of all the plant species living in the rain forest, approximately 25 percent of all prescription drugs come from those plants.[10]

The government's National Cancer Institute devotes resources to screening thousands and thousands of plants for potential anti-cancer activity. Think of all the plant species being destroyed at this moment that have not yet been studied and that may have powerful medicinal properties we will never know about. Are we destroying species that may hold the cure for cancer or AIDS—all for the sake of a hamburger? The National Accounting Office maintains that more plant species are eliminated or threatened by livestock grazing than by any other single factor.[11]

Water

More than one-third of all the water used in the United States is used to irrigate land just to grow food.[12] The amount of water used to produce food for direct human consumption is a drop in the bucket compared with the amount used to produce food for a farm animal. For example, it takes just twenty-four gallons of water to produce a pound of potatoes; it takes more than two thousand gallons to produce a pound of beef when you calculate what is needed to grow feed for the steer.[13] Water is perhaps the earth's most precious resource—and is likely to become very scarce. Changing to a vegetarian diet can decrease your water consumption more dramatically than anything else you can do.

Fuel

According to the Worldwatch Institute, it takes about forty-eight gallons of gasoline to produce the red meat and poultry typically eaten each year by an American.[14] More than one-third of all raw materials used, including fossil fuels like petroleum, are devoted to the production of animal foods. Fuel is used in a myriad of ways in farming—to run farm machinery as well as to support highly mechanized factory farms, which require artificial heating, lighting, and cooling. It stands to reason that when we switch from a meat-based diet to a plant-based one, we decrease the amount of food

Figure 4.2 Primary Sources of River Pollution

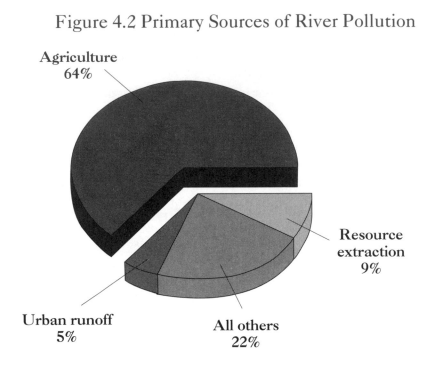

Agriculture
64%

Resource
extraction
9%

Urban runoff
5%

All others
22%

that has to be grown and the amount of fuel needed to feed people.

Beef production is the most devastating in terms of land, water, and fuel use and the destruction of the world's forests. Pork, chicken, eggs, and dairy all require less of these resources than does beef. But they still are highly inefficient compared with the production of vegetable foods.

There is another side to the environmental effects of animal agriculture. Besides being wasteful, it is polluting. Agriculture accounts for 64 percent of all river pollution and 57 percent of all lake pollution.[15] Animal excrement is one of the biggest pollutants from this industry. But processing of animal foods can also produce waste. It takes ten pounds of milk to produce one pound of cheese. The waste product in the process is whey. Whey is used extensively by the food industry as a food additive, but much of it is dumped into the sewage system and can end up in rivers, where it is a costly pollutant.

Animal agriculture also contributes to global warming. The two main sources of methane gas, one of the "greenhouse gases," are rice paddies and cattle. The world's cattle, sheep, and goats emit 70 to 80 million tons of methane per year, through manure and belching, amounting to as much as 30 percent of the total amount released into the atmosphere.[16] The destruction of rain forests also contributes to global warming, since the burning of these forests releases copious amounts of carbon dioxide, another greenhouse gas, into the atmosphere.

Toward an Earth-Friendly Diet

It is clear that the effects of animal agriculture are devastating to the environment. Of course, all agriculture—whether it involves animal foods or plant foods—is destructive. It all uses water, fuel, and land and produces pollution. But we need to eat, and therefore we need agriculture. However, it is clearly much more efficient to grow plant foods for humans than to feed these plant foods to livestock to produce meat, milk, and eggs. When we eat a plant-based diet, we can feed people by growing less food and therefore will use less of all natural resources, including land; we also produce less pollution.

Many people are choosing organic meats with a mind toward protecting the environment. This is a good choice, but it is important to remember that all meat, no matter how it is produced, has a destructive impact. A better approach is to eliminate beef from your diet and to greatly reduce all other animal products. The fewer animal products you eat, the more earth friendly your diet. And, of course, choose locally grown organic grains, beans, and produce as often as possible.

Many proponents of animal agriculture point out that animals graze on land that isn't fit for anything else. While that is true, it is also true that there just isn't enough of that land available. That's why ranching continues to encroach on forestland. And while cattle spend much of their lives grazing on rangeland, they are "finished," or fattened, in feedlots, which is where they are fed copious amounts of grain and soy.

Although this grain fed to animals is a variety not suitable for human consumption, it is grown on land, using resources that could be devoted to plant foods for humans.

Feeding a Hungry World

Given the inefficiency of animal agriculture, and the drain on resources, it is clear that this is not the best way to feed an ever-growing population. However, we do have enough land to feed everyone in the world a plant-based diet, since plant foods are so efficiently and cheaply produced.

If more people switched to a plant-based diet, would that free up more grains and beans to feed hungry people? There is some debate about this. On the one hand, it has long appeared that there is presently enough food to feed everyone, with the problem being one of distribution. But we may need to adjust our view of this scenario, as some projections indicate that there may not be enough to go around in the near future. According to a Worldwatch Institute report, our worldwide production of grain has fallen behind population growth, leaving us with less available food per person than we had several years ago.[17] The amount of food that the United States has available for export is also falling.[18]

One thing is certain. We Westerners take more than our share of the available food. In low-income countries, people eat an average of about one pound of grain per day. In the United States, we consume the equivalent of about four pounds a day—including the consumption of animals whose diets heavily rely upon grain. More than a third of the world's grain is fed not to people, but to animals.[19] While people starve to death daily in the world, more than 64 percent of the cropland and 70 percent of the grain in the United States is used for animals.[20] This means that most of our agricultural efforts and resources in this country go toward producing food that most people in the world cannot afford to eat.

As the world's population grows and food production declines, there may be a real need to free up grain to make it available to feed poor people. The only way to do this is for affluent people to eat less of it. The most practical way is to eat the grain directly—not to feed it to food animals.

Of course, freeing up grain is only part of the battle. Getting that grain to hungry nations in the face of poor roads and political upheaval is a big part of the story. But none of that will matter if we don't have enough food.

Choosing a More Humane Diet

A growing number of people are choosing vegetarian diets for ethical reasons. "Ethical vegetarians" may embrace a broad spectrum of beliefs. First, some people believe that it is wrong to kill animals for food. Others believe that animals have inherent rights and that it is not our right to use them for any purpose whatsoever. Therefore, it is wrong to kill animals for food—and even to use them for the production of eggs or milk. A third argument is less philosophical and is easy to support with concrete evidence. That is, animal agriculture involves the inhumane treatment of animals. Ethical vegetarians might argue that it is always wrong to treat animals inhumanely—and especially so when the end products, meat, milk, and eggs, are not dietary necessities and, in fact, should be limited in a healthy diet.

The popular image of a farm is that of a peaceful hillside dotted with contented animals—calves frolicking with each other and nuzzling their mothers, or pigs rooting in the earth or rolling happily in barnyard mud, and a group of busy chickens, clucking and scolding and strutting around the barnyard. The reality is that many food animals never see the outdoors, and most suffer much painful and uncomfortable treatment during their lives.

A common argument in defense of animal agriculture is that farm animals are well treated because it is in the farmer's best economic interest to treat the animals well. There is a certain amount of truth to this. Responsible farmers will protect their investment and their livelihood by keeping animals well fed and medicated and protected against extremes of temperature. However, there are many instances in which efficient farming practices are not the most humane and sometimes are overtly cruel.

The trend today is toward more intensive farming, also known as factory farming. While many American farms may still be small and family run, most meat, eggs, and milk are produced on factory farms. Just over 7 percent of U.S. farms are responsible for nearly 50 percent of all animal-food production.[21]

Chickens and Eggs

Although chickens may not strike most of us

as endearing, cute, or cuddly, they certainly don't deserve the treatment they get down on the farm.

On egg farms, male chicks have no function and are routinely disposed of. Newborn chicks are tossed alive into piles where they suffocate to death—or the live baby chicks are dumped into machines to be ground and made into animal feed.[22] Laying hens spend their entire lives in intense confinement—five chickens crammed together in a cage that measures sixteen by eighteen inches. Because of the stress of this close confinement, chickens tend to peck at one another. Chickens are routinely debeaked, sometimes at one day of age, sometimes later, to reduce the risk of injury.[23] This is achieved by snapping off a portion of the beak with a machine. Studies indicate that debeaked chickens have difficulty eating.[24] There is also evidence that debeaking is not only painful at the time, but produces a chronic state of pain. In fact, one researcher suggests that the reason debeaked birds peck each other less is because they are in constant pain.[25]

Another common practice in egg farming is forced molting. Molting, or the shedding of feathers, increases egg production. On farms, this is achieved by withholding food and water. Chickens may not be fed for as long as ten to twelve days. Agricultural publications suggest that it isn't necessary to remove all of the weaker birds before forced molting, since weaker birds will automatically be culled (that is, they will die) due to the stress of starvation. In fact, approximately 3 to 4 percent of the birds die of starvation during the process.[26]

Veal

No other farming practice has been more criticized than veal production, and with good reason. Two aspects of veal raising make the calf's life miserable.

First, each calf is confined in a crate that measures about 2 by $4\frac{1}{2}$ feet—too small for the calf to turn around or lie down comfortably.[27] Calves are immobilized as much as possible to keep the meat tender and are sometimes chained at the neck. Veal calves are likely to spend their entire lives in these little crates. They are fed an all-milk diet, which is low in iron and produces anemia, to keep their flesh pale. In some cases, when calves are bedded on straw, they are muzzled so that they won't eat the straw.

Second, calves are separated from their mothers between one and three days following birth and are housed sometimes with other calves, but most often alone. Under *natural* conditions calves are rarely alone. They typically spend a great deal of time with other calves in a herd and spend as much as three hours per day being licked by their mothers.[28] On veal farms, these baby animals are most often raised in complete isolation in their tiny crates.

Like many baby animals, calves have a strong sucking reflex. Because they are fed from buckets, they try to frantically suck on anything available, including the bars of their pens. They also crave the iron that is lacking in their diet; one reason that calves are always housed in wooden crates, rather than metal ones, is that they will lick metal bars and increase the iron in their diet, which produces "undesirable" pink flesh.

Over the past several years, the cruel

plight of the veal calf has received a lot of attention. However, farmers have resisted any attempts to improve conditions for these animals. The National Grange, an organization dedicated to the advancement of agriculture, states in its legislative policies: "The National Grange strongly opposes legislation calling for the severe curtailment of the veal industry by such measures as eliminating confinement stalls and crates."[29]

Other Common Farming Practices

Although chickens and veal calves probably suffer the worst abuses, the treatment of all farm animals raises concern. According to *The Stockman's Handbook*, calves to be raised for beef are typically dehorned and castrated without anesthesia at a young age. This handbook offers the following guidelines for dehorning: "Confine or restrain animal to be dehorned in a suitable chute, pinch gate, squeeze pen, or cattle stock. Calves may be handled by throwing, by snubbing them to a fence post or by tying one side of the body against a strong fence or solid wall." For chemical dehorning, instructions are to "rub the chemical over the button until blood appears, protecting the hands while doing so." Because of the stress of dehorning, it generally takes about two weeks for yearling animals to recuperate and regain their original weight.[30]

Other animals are subject to intense confinement for all of their lives. Pigs are most often raised in indoor pens. If the pens have concrete floors, they are likely to suffer joint problems. Slatted floors can result in leg injuries.[31] During the period just preceding slaughter, when pigs are being fattened, they are kept under more crowded conditions with insufficient ventilation, causing aggressiveness, injuries, and infections. On large modern farms, pigs live in row upon row of small stalls, one pig to a stall. Animal husbandry experts recommend just one square foot of space per twenty-five pounds of pig—or about four square feet for a one-hundred-pound pig.[32] Female pigs kept strictly as breeders are often tethered in stalls so small that they can't turn around. Keeping the animals confined makes feeding and cleanup easier. Of course, some family farmers may still avoid some of these practices.

On dairy farms, cows are little more than milk-producing machines. Under natural conditions, cows can live for twenty years and will produce milk for ten to twelve years. But today's dairy cows are forced to produce milk in such great amounts that they can only do so for three or four years. Once she is no longer producing milk, a dairy cow is loaded on the truck and sent off to the slaughterhouse. Because of their debilitated condition these animals are likely to suffer broken bones and leg injuries on the trip. Although severe confinement is less common in the dairy industry than in others, increasingly cows are kept inside barns, where they develop hoof and leg problems from the hard cement floors. Because they are milked by machines and are rarely given a rest from milk production, painful mastitis, or inflammation of the udders, is a common problem for these animals.

All food animals suffer from some inhumane treatment at some point in their lives. At the end of their lives, they are shipped, by truck or train, to the slaughterhouse.

They may spend several days on the truck without food and water and exposed to the elements. There is increasing concern about some practices at the stockyard, especially involving "downers." These are animals that are sick or injured and are unable to walk off the truck. Handlers use electric prods to unload animals, and, although it is an officially condemned practice, downers are sometimes chained and dragged off the truck. In many cases, animals that are too sick to pass inspection are left to die.

With an increase in the population, more meat production, and fewer farms, the face of animal farming has greatly changed. The need for increased efficiency and the fact that farms house such great numbers of animals mean that much less attention can be paid to the welfare and comfort of individual animals. One argument of animal-agriculture proponents is that many of the cruel practices are for the animal's own good. For example, chickens are debeaked to keep them from pecking each other to death. Pigs' tails are "docked" to keep them from biting one another's tails. This rationale ignores the important fact that animals don't normally engage in these kinds of behavior. It is the unnatural conditions of confinement on factory farms that cause the behavior in the first place. Animals who live under more normal conditions don't need to be debeaked or have their tails docked. Animal-science experts note that cannibalism and aggression in animals occur when the animals are kept under less-than-ideal conditions, such as intense confinement.[33]

Because these methods of rearing animals are considered good and efficient animal-

TABLE 4.1 WHY PEOPLE GO MEATLESS	
Health Reasons	46%
Animal Welfare	15%
Influence of family or friends	12%
Other ethical reasons	5%
Concern for the environment	4%
Other	9%
Have always been a vegetarian	4%

Source: Survey of adult Americans conducted by Yankelovich Clancy Shulman for *Time* magazine and CNN, April 1992

husbandry practices, they are not secrets, but are well documented in government and farming publications. On large factory farms, most of these practices appear to be the norm.

WHY GO MEATLESS?

The impact of a vegetarian diet is far-reaching—affecting you personally and the world around you. First, there is a good chance that you will lower your blood cholesterol, slim down, and perhaps lower your risk for certain cancers, heart disease, diabetes, kidney disease, kidney stones, and gallstones. For many people, these are reasons enough to stop eating meat.

But a vegetarian diet is also a humane diet. It makes more food available to everyone in the world. It frees animals from the cruelties of factory farming. Plant-based diets greatly lessen the burden on the planet, saving forests, water, and petroleum. There are few lifestyle changes that you can make that will have as great an impact as eliminating animal products from your diet.

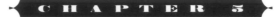

CHAPTER 5

THE POLITICS OF DIET

To change one's diet is to throw into doubt the relationship between gods, men and beast upon which the whole politico-religious system of the city rests . . . to abstain from eating meat in the Greek city-state is a highly subversive act.

—MARCEL DETEINNE, *Dionysus Slain*, 1979

◆

No longer led by a natural instinct in the selection of his foodstuffs as were his remote forebears, [man] finds his dietetic guidance in the advertising columns of the morning paper, and eats not what Nature prepares for his sustenance but what his grocer, his butcher, and his baker find it most to their pecuniary interest to purvey to him.

—JOHN HARVEY KELLOGG, *The Natural Diet of Man*, 1923

◆

Nutrition is more than a science. Whereas the basic principles of nutritional science are clear and straightforward, many factors bias the way this information is presented to you, the consumer, and influence your beliefs about nutrition and diet. It is especially important for vegetarians to recognize these factors. The field of nutrition has a political history that favors the consumption of meat, and this has greatly affected messages and beliefs about vegetarianism.

We receive most of our nutrition advice from government agencies. The United States Department of Agriculture is one of the chief agencies responsible for nutrition education. It has issued a number of food guides over the years, including the old four food groups that most of us were raised on and, more recently, a set of meal-planning guidelines called the food guide pyramid.

The USDA was established by President Lincoln in 1862 with a mandate to serve the interests of farmers and to educate the public about farm products. At that time, farmers made up a substantial part of the population. Because so little was known about nutrition, and the only recognizable problem was undernutrition, consuming more meat and milk seemed to be a sound public health measure. So the USDA managed to promote both the nation's economy and health without conflict. This is no longer true. Today, the USDA continues to support and promote the meat and dairy industries when we now know that these are the very foods we need to reduce in our diet. At the same time, the USDA is supposed to provide consumers with sound nutrition advice.

This dual mandate is basically impossible to uphold, and it greatly shades the type of advice that the USDA provides. It also impacts the advice provided by other government agencies, because federal mandate dictates that government agencies be consistent.

THE FOOD INDUSTRY: NUTRITION EXPERTS?

It is only in the past thirty years or so that the language of government nutrition guidelines has become problematic—problematic for the meat and dairy industries, that is. When the dietary goals for the United States were published in 1977, the meat and dairy groups greatly objected to recommendations to "decrease consumption of meat, eggs, butterfat, and foods high in fat." These powerful industries demanded hearings on the new guidelines; the meat industry in particular won a big battle when the guideline that read "decrease consumption of meat and increase consumption of poultry and fish" was amended to read "decrease consumption of animal fat, and choose meats, poultry and fish which will reduce saturated fat intake." Senator George McGovern, who chaired the select committee on the dietary goals, said that he did not want "to disrupt the economic situation of the meat industry and engage in a battle with that industry that we could not win."[1]

In 1979 the USDA published a booklet called *Food* to help consumers make healthy food choices. The meat, dairy, and egg industries objected to the booklet's advice to cut down on saturated fat and cholesterol. When the booklet was revised for a second printing, the chapter on fat and cholesterol was deleted.[2]

Although evidence of the relationship between animal fat consumption and chronic disease risk is stronger than ever, the government's advice on meat continues to grow weaker. When the USDA released its dietary guidelines in 1980 and again in 1985, the advice about saturated fat and cholesterol had changed from the words "eat less" to the more benign "avoid too much." When the 1990 guidelines were released, the advice about meat had been changed to "have two or three servings of meat for a total of about 6 ounces."[3]

Organizations other than the government have problematic ties to the food industry. The American Dietetic Association (ADA) is a strong voice in the nutrition guidance arena. Because it represents dietitians it is generally perceived as one of the more authoritative voices in the nutrition field. But it is important to remember that this is a professional organization that represents the interests of dietitians. The ADA accepts money from food companies and groups, including the meat industry, to support many of its programs. Some major contributors to ADA programs include McDonald's, Nabisco, the National Dairy Council (NDC), and the National Livestock and Meat Board. Nutrition education materials produced by this organization are routinely sponsored by and reflect the input of the food industry. Can groups like the ADA offer objective nutritional advice without offending the industries that support them? We don't know for certain if there is a true conflict of interest, but there is certainly the appearance of one—something that we consider inappropriate.

The food industry has a profound impact on nutrition education in other ways as well. One of the biggest providers of nutrition education materials to American classrooms is the National Dairy Council. The NDC is a promotional arm of the milk industry that masquerades as a nutrition education organization. The materials that this group distributes showcase and promote dairy foods. A brochure titled *The All-American Guide to Calcium-Rich Foods* lists thirty-five dairy foods, including three different kinds of ice cream, and just seven plant foods that are rich in calcium. According to the NDC, rich ice cream, with twelve grams of fat in a half-cup serving and seventy-five milligrams of calcium, is a better source of calcium than vegetarian baked beans, with less than one gram of fat and the same amount of calcium.[4]

And since the profit to the dairy industry is bigger on higher-fat foods, the NDC rarely emphasizes the importance of choosing nonfat dairy products. In a brochure aimed at elementary-school children, the milk group is touted as containing foods that help build strong bones and teeth. According to the NDC, the foods included in this group are cheddar, Colby, Gouda, and Muenster cheeses; chocolate and white milk; ice cream; pudding; and yogurt, all high in fat.[5]

What Nutritionists Believe About You

There is a prevailing opinion in this country that consumers won't change. As a result, the government and other nutrition professionals only give you the kind of information they believe you can handle, even if that information is less than completely accurate. Nutrition professionals perceive an optimal plant-based diet as too radical or difficult for consumers, and this is one reason they don't recommend it. Instead, dietary recommendations are based on a compromise between what is optimal and what is acceptable.

The National Academy of Sciences' landmark 1982 report on diet and cancer did not recommend a 20 percent fat diet, even though there was a sound scientific basis for doing so. Instead, it opted for recommending 30 percent or less as a compromise between the scientific evidence and its perception of what the public would likely accept.[6] The fear is that consumers will "turn off" to public-health recommendations that are seen as too stringent. While there is an element of truth to this approach, it also denies sound information to those who are willing and who need to change.

Those of us who do provide nutrition counseling admittedly advise many clients who won't change their diet or are willing to make only moderate changes. It's fine to meet those clients halfway and to help them make acceptable changes, but we also need to be honest about the limitations of moderate dietary changes. It is irresponsible to tell a person who is at risk for heart disease that he or she should go on a 30 percent fat diet, when we know that a 10 to 20 percent fat diet could save his or her life, not just prolong it a bit.

Consumers need to know that a 30 percent fat diet that includes red meat and chicken is only going to produce a moderate reduction in blood cholesterol. But a 10 to 15 percent fat diet that is largely plant based is likely to cause significant drops that will greatly lower the risk for heart disease and for other chronic diseases as well. More accurate recommendations are especially important to parents of young children, since they have the chance to develop good lifelong habits before they become more difficult to change.

NUTRITION GOSPEL

Politics and history have a profound effect on how consumers and health professionals have come to view nutrition advice. As a result, the following ideas and approaches have become standard in much of the nutrition community.

Animal Foods and Health

The first meal-planning guide was developed in 1916, and it was aimed at helping Americans to get all of the newly discovered vitamins into their diet. The excitement over the vitamins and the rather limited knowledge about nutrition caused one of the leading nutrition authorities of the day to coin this phrase in 1918: "Eat what you want after you eat what you should."[7] The implication was that as long as you were getting adequate protein and vitamins, whatever else you ate was immaterial.

Although nutritionists recognize the error of this type of thinking, it definitely continues to shade the way some people view nutrition. In the earliest days of nutrition guidance, animal foods were placed at the center of the diet because they were perceived as the best sources of protein, B vitamins, iron, and calcium. Today, we recognize that vitamin deficiencies are a rarity in the United States and Europe (although they are still too common in other parts of the world) and that the true nutrition problems are ones of overabundance—too much fat, protein, and too many calories. Yet some consumers and health professionals still view vegetarianism with suspicion. In this country, where a half-million people die each year from heart disease, many nutritionists still approach low-fat, vegetarian diets—diets that prevent heart disease—with caution for fear that they may be deficient in nutrients.

A 30 Percent Fat Diet

In all fairness, no one is saying that we should be eating a 30 percent fat diet. The recommendation is to eat no more than 30 percent of our calories from fat. But nutritionists recognize that this is not good enough. There is evidence to recommend that consumers lower their fat intake to considerably less than 30 percent, but because many professionals are so convinced that consumers won't eat a low-fat diet, they won't make better recommendations. Of course, throughout the world, many people do eat diets that are well below 30 percent fat. And the dietary advice issued by some governments recommends consuming as little as 20 percent of calories from fat.

In fact, some studies show that lower-fat diets are very acceptable to motivated consumers. Patients who adopted a 10 percent fat diet to reduce cholesterol came to enjoy and prefer their diet after a while.[8] Studies funded by the National Cancer Institute found that women were comfortable with a 20 percent fat diet.[9] In fact, studies at the Purnell Institute in Philadelphia found that when people followed a low-fat diet, the high-fat foods they once enjoyed became completely unappealing.[10]

Unfortunately, when dietitians and other health professionals believe so strongly that consumers won't adopt a low-fat diet, they perpetuate the notion that low-fat eating is unpleasant. Rather than compromising on what is healthy, we need to see more nutritionists taking an aggressive approach toward teaching clients to eat low-fat meals and enjoy them.

The American Heart Association Diet Plan versus a Low-Fat Diet

Unfortunately, heart disease patients frequently receive inadequate advice. People with elevated cholesterol and other risk factors for heart disease need to be very serious about maintaining a good diet. A healthy diet and lifestyle can dramatically reduce an individual's risk of heart disease in most cases. But, instead, recommendations from groups such as the American Heart Association and the National Cholesterol Education Program are to trim the fat from meat, to consume six ounces of meat a day, and to use low-fat dairy products. This provides only small reductions in blood cholesterol levels and almost insignificant reductions in heart disease risk.[11] From a public-health standpoint, it is far too little.

On the other hand, more progressive individuals, beginning with Nathan Pritikin in the 1960s and more recently Dr. Dean Ornish from the University of California, San Francisco, have advocated a low-fat vegetarian eating plan. Dr. Ornish has shown that his dietary program not only lowers blood cholesterol, it actually reverses artery disease by cleaning the plaque right out of arteries.[12] Yet most nutritionists and physicians continue to advocate the watered-down, halfway measures for dietary modifications.

No Good Foods or Bad Foods?

One philosophy that comes directly from the USDA—that there are no good foods or bad foods—has been enthusiastically embraced. The idea proposes that all foods can fit into a healthy diet and that no foods are inherently bad. The food industry loves this philosophy, which allows it to proudly parade any of its unhealthy foods and demonstrate how they can fit into a healthy diet. While there is one small spark of truth in this philosophy, that you can work the unhealthiest food into your diet and still have a healthy diet, it is only true as long as most of what you eat is low-fat, whole plant foods.

In fact, along with the USDA, we don't especially like the terminology "bad foods," because it sets people up for guilt when they eat these foods. Because the majority of our own diet is based on very healthy foods, we suffer absolutely no guilt when we occasionally indulge in less healthy ones, such as French fries, potato chips, or brownies.

However, there is just no getting around it: some foods are better for you than others. You can build a healthy diet on grains, beans, fruits, and vegetables. But you can't build a healthy diet on meat and milk. The important thing to remember is that not all foods are desirable and many foods need to be minimized in your diet if optimal health is your goal.

Another term you'll hear frequently linked to diet is "moderation." The USDA dietary guidelines define "moderation" as "avoiding extremes in diet." "Moderation" is frequently used in nutrition literature and advice, and it is a highly popular and political term. It lets food companies promote their products as having a role in a healthy diet (when "used in moderation"), and it allows nutritionists to give advice without offending anybody—the food industry or their clients.

The food industry likes this concept because, according to nutrition wisdom, any food can be consumed as long as it is consumed moderately. And happily for it, no one really has any idea what "moderate" means when it comes to diet. It is a purposefully vague term that poses as responsible nutrition advice while allowing you to believe that you can eat whatever you please—as long as you judge the amounts to be moderate.

Most of us are able to judge what is moderate only in cultural terms. To someone who lives in a culture where meat is consumed just once or twice a week in one- or two-ounce portions, a moderate consumption of meat will mean something very different than it does to an American who grew up eating twelve ounces of meat a day. For Americans, who eat, on average, a 36-percent-fat diet, getting just 30 percent of

their calories from fat could be called moderate. But we also know that this moderate fat consumption is probably too much fat.

Beware: "Everything in moderation" is a dangerous, unhealthy concept. What if you defined "moderation" as two servings a week, and you decided that you would eat ice cream, sausages, beer, hamburgers, whipped cream, French fries, potato chips, cream cheese, apple pie, and doughnuts—but only in moderation? Well, if you ate all of those things in moderation, you certainly would end up with an unhealthy diet.

The nice thing about following guidelines like the ones in this book is that there is little need to worry about moderation. When you base your diet on whole plant foods with little added fat, eliminate meat, poultry, fish, and fatty dairy products and eggs, and minimize your use of processed foods, you don't need to worry about eating any of the foods included in the guidelines in moderation.

NUTRITION GUIDANCE IN THE 1990S
Food Pyramids
In 1991, the United States Department of Agriculture unveiled its latest food guide for meal planning, the food guide pyramid. This was the first tool in the history of food guidance to tell consumers what savvy nutritionists had long since known: healthy diets emphasize plant foods and deemphasize animal foods. But although many were happy to see the new guide, it was steeped in controversy from the start. One day after its release, it was yanked from the hands of educators and health professionals. The reason? Well, the USDA said that the tool

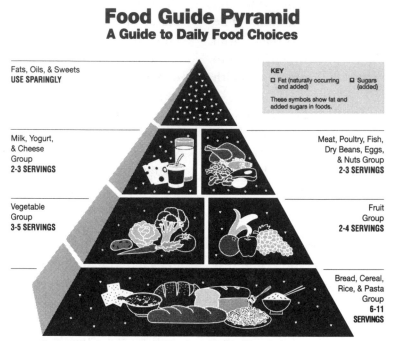

Food Guide Pyramid
A Guide to Daily Food Choices

Fats, Oils, & Sweets
USE SPARINGLY

KEY
□ Fat (naturally occurring and added)   ▽ Sugars (added)

These symbols show fat and added sugars in foods.

Milk, Yogurt, & Cheese Group
2-3 SERVINGS

Meat, Poultry, Fish, Dry Beans, Eggs, & Nuts Group
2-3 SERVINGS

Vegetable Group
3-5 SERVINGS

Fruit Group
2-4 SERVINGS

Bread, Cereal, Rice, & Pasta Group
6-11 SERVINGS

Source: U.S. Department of Agriculture/U.S. Department of Health and Human Services

hadn't been adequately tested to see if it was appropriate for low-income groups—this despite the fact that the pyramid was the result of three years' worth of research.[13]

The more likely reason was that the meat and dairy industries were up in arms due to the position of their products in the pyramid. Apparently the meat industry, in particular, was taken by surprise with the release of the food pyramid. Days after its release, meat industry leaders met with the secretary of agriculture to voice their unhappiness. Several days after that meeting, the American Meat Institute complained via a letter to the USDA that it had "neither seen the pyramid nor been consulted about it" and that the USDA should reject adoption of the food guide pyramid.[14]

Of course, you might wonder why the American Meat Institute should be consulted about the pyramid or any other nutrition education piece. But the USDA saw differently. The pyramid was pulled and retested. In the final analysis, after all the controversy died down, the USDA released the pyramid again—with a number of minor changes. One big victory for the meat and dairy people was that the new guide displayed numbers of servings outside the pyramid where they would be more visible, so that it was clear that consumers were still supposed to eat two or three servings a day each of meat and dairy foods. The delay cost the American taxpayers nearly $1 million.

Perhaps the most significant effect of the

food pyramid was that amidst the controversy surrounding its release nutritionists and consumers got a real look at how the USDA works. It became clear that much more than nutrition science was influencing the information we receive.

But what about the pyramid itself? Is it helpful information for vegetarians or for any consumers? Although we agree that it is a vast improvement over former food guide systems, it still has a number of serious flaws.

First, the pyramid sticks with old-fashioned ideas about what we need to include in our diet. It is of absolutely no use to vegans because it includes a milk group. And according to the USDA, you can't be healthy if you don't drink milk. The pamphlet that accompanies the pyramid states: "No one food group is more important than another—for good health, you need them all."[15] Nowhere in the materials accompanying the pyramid does the USDA note that people can get calcium from foods other than dairy products.

Second, food groupings sometimes make no sense in the food pyramid. Dried beans and nuts are grouped with meat, fish, poultry, and eggs. Granted these foods are all rich in protein and minerals, but any resemblance ends there. Dried beans and nuts are both high in fiber, where meat and other animal foods have none. Dried beans are almost fat free, whereas meat, poultry, and eggs are the biggest contributors of fat in the diet.

The pyramid also makes no provisions for vegetarian foods in the diet. Tofu and meat analogues aren't mentioned as possible alternatives to the meat group. In fact,

beans and nuts are barely mentioned in the text of the pyramid, which goes to great lengths to describe how to include leaner meats in the diet and refers to this food group as "the meat group."

In short, we consider the food guide pyramid a step in the right direction toward teaching people how to eat a more plant-based diet, but it still doesn't spell out an optimal diet for anyone. It allows for far too much meat for good health, and it encourages people to believe that only diets that include dairy products are healthy.

The pyramid is a blend of scientific information about nutrient needs, outdated ways of grouping foods, and political compromises. The food guide pyramid is of limited use to vegetarians. In fact, it doesn't pretend to be useful, since the literature doesn't mention the word "vegetarian." We think there are some other sets of guidelines available that are much more helpful for vegetarians or anyone who wishes to eat a healthy diet.

The Mediterranean Food Pyramid

In the spring of 1994, a joint project of Harvard University, the World Health Organization (WHO), and the Oldways Preservation and Exchange Trust produced a set of meal-planning guidelines based on the style of eating that was once common in Mediterranean countries. In those countries, meals traditionally were rich in plant foods and low in animal products. The main fat used was—and still is—olive oil. This Mediterranean diet is probably one reason for the low rates of chronic diseases in these countries and the greater life expectancy—although as food habits change in this area of the world, the risk for these diseases is on the rise.

In short, the Mediterranean food pyramid recommends the following: limit red meat to a few servings per month and poultry, fish, sweets, and eggs to a few times per week. Small amounts of dairy products and olive oil can be consumed daily, while the bulk of meals should come from beans, vegetables, fruits, nuts, and grains. The guidelines allow for wine in moderation and encourage daily physical activity. In essence, this is a semivegetarian diet. Surprisingly, the amount of fat allowed in this eating plan is rather high. But because both saturated fat and cholesterol are kept to a minimum, and most of the fat is monounsaturated, it still represents a healthier eating style than the USDA's food guide pyramid. For those who follow the Mediterranean food pyramid, we would still recommend keeping an eye on your olive oil intake if you struggle with a weight problem.

We have some concern over the fact that the Oldways organization receives funding from the food industry—including the olive oil, wine, produce, and nut industries. These are all foods that are mentioned in the pyramid. Regardless of these influences, the Mediterranean food pyramid is an improvement over the USDA's food pyramid, since it promotes more sound ideas about optimal nutrition. Although these guidelines are much more in tune with principles of good nutrition, government and professional organizations have not rushed to embrace them, but have stuck firmly to their endorsement of the food guide pyramid.

The Vegetarian Food Pyramid

It should come as no surprise that this is our favorite food guide of all. Developed by the Health Connection, a Maryland-based nutrition-education group, this guide is based on the USDA's pyramid and is similar in format. The difference is that food choices are all vegetarian. It offers consumers guidelines for fitting a variety of vegetarian products—including tofu and meat analogues—into a healthy diet. It also offers alternatives to dairy milk. In fact, you'll note that the pyramid looks quite similar to our guidelines in chapter 10.

For information on getting copies of either the Mediterranean or vegetarian food pyramids, see the resource section at the back of this book.

THE RECOMMENDED DIETARY ALLOWANCES

To understand how to determine whether vegetarians and others meet nutrient needs, we should know something about the recommended dietary allowances, or RDAs. The RDAs are believed by many to be minimal amounts of nutrients that they should receive every day. Actually, the RDAs are probably quite a bit higher than what most individuals need. They were developed for evaluating plans for group meals; for example, they are used to evaluate the nutritional adequacy of school lunch programs. They are much less useful for evaluating the needs of individuals, since those needs vary considerably.

There is actually a group of RDAs for each of the nutrients because needs vary depending on age and sex. So the RDA for calcium for a toddler is quite different than that for a grown man.

RDAs are sometimes expressed in two ways. Often, nutrient needs are determined in relation to body size, calorie intake, or some other factor. For example, our need for vitamin B_1 is largely dependent on our calorie intake. We need about a half milligram of B_1 for every thousand calories we consume. But all RDAs are also expressed as absolute numbers to simplify matters. So the B_1 RDA is 1.5 milligrams for all adult men regardless of how many calories they consume. This makes it easier to talk about the RDAs, because it gives us a number rather than a mathematical equation to use.

For labeling purposes, a figure called the RDI is used. For any given nutrient, this is the highest RDA from all the different age groups, excluding the one for pregnant or

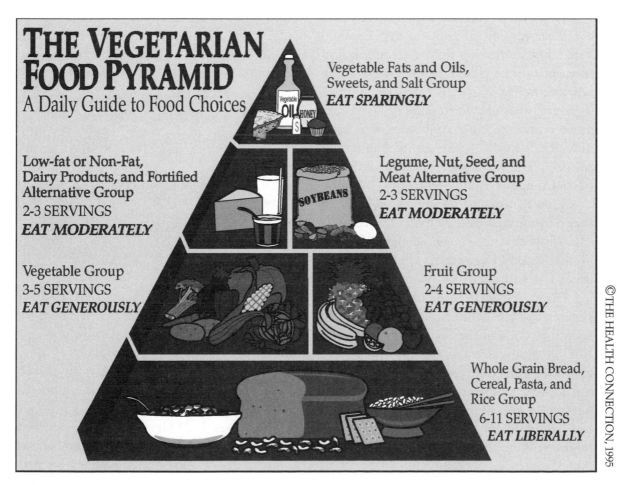

THE VEGETARIAN FOOD PYRAMID
A Daily Guide to Food Choices

Vegetable Fats and Oils, Sweets, and Salt Group
EAT SPARINGLY

Low-fat or Non-Fat, Dairy Products, and Fortified Alternative Group
2-3 SERVINGS
EAT MODERATELY

Legume, Nut, Seed, and Meat Alternative Group
2-3 SERVINGS
EAT MODERATELY

Vegetable Group
3-5 SERVINGS
EAT GENEROUSLY

Fruit Group
2-4 SERVINGS
EAT GENEROUSLY

Whole Grain Bread, Cereal, Pasta, and Rice Group
6-11 SERVINGS
EAT LIBERALLY

lactating women. As a result, the RDI is often much higher than what most people need.

As we explore the nutritional makeup of vegetarian diets, keep the following in mind. All of the RDAs include a substantial safety factor. Nutrient needs vary a lot among individuals, and this safety factor ensures that even those with the highest needs will be covered.

You don't need to meet the RDA for every nutrient every day. What is important is that your average intake over time comes close to the RDA.

RDAs are reasonable estimates that are based on varying amounts of experimental data. They are not carved in stone and should never be viewed as the final word on nutrient needs. Nutrient needs are affected by overall diet and lifestyle. The RDAs are based on the needs of Americans, who eat a diet that includes considerable amounts of animal foods. Vegetarians may have different nutrient needs than omnivores. In some cases, their nutrient needs are most likely lower; in a few cases they might be higher. It is possible that the recommendations of the World Health Organization, which establishes nutrient needs for people in developing countries, are closer to the needs of vegetarians. But while we don't necessarily favor the RDAs as the final word for vegetarians, we also aren't ready to cast them aside in favor of the WHO criteria. Genetics, physical activity, and lifestyle all impact nutrient needs. People living in developing countries, where diets are primarily plant based, might still have different nutrient needs than Western vegetarians.

MEASURING NUTRIENTS

Scientists, including nutritionists, use the metric system to measure nutrients. You don't need to understand this system inside and out to learn about nutrition, but it helps to have a working knowledge of the units of measurement and their abbreviations. In nearly all cases, nutrients are measured in grams, milligrams, and micrograms. The following will help you to put these amounts into perspective:

1 kilogram (kg.) = 1,000 grams

1 gram (g.) = 1,000 milligrams (mg.)

1 milligram = 1,000 micrograms (mcg. or ug.)

FOR COMPARISON PURPOSES

1 kilogram = 2.2 pounds

1 ounce = 28 grams

1 teaspoon dry powder = about 5 grams

When we talk about body weight, we often use kilograms. So to convert your own weight to kilograms, just divide it by 2.2.

Although much of the criticism of the RDAs focuses on the idea that they are too high for most people, there is another viewpoint. The RDAs focus on avoiding deficiency diseases, which are acute conditions. But they don't give any attention to the amount of a nutrient needed to promote optimal health. While it takes just ten milligrams of vitamin C a day to prevent scurvy, it may take many times that amount to ensure that the immune system is operating optimally or to reduce the risk for cancer. The RDAs don't address this question at all.

We are faced with a real dilemma. Vegetarians may need less of many nutrients than the RDAs specify. But for some nutrients, everyone may do well to consume more than the RDA. We don't have enough information to be precise. We would love to tell you exactly how much calcium vegetarians need and how much vitamin B_{12} is really necessary in a vegan diet, but these answers are not yet available. The best advice is to eat a good variety of plant foods, and to use the RDAs for what they are—imperfect guidelines.

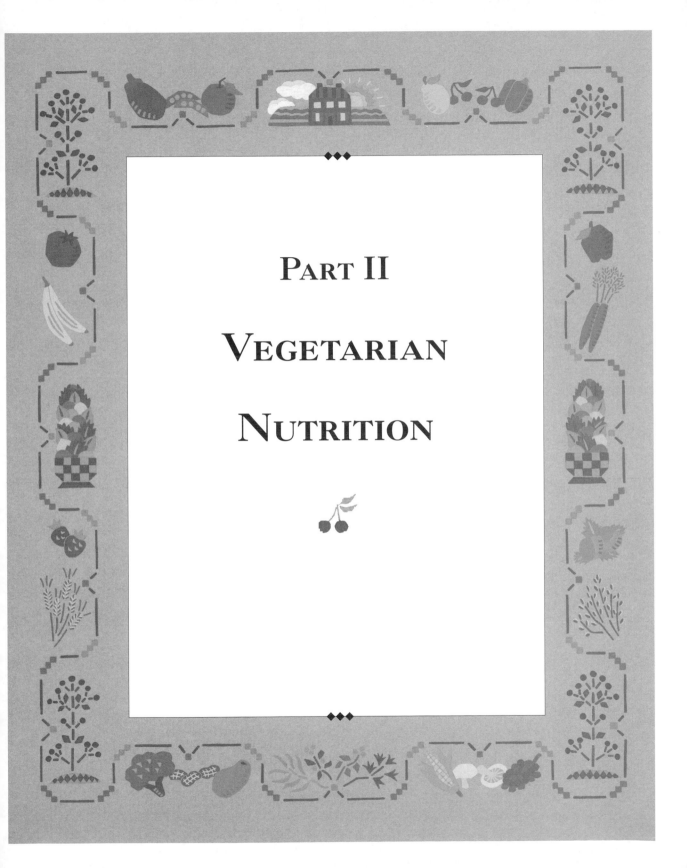

Part II

Vegetarian

Nutrition

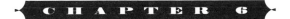

CHAPTER 6

PROTEIN IN VEGETARIAN DIETS

I don't think we need to worry about "high" protein. If we get "some" protein in most of the foods we eat, we'll easily meet our protein needs.

—FRANCES MOORE LAPPÉ,
Diet for a Small Planet, 1982

◆

It is of course possible to eat meat dishes less frequently or to omit meat from the diet altogether, for it has been determined that all the necessary protein and energy may be obtained from other materials.

—C. F. LANGWORTHY, PH.D., AND
CAROLINE L. HUNT, US DEPARTMENT OF
AGRICULTURE CIRCULAR, 1916

◆

While vegetarians do need to be aware of some nutritional requirements, many are needlessly concerned about protein. Believe it or not, it is almost impossible for a vegetarian to be protein deficient.

When scientists first isolated protein from food in the nineteenth century, they gave it a name based on the Greek word *prōteios,* which means "primary." They did so for good reason. Protein is of primary importance to good health—it plays varied and crucial roles in every cell of the body. Enzymes that are central to every biological reaction are proteins. Antibodies, many hormones, muscles, and bones all contain protein. When there isn't enough protein in the diet, people suffer devastating consequences.

Protein's value has always been recognized, but the importance of consuming animal protein has been greatly overemphasized throughout history. Even two thousand years ago, meat was thought to provide the key to optimal health and strength.[1] In 1939 the nutritionist J. S. McLester declared in his book *Nutrition and Diet in Health and Disease* that consumption of large amounts of animal protein contributed to the accomplishments of Western civilization.[2] Not everyone agreed. Dr. John Harvey Kellogg warned that abundant animal protein was, in fact, killing us. He credited diets high in meat protein as contributing to "an unnecessary tax on the liver and kidneys, which contributes to their premature failure and the development of disease in these important organs."[3] Kellogg was certainly closer to the truth. People who limit animal proteins in their diet are healthier. And vegetarians, even those who avoid all animal foods, are not at risk for protein deficiency. Over the years, as science has unraveled the mysteries of this complex nutrient, the following facts have become clear:

• When calories are adequate, protein deficiency is virtually nonexistent. This is because protein is so abundant in the food supply. Grains, vegetables, beans, nuts, and seeds are all rich in protein. Only fats and alcohol are lacking in this nutrient. In underdeveloped countries, protein deficiency is sometimes seen, but it is nearly always due to a lack of adequate amounts of foods, not to the use of low-protein foods. Because plant foods are rich in protein, deficiency is rare in Western vegetarian populations. Vegetarians consume less protein than omnivores, but they easily meet their needs.

• Contrary to old beliefs, vegetarians don't need to consume carefully planned food combinations at meals to meet their protein needs. Meeting protein needs doesn't require any particular meal-planning approach other than this: eat enough calories to maintain ideal weight and include a variety of plant foods in your diet.

• Plant proteins may be healthier than animal proteins, since animal proteins are associated with increased heart disease, loss of calcium from bones, and poorer kidney function.

One reason that people have become so fixated on protein is that foods typically associated with protein—meat, poultry, fish, eggs, and milk—are expensive, and that makes them more socially desirable. Production of these foods requires more land, water, and natural resources, which makes them more costly. For this reason most people in the world can't afford to eat animal foods very often. Historically, this has made animal proteins somewhat of a status symbol. In developing countries, a rise in the standard of living is often accompanied by lifestyle and dietary changes—people begin to emulate the eating habits of North Americans and northern Europeans by consuming more protein-rich animal foods. The World Health Organization recently warned against this trend because it will lead to the same risks of chronic disease that plague Westerners.[4]

PROTEIN CHEMISTRY

For an understanding of protein needs, and especially of the myths that persist about these needs, it is helpful to look at protein chemistry. A protein molecule consists of long, twisted strands, or chains, of amino acids, the building blocks of protein. Every amino acid contains nitrogen, which, for the most part, is found only in amino acids. Our protein requirement is actually a requirement for nitrogen and for certain amino acids. While the foods we eat only contain about twenty different amino acids, our body can produce thousands of proteins by linking amino acids together into different sequences. Each cell of the body contains specific sets of instructions—carried in our DNA—to make the proteins that it requires. The body can also produce its own amino acids. Of the twenty amino acids, we can make eleven of them in our body. These are called nonessential amino acids. The other nine are called essential amino acids (EAA), because we must get them from food. Table 6.1 lists the essential amino acids.

All proteins, whether from meat, milk, eggs, beans, nuts, grains, or vegetables, contain all of the essential amino acids. However, plant proteins tend to be a little short in one or more of the EAAs. These are called limiting amino acids. Historically, the fact that plant proteins are somewhat limited in some EAAs has caused them to be viewed as "incomplete proteins." It's true that the limiting amino acid does impact the overall quality of a protein. But we will see a little bit later that the concept of "completeness" doesn't hold up too well.

Protein quality also depends on how well a food is digested—that is, on how easily a particular protein is broken down to its individual amino acids. Diets based on plant proteins are about 85 percent digestible, whereas those based on animal proteins are about 95 percent digestible.[5] That's a pretty small difference, and it shows that most proteins are actually digested very well.

How Much Protein Do We Need?

Many factors, including age, body size and composition, climate, activity level, emotional state, and overall health, affect our protein needs. The number of calories in the diet also affects protein needs. When calories are too low, the body burns protein for energy, and the overall protein requirement goes up. Our comments here apply to the protein needs of healthy, nonpregnant adults.

Scientists generally assess protein needs by performing nitrogen balance studies. These measure the amount of nitrogen a person loses each day through the urine, feces, and sweat. Because nitrogen is sup-

Table 6.1 Essential Amino Acids	
Histidine	Phenylalanine
Isoleucine	Threonine
Leucine	Tryptophan
Lysine	Valine
Methionine	

plied to the body by dietary protein, some simple arithmetic reveals how much protein a person needs to eat to replace the lost nitrogen.

Under normal, healthy conditions, adults should be in nitrogen balance. That is, the amount of protein they retain equals the amount that is lost from the body. During periods of growth, such as in children, pregnant women, and bodybuilders, people should be in positive nitrogen balance. This means that the body holds on to extra nitrogen to build new tissues. The amount of nitrogen consumed is actually greater than the amount lost. When people are in negative nitrogen balance, they are not consuming enough protein to replace the nitrogen they are losing; their diet is too low in protein. Negative nitrogen balance is protein deficiency, and it is never healthy or normal.

Balance studies tell us how much protein people must consume to meet their nitrogen needs. They are among the best and most traditional methods for doing so. However, they aren't perfect. Some scientists feel that the studies underestimate real protein needs, so we need to bring a little caution to the interpretation of their results.

Balance studies have been used to establish the protein RDA. This is usually stated in two ways. First, the RDA for protein is 63 grams for an adult male and 50 grams for an adult female. These are reference figures thought to cover the needs of most American adults. But it is more helpful to calculate individual protein needs because these needs vary so much depending on body size. Protein requirements are based on ideal body weight, not actual weight. If you weigh 170 but would be healthier at 150, then your protein needs are based on 150 pounds.

The more specific RDA for protein is 0.8 grams of protein for every kilogram of ideal body weight.[6] A kilogram is equal to 2.2 pounds. So to find your individual protein need you can use this calculation: ideal body weight (in pounds) × 0.8 ÷ 2.2. A faster method to give you a rough estimate of protein needs is to simply divide your ideal weight in pounds by 3.

These calculations include a big safety factor so the RDA will almost always be higher than what an individual actually needs. In the case of protein, the RDA exceeds the protein requirement of 98 percent of the American population. However, because protein needs vary so much from person to person—one estimate is that they vary as much as fourfold—we think it is a good idea for all people to strive to meet the RDA.[7] It isn't too difficult to do this, as the average American male consumes about twice as much protein as is needed.[8] Vegetarians usually have diets that are lower in protein, but they also easily meet the protein RDA.[9] An important question, however, is whether the RDA should be different for vegetarians. That is, do vegetarians need more protein than omnivores?

VEGETARIANS AND PROTEIN

We mentioned that protein needs vary depending on factors such as age, health, activity, and others. But an additional factor affects protein needs—the quality of the proteins you eat. The RDAs assume that most people eat a mixture of plant and animal proteins. We've already noted that plant proteins tend to be of somewhat lesser quality for two reasons: first, they are slightly less digestible than animal proteins, and, second, they contain limiting amino acids. When you eat lesser-quality proteins, you need somewhat more protein in your diet.

Laboratory studies confirm that people who consume only plant proteins require increased protein. This is particularly true for vegetarians who get most of their protein from beans and whole grains. However, it is somewhat less true for those who consume some foods that are better digested, such as tofu, soymilk, and some refined foods. Lacto-ovo vegetarians, who eat very high-quality proteins in eggs and dairy products, are likely to have protein needs similar to those of omnivores. A better RDA for vegans might be 1.0 gram of protein per kilogram of body weight (compared to the 0.8 that is recommended for the general population). But, as is true for most RDA values, this includes a generous safety factor and is more than what most vegans will need.

Vegetarians consume somewhat less protein than omnivores. A typical vegan diet gets about 11 to 12 percent of its calories from protein, and lacto-ovo vegetarians typically eat a diet that is about 13 percent protein.[10] An omnivore diet is about 15 to 17 percent protein.[11] But despite vegans' somewhat higher needs and lower intake, surveys show that they get plenty of protein. You don't need to do anything special to meet your protein needs. Just eat enough calories to maintain your ideal weight and include a variety of plant foods in your diet. (See table 6.2 for sample menus that provide adequate protein.) By doing so, vegetarians easily meet their needs. In fact, vegetarian protein intake is more desirable than that of omnivores. Meat-based diets are too high in protein, and we will see shortly that this is unhealthy.

PLANT FOODS ARE RICH IN PROTEIN

You can see from table 6.3 that plant foods are much richer in protein than many people suspect. Foods that are typically not viewed as protein rich are actually quite high in this nutrient. For example, broccoli, with 2.8 grams of protein and 27 calories in a half cup, is 40 percent protein. This means it is more protein dense than ground beef, although it is lower in total protein.[12] Diets that are 10% protein are sufficient to meet protein needs.

Given the high amount of protein in plant foods, why is it that animal foods get all the credit for their protein content and plant foods get ignored? One answer has to do with a very fundamental mistake in the nutrition research that has been used to evaluate food sources of protein. Since 1919, the official procedure for evaluating

TABLE 6.2 SAMPLE VEGETARIAN MENUS

VEGAN		Protein (grams)
Breakfast	1 cup Shredded Wheat	3.0
	1 cup soymilk	10.0
	Slice toast	2.4
	½ sliced banana	1.2
Lunch	1 whole wheat pita	4.0
	½ cup hummus	6.0
	½ cup romaine lettuce	0.5
	½ cup raw broccoli	1.3
	2 tablespoons sunflower seeds	5.0
	2 tablespoons dressing	—
	Peach	0.6
Dinner	1 cup vegetarian baked beans	12.0
	Baked potato	4.7
	1 cup steamed kale	1.2
Snack	Milk shake (½ cup strawberries, 1 cup soymilk)	11.0
TOTAL		62.9
LACTO-OVO		
Breakfast	1 cup Shredded Wheat	3.0
	1 cup 2% milk	8.0
	Slice whole wheat toast	2.4
	½ cup orange juice	1.7
Lunch	2 slices whole wheat bread	4.8
	2 ounces American cheese	12.6
	½ cup steamed broccoli	2.3
Dinner	½ cup curried tofu	20.0
	1 cup brown rice	4.9
	1 cup steamed collards	5.0
TOTAL		64.7

TABLE 6.3 PROTEIN CONTENT OF SELECTED PLANT FOODS

Food	Serving Size	Protein (grams)	Calories from Protein (%)
Spinach, cooked	½ cup	2.5	48.0
Broccoli, cooked	½ cup	2.5	45.6
Tofu, firm	½ cup	20.0	43.6
Tofu, regular	½ cup	10.0	42.4
Soybeans	½ cup	15.0	39.0
Lentils, cooked	½ cup	9.0	31.2
Soymilk	1 cup	10.0	26.0
Chickpeas, cooked	½ cup	7.5	22.4
Quinoa, cooked	½ cup	5.5	18.8
Whole wheat bread	1 slice	2.5	18.0
Peanut butter	2 tablespoons	8.0	17.2
Potato	1 medium	4.5	8.0

protein quality has been the protein efficiency ratio, or PER. The PER most commonly measures the rate at which young rodents grow when they are fed proteins from different foods. Proteins that produce slower growth are considered to be of lesser quality.

We now know that the PER vastly underestimates the quality of some proteins. The reason is that rats have higher protein needs and different amino acid needs than humans. For example, the amino acid pattern in beans is not well matched to a rat's needs; so when rats are fed bean protein, they grow poorly.[13] But because the amino acids in beans are a good match for human needs, beans are an excellent source of high-quality protein for us. For years, this faulty research led us to greatly undervalue the protein in beans.

Recently, the Food and Drug Administration and the World Health Organization adopted a new technique for assessing protein quality.[14] It has a rather cumbersome name—the protein digestibility corrected amino acid score, or PDCAAS—but it gives much more reliable results than animal experiments do because it is based on human needs.[15] As a result, plant foods—beans in particular—have received a boost up the protein-score ladder to take their rightful place as good-quality protein sources.

THE MYTH OF PROTEIN COMBINING

The myth that has died hardest is the idea that we need to eat plant foods in certain combinations at each meal to get adequate protein. This idea, called protein combining or protein complementing, was popularized in the 1970s by Frances Moore Lappé in *Diet for a Small Planet*.[16] Lappé made a significant contribution to the way people thought about protein in the diet. She proved that plants could easily meet protein needs and revealed the environmental costs of a meat-based diet. Her book taught millions of people how to switch to a healthier, more environmentally friendly diet.

Unfortunately, she made one mistake at the time that stuck in the consciousness of many vegetarians. She taught that in order to achieve adequate protein intake from plant foods, one had to eat them in certain combinations.

Plant foods are often considered "incomplete" because they contain limited quantities of one or more of the essential amino acids. She believed that if you match the strengths of one plant food to the weaknesses of another, you produce a complete protein. That is, if one protein is lacking in amino acid A but is high in amino acid B, you can eat it with a food that is abundant in amino acid A, but a little short on amino acid B. The beauty of the system is that you don't really need to know anything about nutrition to follow it. It turns out that any legume pairs up perfectly with any grain or nut or seed to make a complete protein.

Dr. Lappé's theory was a sound one. In fact, it was not only scientifically correct, it was also completely practical. Most of the world's people have never heard of protein combining, but they've been doing it anyway since the earliest times. A look at some of the best-known plant-based world cuisines bears this out. In Latin American countries, beans and grains are central to the diet in the form of pinto beans wrapped in corn tortillas or black beans served on rice. In Asia, most meals include rice, corn, or noodles and soybean products such as tofu. In Africa, peanuts, which are actually in the legume family, are often paired with grains like millet or corn.

Where Dr. Lappé went wrong was in her carefully spelled out rules for combining foods in precise amounts at each meal. In the tenth-anniversary edition to her book she corrected earlier ideas about protein combining when she said, "In combatting the myth that meat is the only way to get high-quality protein, I reinforced another myth. I gave the impression that in order to get enough protein without meat, considerable care was needed in choosing foods. Actually it is much easier than I thought."[17]

Although Dr. Lappé went too far in her rules for protein combining, she was right about one thing: combining plant sources of protein does seem to improve their protein quality. And the better the quality of the protein in a diet, the less protein you need to meet protein needs. In fact, in countries where food is in short supply and the diet is unvaried, protein combining may make it easier to meet protein needs.

But since *Diet for a Small Planet* was published, we've learned some additional things about protein nutrition. One is that complementary plant proteins don't need to be consumed at the same meal. According to the American Dietetic Association, "Intakes of different types of protein that complement one another should be eaten over the course of the day . . . it is not necessary that complementation of amino acid profiles be precise and at exactly the same meal."[18]

That is, proteins eaten at one meal can combine with proteins eaten at the next meal to improve the quality of the protein. There is some debate about how far apart those meals can be to gain the maximum effect. Timing is probably more important to children, who have higher protein needs, than to adults.[19] We address this issue in more detail in chapter 13.

One reason for this more relaxed approach to protein combining is the discovery that our bodies have a storage pool of essential amino acids.[20] These EAAs, which always seem to be on tap, can be used to complement any incomplete proteins that come into the body from our diet. This newer understanding of protein combining simply means that people need to eat a variety of protein sources throughout the day, not combine them at each meal. This is still protein combining in a sense; it is just a more relaxed but equally as effective approach. It's doubtful that this has had any real impact on the way people eat. Most people unconsciously combine proteins at meals anyway. They eat peanut butter on bread, bean soup with pasta, and soymilk poured over morning bran flakes—all examples of unintended but effective protein combining.

Although some degree of protein combining seems to be helpful, is it absolutely necessary for meeting protein needs? Actually, it isn't. To understand why, we have to take a critical look at the whole concept of complete and incomplete proteins.

The completeness of any individual food protein isn't a yes-or-no proposition. It's really more a matter of degree. Some proteins come closer to meeting human amino acid needs than others, but there is a whole range of patterns. In practical terms, no precise line divides complete proteins from incomplete ones. All food proteins (except gelatin) contain all nine of the essential amino acids, so in a very real sense, all proteins are complete. When the protein in a food has a limited supply of one or two amino acids, you just have to eat more of that food to meet your needs. This means that you can meet your protein needs from a single plant food, if you eat enough of that food.

In a 1968 study, called the Michigan State University Bread Study, university students ate a diet for fifty days that provided 90 to 95 percent of its protein from wheat. The rest came from vegetables. Even on this restrictive diet, the students met their protein needs.[21] Other studies on wheat, including some in children, have shown similar results.[22]

Another study used rice as the sole source of protein and showed that rice alone was able to keep subjects in nitrogen balance.[23] In fact, when the researchers added chicken to these diets, which raised protein intake considerably, there was no improvement in protein status. The subjects did just as well with an all-rice diet. Potato protein also meets protein needs by itself, and so does corn.[24]

Although these laboratory studies are interesting and allay some fears that vegetarians may have about meeting protein needs, they have only limited practical value. We can't recommend that you meet all of your protein needs through either wheat or rice. For one thing, it can take a huge amount of these foods to meet needs. The Michigan Bread Study showed that adult males would need to eat twenty-eight slices of bread a day to meet their protein needs. That's nearly two thousand calories from bread alone. It doesn't leave much room in the diet for other foods that are necessary to meet other nutrient needs.

Also, in the Michigan Bread Study and other studies, there was a period of adaptation. Subjects didn't meet protein needs during the first part of the study, but they eventually adapted to a lower protein intake so that they were in positive nitrogen balance. Scientists have long known that humans can adapt to a low protein intake. This is a defense mechanism. In severe protein deficiency, many of the body's reactions involving protein slow down in order to save protein for only the most essential functions. Although the body is in nitrogen balance, it may not be operating at an optimal level. It's surviving, but it may not be thriving.

In nitrogen-balance studies in which subjects adapt to a low protein intake or to proteins of lesser quality, nothing close to starvation is taking place. But possibly some very subtle changes are occurring in the way the body is using proteins, and these changes represent a less-than-ideal situation.

So what can we conclude from these studies? Well, the important fact is that grains contain high-quality protein that can meet human protein needs without food combining. What isn't clear from these stud-

ies is how much of a grain it takes to do this. Eating a variety of protein-rich foods throughout the day is still best; this allows protein to be used more efficiently so that we can meet our needs on smaller amounts of food. This is especially important for people with very high protein needs, such as pregnant women, children, and athletes, and for people with a low calorie intake.

PROTEIN: THE VEGETARIAN EDGE

It's enough to know that vegetarians can meet their protein needs with little effort. But there are some real advantages to meeting protein needs through plant foods. Plant proteins are healthier for you.

First, as we saw in chapter 2, replacing animal protein with plant protein may lower blood cholesterol levels. In fact, one of the first proposed explanations for heart disease focused not on fat, but on animal protein. In 1908, the Russian physician Ignatowski suggested that the high rate of heart disease among the Russian aristocracy was due to its excessive use of meat.[25] This may be one of the reasons that traditional heart-healthy diets, which make liberal use of lean meats, reap only moderate benefits in lowering blood cholesterol. People who have been following these diets can lower their cholesterol further by trading their skinless chicken and fish for a vegetarian meal. This dietary change reduces fat intake and has the added advantage of replacing animal protein with plant protein.

Of course, there are some other heart-healthy attributes of plant proteins. These foods tend to be much lower in saturated fat than meat, eggs, and dairy, and they are

IS TAURINE AN ESSENTIAL NUTRIENT?

Although we need only nine amino acids in the diet, there are many others that our body needs in order to function healthfully. Whether or not we get these other amino acids from food is immaterial, however, since the body can synthesize them itself. One amino acid that has been under scrutiny is taurine. It isn't found in any plant foods, so vegans don't consume it.

Taurine has many functions, especially with respect to the cardiovascular system, blood platelets, muscle contraction, and also to eyesight and the nervous system.[26] This amino acid is found in nearly every cell in the body. For animals that can't make their own taurine, the effects of a deficiency can be devastating. Cats can't make taurine and will go blind if they don't have it in their diet. That's one reason that a meat-based diet makes sense for cats.

But concern over the taurine content of the human diet is unfounded. While it was once believed that humans might not make this amino acid in sufficient quantities, this isn't true. Studies show that humans have no trouble producing plenty of taurine.[27] In vegans, the levels of taurine in the blood are only slightly lower than levels in omnivores.[28]

In order to make enough taurine, we need to consume the essential amino acid cysteine. A taurine deficiency has been seen in hospitalized patients who receive tube feedings that contain neither taurine nor cysteine.[29] However, vegetarians get plenty of cysteine and are able to make their own taurine. Also, if taurine levels drop, the kidney excretes less and conserves it.[30]

Although infants, especially preterm infants, have a reduced ability to make taurine, this doesn't seem to present any problems. Adding taurine to formulas doesn't affect the development of preterm infants.[31] And although the breast milk of vegan mothers is lower in taurine than the breast milk of omnivores, both are much higher than cow's-milk infant formula.[32]

There is no indication that taurine is essential in the diet of humans.

always cholesterol free. Diets based on plant proteins are always the best choice for preventing a heart attack or stroke.

Also, as we will see, too much protein in general, and too much animal protein in particular, may increase the risk for osteoporosis. Animal protein causes bones to lose calcium. Since plant-based diets are lower in total protein, and since the protein in legumes doesn't appear to increase calcium loss as much, vegetarian diets may be better for bone health. Finally, excess protein is unhealthy for people with kidney disease and may actually hasten this disease in susceptible people.

There is one final reason that plant proteins are always a better choice. They are much more efficiently produced. An acre of farmland devoted to soybeans will provide roughly thirty times more protein than an acre devoted to cattle grazing. Because plant protein provides adequate nutrition and is efficiently produced, we can feed more people with less water, petroleum, and pollution when we depend on grains and beans rather than meat. In a world with ever-dwindling resources, this may be plant protein's most important claim.

PROTEIN IN PERSPECTIVE

We've seen that vegetarians can relax about meal planning and meeting protein needs. Protein is a complex issue, though, and we've presented some complex ideas in this chapter. Summing up the main points might simplify things a little.

First, old ideas about the "completeness" of proteins really don't hold up under scrutiny. Plant proteins contain all of the essential amino acids, which makes them as complete as any other protein. Although plant proteins tend to be a little short in one or two of the amino acids (the limiting amino acids), that just means that it takes more of an individual plant food to meet protein needs. Studies show that people can actually meet their protein needs by consuming just rice or wheat or potatoes, if they consume enough of those foods. However, we aren't certain how much of those foods it takes to meet those needs, and it is doubtful that children could meet their needs by consuming just one of those foods.

Eating plant proteins in certain combinations greatly optimizes the way proteins are used. Remember, the better the quality of the protein, the less of that protein you need to meet your needs. So when grains are eaten in combination with beans, or beans are paired up with nuts or seeds, the protein quality escalates so that protein needs are met with just small amounts of plant foods. Scientists have known this for decades and have called it protein combining.

More recently we've learned that protein combinations don't have to be consumed at the same meal. The grains you eat for breakfast will hook up with your lunchtime beans to produce the same effect as if you had eaten them together. As a result, when vegetarians eat a variety of plant foods throughout the day and are consuming adequate calories, it is virtually impossible to be deficient in protein. In fact, protein is essentially a nonissue for vegetarians. The only way you can become deficient in this nutrient would be if you based your diet on foods that are nearly devoid of protein—fruits, juices, fats, and alcohol.

Plant protein is more than adequate. It is healthier for you. People who rely on plant foods to meet their needs may have lower risks of heart, bone, and kidney disease. After decades of worrying about how vegetarians can meet their protein needs, we are finding that vegetarians have the edge when it comes to protein nutrition.

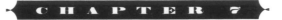
MEETING CALCIUM NEEDS ON A PLANT-BASED DIET

The minimum calcium requirement of adult males is probably so low that deficiency is unlikely on most natural diets.

—MARK HEGSTED, PHD, *J Nutrition*, 1952

◆

Calcium is abundant in plant foods. Foods rich in this mineral include beans, soy products (tofu, textured vegetable protein, or TVP, soymilk, tempeh), dark green leafy vegetables, sea vegetables, and many seeds and nuts. Consuming four or five servings of these calcium-rich plant foods will help to meet the RDA of eight hundred milligrams. But the calcium needs of Americans and especially of vegetarians are an issue of heated debate. And myths about calcium, dairy foods, and bone health abound and are reinforced by the dairy industry and even nutrition professionals.

If you are like most Americans you probably believe that osteoporosis—a disease of weakened, easily fractured bones—is caused by a deficiency of calcium in the diet. And the best way to prevent it is to consume plenty of calcium-rich foods, like milk, and perhaps to take a calcium supplement every day. So it might surprise you to know that throughout the world people who consume the most calcium actually have the poorest bone health. Figure 7.1 shows a striking relationship between calcium intake and osteoporosis. Populations with the highest calcium intake have the highest rates of hip fracture, which is a symptom of osteoporosis.

Osteoporosis, like heart disease, cancer, diabetes, and obesity, appears to be a disease of affluence and excess, rather than one of deficiency. The more scientists learn about osteoporosis, the more they realize that it is an extremely complex disease related to overall lifestyle, a big part of which includes diet. The idea that dosing yourself with calcium will automatically keep your bones in good shape is just plain wrong.

WHO NEEDS MILK?

The dairy industry promotes milk and other dairy foods as "calcium the way nature intended it." The facts suggest otherwise. About two-thirds of the world's adult population has trouble digesting milk.[1] These people lack an enzyme called lactase, which is needed to digest lactose, the sugar in milk. Undigested lactose travels down to the colon, where bacteria metabolize it, producing gas in the process. The result can be cramps, flatulence, nausea, and diarrhea.

All mammals, including humans, are

Figure 7.1 Relationship between Hip-Fracture Rate and Calcium Intake

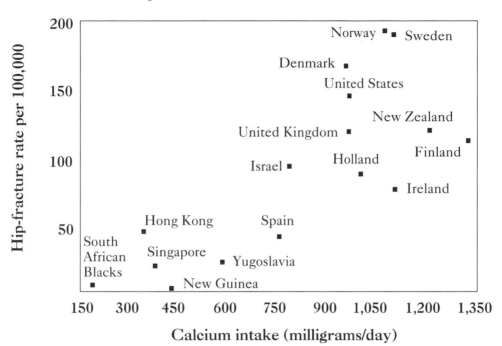

Albew BJ, Holford TR, Insogna KL. Cross-cultural association between dietary animal protein and hip fracture: a hypothesis. *Calcif Tissue Int* 50:14–18, 1992.

normally born with plenty of the enzyme lactase. This allows them to easily digest their mother's milk, which is rich in lactose. But throughout most of the world, the activity of this enzyme decreases with age and declines dramatically by age five.[2]

This inability to digest lactose is called lactose intolerance. Although the name suggests it is some type of a disease, it is actually the norm for human adults. In fact, nutritional anthropologists believe that until ten thousand years ago or so, all human adults were lactose intolerant.[3] Apparently, a genetic mutation occurred among northern Europeans allowing them to continue digesting milk sugar into adulthood. The rest of the world, including Asians, native North and South Americans, Africans, and Mediterranean groups, continued to develop normally; that is, they continued to lose their ability to digest milk as they matured. Figure 7.2 shows the extent of lactose intolerance among different cultural groups.

Not surprisingly, people living in countries where lactose intolerance is common consume relatively few dairy foods. They also tend to have a lower calcium intake than North Americans and northern Europeans, though this doesn't seem to adversely affect their bone health.

It is obvious that milk may not be quite as

Figure 7.2 Estimated Prevalence (%) of Lactose Intolerance in Different Populations

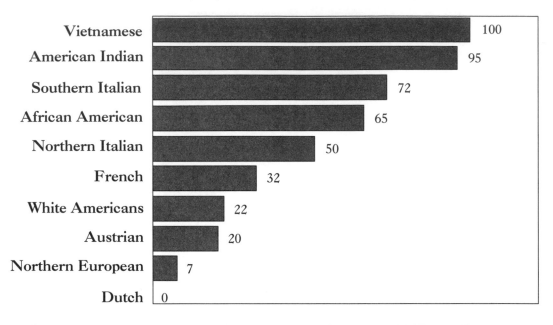

Population	Prevalence (%)
Vietnamese	100
American Indian	95
Southern Italian	72
African American	65
Northern Italian	50
French	32
White Americans	22
Austrian	20
Northern European	7
Dutch	0

Flatz G. Genetics of lactose digestion in humans. In *Advances in Human Genetics*. Harris H, Hirschorn K, eds. Plenum, New York: pp 1–77.

"natural" as it is made out to be. Vegetarians who avoid dairy products may seem to be choosing an unusual diet by Western standards, but are actually choosing a typical diet by world standards. The belief that milk is essential in the diet is clearly incorrect. In part, this belief is due to promotional efforts of the dairy industry and of the United States Department of Agriculture, which represents the interests of the dairy industry. Unfortunately, even many nutritionists continue to promote milk as an essential food.

People who are lactose intolerant often add special enzymes to their milk to make it more digestible. But there is no reason to consume a food that is unsuited to the physiology of most of the world's people. We can get plenty of calcium from nondairy foods. Our earliest ancestors got most of their calcium from wild plant foods, and anthropologists believe their calcium intake was higher than that of modern people.[4]

CALCIUM AND BONES

Although milk is not essential in the diet, calcium certainly is. The adult human body contains about three pounds of calcium. Approximately 99 percent of this calcium is found in our bones and teeth. Most of the remaining 1 percent is found in the bloodstream. Maintaining normal levels of blood calcium is actually more important than keeping it in the bones. In fact, the bones are a storage place for calcium that is used to replenish calcium in the blood when levels get too low.

Blood calcium is needed for muscle contraction—which includes the beating of your heart and the moving of your diaphragm, allowing you to breathe. It is also necessary for nerve transmission and blood clotting. The amount of calcium in the blood is very tightly controlled by hormones and other factors, since too much or too little can be fatal. Some calcium is lost from the body as blood is continuously filtered by the kidneys. The kidneys return almost all of the calcium to the bloodstream, but some is excreted in the urine. Calcium is also lost in the feces, and smaller amounts are lost through sweat. When blood calcium levels drop due to these losses, the bones release calcium into the blood. As a result, blood levels of calcium stay pretty constant; a blood sample won't tell you very much about how much calcium is in your bones.

Bones themselves are very dynamic. They are constantly breaking down to replenish blood calcium and building back up again. We need a source of calcium in the diet to replenish what is lost every day.

Bones grow in length during the early part of life and then continue to get heavier and more dense until about the age of thirty. Somewhere between age thirty and thirty-five, peak bone mass is reached. This means that bones are at their greatest density and have stopped growing. The more dense your bones are at this point, the less your chance of developing osteoporosis later in life.[5]

Between the ages of thirty-five and forty-five, peak bone mass is generally maintained. But around the late forties bones begin to break down faster than they can be rebuilt. After the age of forty-five, humans lose as much as 0.5 percent of their total bone mass every year.[6] Over a period of thirty years or so, this bone loss can significantly affect bone health.

For women, bone loss really steps up after menopause. This is because they stop producing estrogen, a hormone that protects bones. Women can lose 15 to 50 percent of their bone mass in the first ten years following menopause.[7] Loss of bone mass leads to smaller, more porous and brittle bones and eventually to osteoporosis. Osteoporosis, which literally means "porous bones," makes the bones more susceptible to fractures.

Between 15 and 20 million Americans have osteoporosis, and one out of every five American women over the age of sixty-five has had one or more fractured bones.[8] In severe osteoporosis, bones can fracture spontaneously just because they can't support the weight of the body. Even the impact of a sneeze can cause small bones to splinter. Osteoporosis is more serious than the inconvenience of breaking a leg; about fifty thousand Americans die each year from complications related to this disease.

Everyone loses bone mass in the later years. Whether or not that bone loss leads to osteoporosis depends on many factors. Genetics certainly plays some role here. For example, men have heavier bones than women, and African Americans have denser bones than Caucasians.[9] You can inherit good bones to some degree, since the bone density of parents influences that of their children.[10]

Calcium is always essential in the diet, but a high calcium intake generally won't increase the strength of bones once they have stopped growing. However, it is possible to slow the rate of calcium loss from bones and to keep bones from getting weaker. We'll see later in this chapter that lifestyle and diet have a lot to do with this.

BONE HEALTH IN VEGETARIANS

Unfortunately, scientists don't have a very clear picture of the bone health of Western vegetarians. There is no difference in bone densities of vegetarians and nonvegetarians, for men or younger women.[11] Some studies show that lacto-ovo vegetarians have denser bones than meat eaters.[12] Older lacto-ovo vegetarian women may actually lose less bone than omnivores, although one recent study disputes this.[13] But whether or not lacto-ovo vegetarians have stronger bones, it is clear that their bones are at least as strong. This isn't surprising, since lacto-ovo vegetarians often consume dairy products in place of meat and they generally consume as much calcium as omnivores or perhaps even more.[14]

But what about vegans? There is very little information about calcium intake and bone health in strict vegetarians. The few available studies show that Western vegans consume considerably less calcium than both lacto-ovo vegetarians and meat eaters,[15] although one study found vegetarians are more efficient than omnivores at absorbing calcium.[16] But we don't know if this increased absorption compensates fully for the lower intake. Only one study has looked specifically at osteoporosis in Western vegans. And although it showed that older vegans had lower bone density than lacto-ovo

vegetarians, the study had too many shortcomings to allow us to draw any real conclusions from this finding.[17] It involved only eleven vegans, and they had followed a vegan diet for only a very short time.

We do know that on a worldwide basis, populations with largely plant-based diets and low calcium intakes are not more likely to get osteoporosis. In fact, they may have less osteoporosis. This is because many factors other than calcium intake affect bone health. Vegetarians may actually need less calcium than omnivores. To understand the controversy over this issue, we need to first understand the assumptions about calcium needs.

ASSUMPTIONS ABOUT CALCIUM REQUIREMENTS

Among the nutrients, calcium is a giant. The 800-milligram RDA is more than seventeen times the requirement for vitamin C and more than fifty times that for iron.[18]

Most American males meet the calcium RDA, while women—especially teenage girls—tend to fall short of it.[19] This may or may not be a problem. Like all the RDAs, the one for calcium includes a generous safety factor. On the other hand, some experts consider the RDA for calcium to be too low.[20]

The RDA for calcium is based on two assumptions. One is that the average person typically loses between 200 and 250 milligrams of calcium from the body each day through urine, feces, and sweat. The second assumption is that the average person absorbs 30 to 40 percent of the calcium in his or her diet. If a person consumes 800 milligrams of calcium, then he or she can expect to actually absorb between 240 and 320 milligrams of calcium, which is enough to replace the amount lost.

But the actual amount of calcium absorbed varies a lot, depending on many factors. Both the need for calcium at a particular time and the amount of calcium in the diet will affect how much calcium is absorbed. For example, if calcium intake is very high—above 800 milligrams a day—only about 15 percent is absorbed.[21] When people consume smaller amounts of calcium, absorption rates go up. They also go up when needs are high; for example, children can absorb as much as 75 percent of the calcium in their diet.[22] Also, when calcium intake is low, less is lost in the urine.[23] By absorbing more and excreting less, the body can adapt to relatively low calcium intakes.

There is also some individual variation in amounts of calcium absorbed that has nothing to do with the amount in the diet. Most people appear to do well when they consume between 400 and 800 milligrams of calcium per day. In one study, for example, bone health was affected only when women consumed fewer than 405 milligrams of calcium or more than 777 milligrams.[24] However, although most people fall in that range, some people have much higher needs—perhaps as high as 1,500 milligrams per day.[25]

So far, we've talked only about the absorption rates of calcium. But there is another side to the equation that affects calcium needs. This is the amount of calcium that we lose from the body. We said that the average person loses between 200 and 250 milligrams of calcium each day. But these figures are for the average omnivore. Vegetarians may lose quite a bit less because of the amount and type of protein in their diet.

PROTEIN AND CALCIUM

Since it is difficult and expensive to directly measure bone density, researchers often estimate the rates of osteoporosis by counting the number of hip fractures in a population. A rather striking observation is that populations that eat the most animal protein tend to have the highest rates of hip fracture.[26] Interestingly, where protein intake is high, calcium intake is high as well. This makes sense. People who can afford to eat protein-rich diets based on plenty of animal foods are North Americans and northern Europeans—many of whom can also digest dairy products. So the higher hip-fracture rate occurs in people with high-protein diets despite the fact that they also consume a lot of calcium. You can see that figure 7.3, which shows the relationship between protein intake and hip-fracture rate in several countries, looks quite similar to figure 7.1, which shows the relationship between calcium intake and hip-fracture rate.

There may be a very straightforward explanation for this. As long ago as 1920, scientists observed that a diet high in meat caused huge increases in the amount of calcium excreted in the urine.[27] More than twenty-five years ago, researchers first proposed that this could lead to weakened bones.[28]

Why would meat have this effect? Scientists think they have the answer. Meat and animal protein in general produce a potentially dangerous acid condition in the blood. Fortunately, the body has a variety of ways to neutralize this acid. One of these

Figure 7.3 Relationship between Hip-Fracture Rate and Animal Protein Intake

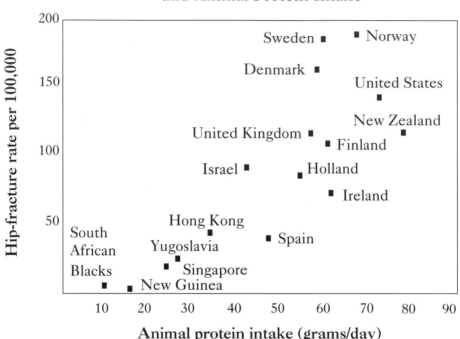

Albew BJ, Holford TR, Insogna KL. Cross-cultural association between dietary animal protein and hip fracture: a hypothesis. *Calcif Tissue Int* 50:14–18, 1992.

defenses results in the release of calcium from the bones. The calcium involved in the process is eventually excreted in the urine. So anything that causes the blood to become more acidic ultimately results in calcium loss. The effect of protein intake on calcium loss can be profound, as studies show.

Researchers at Tufts Medical School showed that when acidosis (acid buildup) was produced in subjects' bloodstreams, they lost three times more calcium than under normal conditions.[29]

Diets that contain meat produce more acid than vegetarian diets, and lacto-ovo-vegetarian diets produce more acid than vegan diets.[30]

When people switched from a lacto-vegetarian diet (no eggs or meat) containing a low but adequate amount of protein to a diet that included meat and eggs and twice the protein, acid levels increased about fivefold. As expected, the amount of calcium excreted in the urine also increased dramatically.[31]

In a study at the University of Wisconsin, when subjects increased their protein intake from 48 grams a day, which is close to the RDA, to 95 grams a day, which is close to what most omnivores consume, it caused 50 percent more calcium to be lost.[32] When protein intake was very high—142 grams—it became impossible to keep the body in calcium balance even when the subjects consumed 1,400 milligrams of calcium—nearly twice the RDA.

Young men were in calcium balance on just 600 milligrams of calcium a day when their diet was low in protein. As meat was added to their diet, they slipped into negative calcium balance; that is, they lost more calcium than they retained.[33]

Generally, doubling your protein intake will cause the amount of calcium you lose to double as well.[34] Researchers at the University of Connecticut found that increasing a person's protein intake by 50 grams caused an extra 60 milligrams of calcium to be lost.[35] Over a thirty- to forty-year period, this could add up to an entire pound of calcium loss, or one-third of a person's bone mass!

Researchers speculate that when protein intake is 50 percent higher than protein needs, it could account for the 1 to 1.5 percent loss of bone per year that is typically seen in postmenopausal women.[36]

Since bones are constantly absorbing and releasing calcium, it is normal to lose some calcium in the urine and feces. But anything that increases that loss can have a detrimental effect on bone health. In fact, research from hundreds of subjects indicates that urinary calcium loss is actually three to four times more important in determining calcium balance than calcium intake.[37] In Western populations, a protein intake higher than 75 grams a day is likely to produce negative calcium balance.[38] People who eat meat typically consume more protein than this.

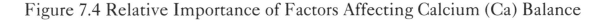

Figure 7.4 Relative Importance of Factors Affecting Calcium (Ca) Balance

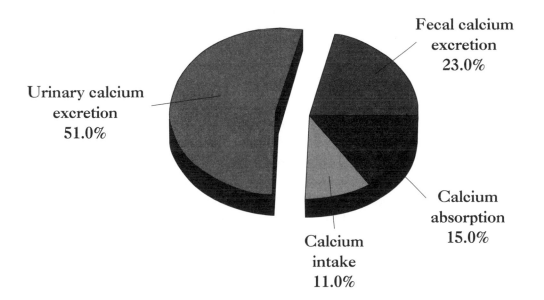

Heaney RP. Cofactors influencing the calcium requirement—other nutrients. NIH Consensus Development Conference on Optimal Calcium Intake. NIH Consensus Development Conference, June 6–8, 1994, pp 71-77.

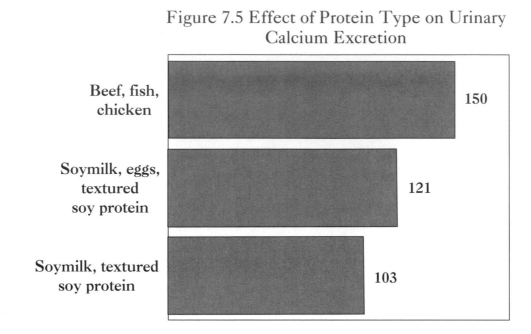

Figure 7.5 Effect of Protein Type on Urinary Calcium Excretion

Beef, fish, chicken — 150

Soymilk, eggs, textured soy protein — 121

Soymilk, textured soy protein — 103

Calcium excretion (milligrams/day)

But not so the average vegetarian. Vegetarians consume less protein than non-vegetarians. Perhaps of equal importance, they consume a different kind of protein.

NOT ALL PROTEIN IS EQUAL

Protein from legumes may not have the same effect on calcium loss as that from animal protein. In a study at the University of Texas Health Science Center, subjects ate diets that contained the same amounts of calcium and protein, except that the protein came from three different sources.[39] One diet contained protein from meat and cheese; another included soyfoods, cheese, and eggs; and the third included protein from soyfoods only. When the subjects consumed protein from meat and cheese, they excreted 50 percent more calcium than when they ate soy protein

only. Calcium excretion fell somewhere in the middle when they consumed soyfoods, cheese, and eggs.

These different effects are most likely due to the amino acid makeup of different proteins. You may remember from chapter 6 that amino acids are the building blocks of protein. Protein from soy and other beans is relatively low in the amino acids methionine and cysteine, which contain the element sulfur. Sulfur-containing amino acids seem to be the real culprits in producing the acid conditions associated with high-protein diets. Also, they produce compounds that may directly inhibit the kidneys' reabsorption of calcium, so that even more is lost in the urine.[40] In comparison with legumes, animal proteins are especially high in sulfur.

For healthy bones, what seems to be most important is how much calcium you consume relative to how much protein (especially animal protein) you consume.[41] The ideal ratio, according to some researchers, is 16:1. That is, people should consume 16 milligrams of calcium for every 1 gram of protein in their diet.[42] Omnivores do very poorly in this regard. Their ratio is 9–12:1, which is much too low. To make matters even worse, most of their protein is from animal foods, which worsens calcium balance. Lacto-ovo-vegetarians have much better ratios and a higher intake of plant protein. Vegans consume less calcium, but because of their lower protein intake their calcium-to-protein ratio is about the same as that of omnivores.

So lacto-ovo-vegetarian diets are more likely to produce conditions that favor bone health. Bear in mind, however, that the protein in grains is quite high in sulfur amino acids. Per gram of protein, it is as high in these amino acids as meat. But because vegetarians eat less total protein, and get some protein from legumes, they have a definite advantage.

This lower protein intake clearly results in a reduced calcium requirement. But bone health is complex. A whole host of factors affects its outcome, and we need to consider all of them in establishing the calcium needs of vegetarians.

OTHER FACTORS THAT AFFECT CALCIUM NEEDS

Sodium

Sodium greatly increases calcium excretion in the urine and might increase the risk of osteoporosis.[43] One study showed that people lose as much as 80 milligrams of calcium for every 2,300 milligrams of sodium they consumed.[44] Americans consume between 4,000 and 5,800 milligrams of sodium per day, although our requirement is for just 500 milligrams under normal conditions. Highly salted processed foods contribute to the risk for osteoporosis just as much as animal protein. Women who consume high-protein, high-sodium diets may need as many as 2,000 milligrams of calcium to stay in calcium balance, but they may need as few as 450 milligrams of calcium when their diet is low in both protein and sodium.[45] Worldwide, sodium intake varies as much as a thousandfold, so it could be an important factor in the varying risk of osteoporosis among countries.[46] In fact, a single fast-food burger, because of its high protein and sodium and low calcium, can cause you to lose 22 milligrams of calcium, which means you have to consume 100 milligrams more of calcium to make up for that burger.[47]

Phosphorus

Diets with too much phosphorus relative to calcium intake might also cause bone loss.[48] This could be especially important for young women who typically have a low calcium intake but drink a lot of soft drinks, which are high in phosphorus.[49] Animal foods—particularly meat—are generally high in phosphorus. This area is still one of debate, however, because some studies don't show any effect of phosphorus on bone health.[50] It is interesting to note that phosphorus causes less calcium to be excreted in the urine, but it also causes more to be excreted in the feces.

Other Nutrients and Nondietary Factors

Bone health is affected by many different dietary factors, so that the quality of the whole diet has an impact. Nutrients that are necessary to maintain healthy bones include vitamin D, vitamin K, and the minerals potassium, magnesium, and boron.

Caffeine also causes you to lose calcium. A six-ounce cup of coffee containing caffeine causes a loss of about five milligrams a day.[51]

There are also many nondietary factors that affect bone health. Countries with the highest rates of hip fracture are populated by people of northern European ancestry, who are at a higher genetic risk for osteoporosis. Genetics affects bone health to varying degrees, since people of different ethnic backgrounds actually process calcium differently even on similar diets.

Childbearing practices may be important, too. Both pregnancy and breast-feeding may lower the risk of osteoporosis, although a few studies dispute this.[52] In developing countries, where osteoporosis is less common, women tend to have more pregnancies and to breast-feed for a much longer time.[53]

Of all the factors that affect bone health, exercise or physical activity is one of the most important. Undoubtedly, this also works in favor of those who live in developing countries, where physical activity is a normal part of daily life. Exercise might actually be more important than calcium for bone health and might explain the differences in rates of osteoporosis throughout the world.[54]

The relationship of activity to bone health is easy to demonstrate. Hospitalized patients who are bedridden for long periods lose significant amounts of calcium.[55] Tennis players have bones that are a third thicker in the arm they use to play tennis than in their nondominant arm.[56] Exercise doesn't have to be intense to improve bone health; in post-menopausal women, simply walking between 1 and 1.5 miles per day was associated with a reduced rate of bone loss.[57] Even in older people, exercise can not only slow bone loss, but can actually increase bone density.[58]

Some researchers believe that the rate of hip fracture is not entirely related to the calcium content of the bones. Groups of people with similar bone density can have very different rates of hip fracture.[59] It is possible that some people are just more likely to fall and therefore to break bones more frequently.[60] There could be any number of reasons for this. In certain cultures, women may leave the house less often. Also, hip fractures are more common in northern Europe and North America—areas where slippery snow and ice are most likely to be a problem.

Even height seems to affect hip fracture. Men over six feet tall are twice as likely to have a hip fracture as men who are five feet ten inches or shorter.[61]

DO VEGETARIANS NEED LESS CALCIUM?

We can make a good argument for a lower calcium RDA for vegetarians because their lower intake of total protein almost certainly spares calcium. The World Health Organization recognizes that people who consume plant-based diets need less calcium. Its calcium recommendations for people in developing countries are about two-thirds those for people in the United States.[62] In fact, you can see in table 7.1 that U.S. calcium requirements are quite high compared with the guidelines established by other countries.

It is especially tempting to speculate that

	Children	Adolescents	Adults	Pregnant Women
TABLE 7.1 RECOMMENDATIONS FOR CALCIUM INTAKE (IN MILLIGRAMS)				
United States	800	1,200	800	1,200
Canada	550–700	1,000–1,100	700–800	1,200
United Kingdom	600	700	500	1,200
Japan	400	900	600	1,000
Korea	500–700	800	600	1,000
WHO	450	650	450	1,100

Western vegans need less than the RDA for calcium, since they consume less total protein and no animal protein. We believe that vegans probably do need less calcium than omnivores. But we just don't have enough information to say with any certainty how much calcium Western vegans need. We've seen that calcium needs are impacted by many factors—not just protein. We need to consider all of these before we can say with any certainty what lacto-ovo-vegetarian and vegan calcium needs are. No one has studied the specific needs of Western vegetarians. Until researchers actually determine the calcium needs of vegetarians, we recommend that vegetarians—including vegans—continue to use the RDAs as guidelines. This is admittedly a conservative recommendation, and we recognize that many vegans may need less calcium than this. But children, teens, and young adults, in particular, should probably strive to meet the RDAs because adequate calcium is so important at these stages. In the case of early bone development, we prefer to err on the side of being too conservative.

Fortunately, the calcium RDA is easy to meet on vegan diets because plant foods are rich in calcium.

VEGETARIAN CALCIUM SOURCES

Even nonvegetarian Americans get quite a bit of their calcium from plant foods. In fact, about 40 percent of the calcium in the American diet comes from plants.[63] Many foods are good sources of calcium. But the amount of calcium in a food is only part of the story. The amount that is actually absorbed varies quite a bit among foods. Some compounds in plant foods can interfere with calcium absorption. Three are of potential interest in vegetarian diets: fiber, phytates, and oxalates.

Fiber might bind calcium, making it unavailable to the body. The true effects of fiber aren't very clear. Some studies show it has a negative effect on calcium absorption, and others show no effect.[64]

Phytates, found in whole grains, can bind to calcium and interfere with its absorption. However, when grain products are leavened with yeast, the yeast breaks apart the bond between the phytate and calcium, freeing the calcium for absorption. This means that yeast-

TABLE 7.2 AVAILABILITY OF CALCIUM FROM SELECTED PLANT FOODS

Food Source	Calcium Content (milligrams)	% Absorbed	Calcium Absorbed
Beans, Pinto (½ cup)	45	17	7.6
Broccoli (½ cup)	35	53	18.4
Brussels sprouts (½ cup)	19	64	12
Cabbage, Chinese (½ cup)	79	54	43
Cabbage, Green (½ cup)	25	65	16
Kale (½ cup)	47	59	28
Mustard greens (½ cup)	64	58	37
Sesame seeds (1 ounce)	28	21	7.7
Tofu, raw, firm (½ cup)	258	31	80
Turnip greens (½ cup)	99	52	51
Cow's milk (1 cup)	300	32	96

Source: Weaver CM and Plawecki KL. Dietary calcium: adequacy of a vegetarian diet. Am J Clin Nutr 59(suppl):12385–415, 1994.

raised breads are better sources of calcium than are flat breads. But surprisingly, the calcium in even unleavened bread products is better absorbed than that in milk.[65] So phytates may not be as important as we once thought.

Oxalates, found in some vegetables, can also bind calcium. The calcium in spinach, Swiss chard, beet greens, and rhubarb is poorly absorbed because of the presence of oxalates.[66]

But overall, calcium from plant foods is very well absorbed. Perhaps the most important observation is that osteoporosis is less common in countries where diets are high in both fiber and phytates. And recent laboratory studies from Purdue University show that the calcium in many plant foods is actually better absorbed than the calcium in milk. For example, more than 50

TABLE 7.3 PLANT SOURCES OF CALCIUM

	Calcium (milligrams)		Calcium (milligrams)
GRAINS		Lima beans	52
Corn bread (2 ounces)	133	Navy beans	128
Corn tortilla	53	Pinto beans	82
English muffin	92	Vegetarian baked beans	128
Pita (1 small pocket)	31		
		NUTS AND SEEDS (2 tablespoons)	
VEGETABLES (½ cup cooked)		Almond butter	86
Bok choy	79	Almonds	50
Broccoli	89	Brazil nuts	50
Collard greens	178	Sesame seeds	176
Kale	90	Tahini	128
Mustard greens	75		
Squash, butternut	42	**SOYFOODS**	
Sweet potatoes	35	Soybeans (1 cup cooked)	88
Turnip greens	125	Soymilk (1 cup)	84
		Soymilk, fortified (1 cup)	200–300
FRUITS		Soy nuts (½ cup)	252
Figs, dried (5)	258	Tempeh (½ cup)	77
Orange (1 medium)	56	Textured vegetable protein	
Orange juice, calcium fortified		(½ cup rehydrated)	85
(6 ounces)	200	Tofu (½ cup)	120–350
Raisins (⅔ cup)	53		
		OTHER FOODS	
LEGUMES (1 cup cooked)		Blackstrap molasses (1 tablespoon)	187
Black beans	103	Rice Dream, fortified (1 cup)	300
Chickpeas	78	Take Care (1 cup)	300
Great northern beans	121	Vegelicious (1 cup)	300
Kidney beans	50		
Lentils	37		

percent of the calcium in kale, broccoli, and turnip greens is absorbed, compared with about 30 percent of the calcium in milk.[67] Table 7.2 shows several plant sources of calcium with the amounts of calcium that are actually absorbed by the body.

Generally speaking, dark-green leafy vegetables, cooked dried beans, soy products, and some nuts, seeds, and dried fruits are all good sources of calcium. Calcium-fortified foods, such as fortified soymilk or orange juice, are also excellent sources of this mineral, and calcium is found in very high amounts in sea vegetables.

Vegans can generally meet the calcium RDA by including four or five servings of calcium-rich foods every day in their diet. If foods that are very rich in well-absorbed calcium are used frequently—such as tofu, broccoli, soymilk, or blackstrap molasses—then fewer servings would most likely be needed. We assume that most vegans will get their calcium from a variety of plant foods, including some that contain less calcium than calcium-set tofu or broccoli and some in which the calcium is not as well absorbed. Table 7.3 lists plant foods that are rich in calcium, although in most cases we don't know how much of that calcium is absorbed. Since these foods are not high in oxalates, however, it is a safe assumption that the calcium is fairly well absorbed.

Consuming a variety of foods makes diets more interesting and healthy. Therefore, it is actually a good idea to meet calcium needs from many different foods. We don't recommend relying on just one or two foods such as broccoli or milk to meet those needs. Lacto-ovo vegetarians should explore ways to use more plant sources of calcium in their diets. The vegan menu plans throughout this book illustrate how easy it is to meet calcium needs with plant foods.

Beyond Osteoporosis

We have talked about the need for calcium only in relation to bone health and osteoporosis. A number of studies show that high-calcium diets might lower blood pressure and reduce colon cancer risk.[68] However, vegetarians have lower risks of both hypertension and colon cancer compared with omnivores. Worldwide, populations that consume low levels of calcium tend to have some of the lowest rates of colon cancer, most likely because they eat a plant-based diet. In fact, rural South African blacks, who consume fewer than two hundred milligrams of calcium a day, have almost no colon disease of any kind.[69]

Dosing up on huge amounts of calcium is probably helpful only when people are eating the unhealthy diets that produce hypertension and colon cancer. It is better to eat a healthy plant-based diet that protects against disease. This diet will supply enough calcium to meet the moderate needs of healthy people.

Calcium in Perspective

Getting plenty of calcium is crucial to good bone health. Adequate calcium is especially important for children and young adults, since their bones are growing. Building dense, heavy bones early in life reduces the risk of osteoporosis later in life.

But the idea that people need to consume milk is a myth. Plant foods such as beans, soy products, leafy green vegetables, nuts, and fortified orange juice are rich in absorbable calcium. In addition, vegans may need less calcium than omnivores because high protein intake causes increased calcium loss. However, there is very little information on the bone health of vegans, and there haven't been any studies to show how much calcium vegans actually need. It's probably a good idea to strive to meet the RDA—especially for vegan children—until we know otherwise.

VITAMINS IN VEGETARIAN DIETS

In the matter of vitamins, also, the flesh-abstainer need have no concern.

—JOHN HARVEY KELLOGG,
The Natural Diet of Man, 1923

♦

Vitamins were the last of the six classes of nutrients to be discovered, probably because they are present in foods in such tiny amounts. The discovery of the vitamins in the early part of this century was probably one of the most exciting and important events in nutritional history. Today, we know of thirteen vitamins that are needed by humans. We generally divide them into two classes. Vitamin C and the eight B vitamins are water soluble; we tend to excrete any excess of these vitamins in the urine and don't store them to any great extent (vitamin B_{12} is the exception). Vitamins A, D, E, and K are fat soluble, and we do store these in the body. Because we don't excrete these vitamins very well, there is a danger of toxicity when people overdose on them. Generally, you can only overdose by using vitamin supplements, although vitamin D may be an exception to this.

Fat-soluble vitamins need dietary fat for absorption, so that a diet too low in fat can raise the risk for vitamin deficiency. But the amount of fat you need for all these vita-mins to be absorbed is quite small; getting enough fat for vitamin absorption is unlikely to be a problem except in very extreme cases.

Vitamins function in diverse and numerous ways. But their functions generally fall into a few categories. The water-soluble vitamins are often found as a part of the body's enzyme systems, and so these vitamins are needed to catalyze reactions that sustain life. It takes just the tiniest amount of any vitamin to do this, but when the vitamin is absent, the effects can be widespread and devastating. Fat-soluble vitamins don't function in enzyme systems but have very diverse activities that affect bone health, the immune system, eyesight, and blood clotting.

A few of the vitamins are of particular interest in vegetarian diets. These are vitamin B_{12}, riboflavin (vitamin B_2), vitamin B_6, and vitamin D. We're going to look first at vitamin B_{12} because it is one of the more relevant issues in vegan diets. Then we'll look at each of the water-soluble vitamins followed by the fat-soluble ones.

VITAMIN B_{12}

So much controversy over such a tiny vitamin. One teaspoon of vitamin B_{12} is enough to meet the needs of nearly a hundred people for their entire lives. Our

Table 8.1 Recommendations for Vitamin B_{12} Intake (in Micrograms)

	United States	Canada	United Kingdom	WHO
Children	0.7–1.4	0.5–1.0	1.0	1.0
Adolescents	2.0	1.0	1.5	1.0
Adults	2.0	1.0	1.5	1.0
Pregnant Women	2.2	1.2	1.5	1.4

need for this vitamin is so minuscule that possibly at one time we were able to meet that need by eating food and drinking water that was contaminated with it.

Vitamin B_{12} Requirements

The RDA for B_{12} is just 2 micrograms per day. The World Health Organization says that people need even less—1 microgram per day—and requirements in the United Kingdom fall right in between, at 1.5 micrograms per day. One microgram is about one thirty-millionth of an ounce—just to give you an idea of how tiny our B_{12} requirement is.

Sources of Vitamin B_{12}

All of the vitamin B_{12} in the world ultimately comes from bacteria. Neither plants nor animals can synthesize it. But plants can be contaminated with B_{12} when they come in contact with soil bacteria that produce it. Animal foods are rich in B_{12} only because animals eat foods that are contaminated with it or because bacteria living in an animal's intestines make it. Humans also make B_{12} in their intestines, but whether or not this constitutes a source of the vitamin for us is debatable.

Lacto-ovo vegetarians get plenty of B_{12} from milk products and eggs. A cup of milk contains one microgram of B_{12}, or about 50 percent of the adult RDA. Theoretically, plant foods are completely devoid of B_{12} unless they are contaminated with bacteria. There is some debate over the extent to which this contamination can meet human B_{12} needs. It could be significant in some populations. A study of Iranian vegetarians found that they stayed in good B_{12} status by consuming vegetables that were grown in night soil—which is soil heavily fertilized with human excrement.[1] But generally it is believed that vegans must use foods that are fortified with B_{12}—or take supplements—to meet their needs.

Determining how much vitamin B_{12} is in a food is complicated by the fact that foods also contain B_{12} analogues. These are chemically similar to vitamin B_{12} but have no vitamin activity for humans. They also may interfere with B_{12} absorption. In foods that are rich in vitamin B_{12}, as much as 30 percent of that B_{12} could be analogues.[2] And, in some foods, *all* of the B_{12} is actually analogue.

Old methods of analyzing the B_{12} content of foods didn't distinguish between active

TABLE 8.2 VITAMIN B$_{12}$ CONTENT OF FOODS

Fortification of commercial products can change over time, so it is always a good idea to check the label.

Food and Serving Size	B$_{12}$ (micrograms)
BREADS, CEREALS, GRAINS	
Kellogg's Corn flakes (¾ cup)	1.50
Grape-Nuts (¼ cup)	1.48
Nutri-Grain (⅔ cup)	1.50
Product 19 (¾ cup)	6.00
Raisin Bran (¾ cup)	1.50
Total (1 cup)	6.20
MEAT ANALOGUES (1 burger or 1 serving according to package)	
Loma Linda "chicken" nuggets	3.00
Loma Linda Sizzle Franks	2.00
Morningstar Farms Grillers	6.70
Worthington Stakelets	5.16

Food and Serving Size	B$_{12}$ (micrograms)
FORTIFIED SOY AND VEGETABLE MILKS (1 cup)	
Better Than Milk	0.60
Edensoy Extra	3.00
Sno-E	1.20
Soyagen	1.50
Take Care	0.90
Vegelicious	0.60
ANIMAL PRODUCTS	
Egg (1 large)	0.56
Milk (1 cup)	0.89
Yogurt, plain nonfat (1 cup)	0.60
OTHER FOODS	
Red Star T-6635+ nutritional yeast (1 tablespoon)	4.00

B$_{12}$ and B$_{12}$ analogues. Many plant foods once thought to be good sources of B$_{12}$ actually contain only analogues. These include tempeh, sea vegetables, spirulina, sprouted legumes, miso, and umeboshi plums. Although shiitake mushrooms, sourdough bread, parsley, and barley malt syrup contain tiny amounts of B$_{12}$, eating them doesn't seem to raise the levels of B$_{12}$ in the blood.[3] One recent study did indicate that the seaweeds chlorella and nori contained usable vitamin B$_{12}$, but not in amounts that realistically could be relied upon to provide sufficient levels of this vitamin.

Legumes, including soybeans, might be contaminated with B$_{12}$, since their root nodules can harbor B$_{12}$-synthesizing bacteria. However, studies of soy products like tofu, tempeh, and miso show that they don't contain B$_{12}$.

The only plant foods that are *reliable* B$_{12}$ sources are fortified. Nutritional yeast that is grown on a culture that is rich in B$_{12}$ is a good dietary source. Look for Red Star brand T-6635+ which is the only nutritional yeast that is a reliable source of B$_{12}$. Nutritional yeast is different from regular baking yeast, which is not a good source of B$_{12}$.

Many breakfast cereals are B$_{12}$ fortified. But be sure to read the label carefully. Manufacturers often list their nutrient content for cereal alone and for cereal *plus* milk. Cereal plus milk will always contain some B_{12} because milk contains this vitamin. Make sure that the cereal itself contains B_{12}.

Some meat analogues and soymilks are also B_{12} fortified. If you are a vegan and don't use fortified products, a supplement is a good idea. Keep in mind that the percentage of B_{12} you absorb declines rapidly as the dose goes up. If your B_{12} pill contains fifty micrograms, you are likely to absorb only about one or two micrograms.[4]

Vitamin B_{12} Functions and Deficiency Symptoms

Like all the vitamins, B_{12} plays roles in the body that are crucial to life. It is needed for cell division, and deficiency symptoms show up in the red blood cells, which divide very rapidly. The hallmark of B_{12} deficiency is pernicious anemia, or low red blood cell count, in which the cells are abnormally big. B_{12} deficiency also causes myelin, the sheath that covers the nerves, to break down. This can result in damage to nerves, producing a whole host of symptoms such as decreased sensation, difficulty in walking, loss of bowel and bladder control, vision problems, memory loss, dementia, depression, general weakness, and psychosis.[5] This damage can be permanent.

At one time, nutritionists believed that anemia was the first B_{12}-deficiency symptom to appear. This was considered advantageous, as the anemia could be cured and it served as a warning sign before the more serious neurological symptoms developed. But more recent evidence is that the neurological symptoms can actually occur first. Also, another B vitamin, called folic acid, is involved in cell division and can mask B_{12}-deficiency anemia. This means that if the diet is high in folic acid and low in B_{12}, anemia will not develop, and a person may not know that there is a problem until the more serious neurological symptoms appear. This may be a real concern for vegans, because they consume two to three times as much folic acid as omnivores.

B_{12} Status in Vegetarians

Vitamin B_{12} deficiency in vegetarians is a controversial issue. Some scientists feel that overt B_{12} deficiency is a rarity or that most or all cases are due to absorption problems.[6] There are only a few reported cases of this vitamin deficiency among the world's vegetarians. But other scientists feel that B_{12} deficiency may be more common than we think.[7] For one thing, B_{12} deficiency is most often diagnosed on the basis of anemia. But we noted that this symptom can be covered up by high folic acid intake. So mild B_{12} deficiency can go undetected.

Although actual B_{12} deficiency seems to be uncommon, we think that vegans should not be too complacent about vitamin B_{12}. Research indicates that vegans and even lacto-ovo vegetarians often have suboptimal and marginally deficient levels of vitamin B_{12}.[8] In one study of twenty-six vegans, three of the subjects had levels low enough to qualify as deficiency.[9] The fact that they didn't have anemia may have been due to high levels of folic acid in the diet.

The same was true in a study of vegan members of the Natural Hygiene Society and another of Israeli vegans.[10] It is interesting to note that although the Israeli vegans with the lowest B_{12} levels did not have anemia, they complained of weakness, fatigue, and poor mental concentration, which could all be linked to neurological B_{12} deficiency problems. When they were given B_{12}, their blood levels of B_{12} increased, and their symptoms improved.

Some infants of vegetarian mothers show a tendency toward lower-than-normal B_{12} levels.[11] These low levels are easily raised with supplements of B_{12}, but there still may be long-term consequences of B_{12} deficiency in infancy.[12] One theory is that a mother's stores of B_{12} are not available to the fetus or to a breast-fed infant. Only the B_{12} in the mother's diet reaches the fetus or gets passed into breast milk.[13] Although this theory has recently been challenged, it is absolutely essential to ensure adequate B_{12} intake during pregnancy and lactation and in young children.[14]

Despite these observations, overt B_{12} deficiency still seems to be more the exception than the rule in vegans. If only animal foods provide B_{12}, then the relatively good B_{12} status of vegans is a bit of a mystery.

Why Aren't More Vegans B12 Deficient?

There are a number of possible explanations for the fact that the B_{12} status of vegans seems to be satisfactory:

• Deficiency doesn't seem to show up for at least several years after a person stops consuming food sources of vitamin B_{12}, and it can actually take as long as twenty years. This is because the body stores large amounts of this nutrient in the liver and muscle. There have been very few studies of people who have followed strict vegan diets for twenty or more years.

• Through a complex system, most of the B_{12} in our body—about 65 to 75 percent—is recycled rather than excreted. For this reason people can go for years on diets that are deficient in B_{12} without developing deficiency symptoms. One interesting finding is that B_{12} analogues seem to get excreted while true B_{12} gets reabsorbed.[15]

• We also have our own B_{12}-producing factory in our intestines. The bacteria living in our intestines produce active B_{12}, although much of it ends up in our feces. This B_{12} is thought to be produced too far down in the intestines to be absorbed by the body.[16] The bacteria in the upper intestine also make B_{12}, but it is not clear how much we absorb.[17] Bacteria in the mouth also produce B_{12}, although not enough to meet B_{12} needs.[18]

• Some vegans may get plenty of B_{12} from food that is contaminated with bacteria.

• Many vegans don't become B_{12} deficient simply because they use B_{12}-fortified foods or supplements.

With the exception of using fortified foods, none of these explanations is completely reliable. That is, we wouldn't recommend that vegans depend on B_{12} stores, their own internal B_{12} production, or contaminated food to meet their lifelong B_{12} needs. But taken together, all of these factors might help explain why vegans rarely develop overt B_{12} deficiency.

Although deficiency is uncommon, vegans need to make sure they are consuming adequate B_{12}. Because neurological damage can be the first sign of B_{12} deficiency, our concern is that subtle neurological damage could occur before anemia develops and before a person knows that he or she is deficient. Therefore, the use of fortified foods or B_{12} supplements is the best idea for vegans.

Is a Vegan Diet a Natural Diet?

The question comes up over and over again: How can a vegan diet be a natural way to eat if it doesn't supply all essential nutrients—that is, if it doesn't supply B_{12}?

But in one sense, what we know about B_{12} *supports* the case for a vegan diet. The human body carefully hoards and guards its supply of B_{12}. By storing it so well and recycling it so efficiently, our system can get by on very little B_{12}. This suggests that our "natural" diet was quite low in this vitamin. Once upon a time, people probably ingested all the B_{12} they needed through foods and water naturally contaminated with bacteria that synthesize the vitamin. Perhaps these foods are the true natural sources of B_{12}. But as the food supply and our lifestyle change, we need to consider new sources. For vegans, this simply means consuming foods that are fortified with vitamin B_{12} or using a supplement. If B_{12} is an issue for vegans, it is one that is easily resolved.

THIAMIN (VITAMIN B₁)

Thiamin Requirements

Thiamin is needed for the conversion of carbohydrates to energy, and so our needs are very closely tied to calorie intake. Generally, we need about 0.5 milligram of thiamine for every thousand calories we consume. The RDA—1.5 milligrams for men and 1.1 for women—is set at a fairly high level. These levels decrease a bit for older people, because they generally have a lower calorie intake.

A deficiency of thiamin results in the disease known as beriberi. This disease involves extensive damage to the nervous and cardiovascular systems, resulting in muscle wasting and weakness, mental confusion, and paralysis.

Food Sources of Thiamin

Vegetarians get plenty of thiamin.[19] Whole grains are especially rich in this vitamin. Although it is lost when grains are refined, it is added back when these grains are enriched. Nutritional yeast and brewer's yeast are also good sources of this nutrient.

RIBOFLAVIN (VITAMIN B₂)

Riboflavin, also known as vitamin B_2, is one of the flashier vitamins. It has a bright, fluorescent yellow hue. If you take vitamin pills and notice that they turn your urine bright yellow, it is because of the excess riboflavin being excreted.

Like all the B vitamins, riboflavin acts as a part of enzyme systems. It appears to have more functions in the body than any other vitamin, and so deficiency symptoms show up in varied ways. They can include skin disorders, anemia, a swollen tongue, cracks in the skin around the mouth, and even neurological symptoms.

TABLE 8.3 THIAMIN CONTENT OF FOODS

Food and Serving Size	Thiamin (milligrams)	Food and Serving Size	Thiamin (milligrams)
BREADS, CEREALS, GRAINS		**FRUITS**	
Bagel (1 whole)	0.21	Figs (10)	0.13
Barley, whole-hulled (½ cup)	0.29	Orange (1 medium)	0.12
Bran flakes (1 cup)	0.50	Orange juice (1 cup)	0.20
Cheerios (1¼ cups)	0.37	Pineapple (1 cup chunks)	0.14
Corn bread (2 ounces)	0.10	Watermelon (1 cup cubes)	0.13
Cream of Wheat, cooked (½ cup)	0.12	**LEGUMES (½ cup cooked)**	
English muffin (1 whole)	0.26	Kidney beans	0.14
Grape-Nuts (¼ cup)	0.37	Lentils	0.16
Grits, enriched, cooked (½ cup)	0.12	Lima beans	0.15
Millet, cooked (½ cup)	0.13	Navy beans	0.13
Oatmeal, instant, cooked (1 packet)	0.53	Pinto beans	0.15
Oatmeal, regular, cooked (⅔ cup)	0.19	Soybeans	0.13
Pasta, enriched (½ cup)	0.10	Soymilk	0.15
Pasta, whole wheat (½ cup)	0.07	Split peas	0.15
Pita (6-inch pocket)	0.18	**NUTS AND SEEDS (2 tablespoons)**	
Rice, brown (½ cup)	0.10	Brazil nuts	0.23
Rice, white (½ cup)	0.17	Peanuts	0.28
Rye bread (1 slice)	0.10	Sunflower seeds	0.40
Wheat germ (2 tablespoons)	0.24	Tahini	0.40
White bread (1 slice)	0.11	**OTHER FOODS**	
Whole wheat bread (1 slice)	0.09	Brewer's yeast (1 tablespoon)	1.25
VEGETABLES (½ cup cooked)		Nutritional yeast (1 tablespoon)	5.00
Peas	0.20		
Potatoes	0.13		
Squash, winter	0.17		

Riboflavin Requirements

The RDA for riboflavin is 1.7 milligrams per day for men and 1.3 for women. Some researchers feel that the RDAs for riboflavin are too high. In a study of nutrient intake in the People's Republic of China, Dr. Colin Campbell and his colleagues found that the average intake of riboflavin was well under a

TABLE 8.4 RIBOFLAVIN CONTENT OF FOODS

Food and Serving Size	Riboflavin (milligrams)	Food and Serving Size	Riboflavin (milligrams)
BREADS, CEREALS, GRAINS		**FRUITS**	
Barley, whole-hulled, cooked (1/2 cup)	0.13	Banana (1 medium)	0.11
Bran flakes (1 cup)	0.60	**LEGUMES (1/2 cup cooked)**	
Bread, pumpernickel (1 slice)	0.17	Kidney beans	0.09
Cheerios (1 1/4 cups)	0.42	Soybeans	0.24
Corn flakes (1 1/4 cups)	0.40	Split peas	0.09
Granola (1/4 cup)	0.42	**SOY AND VEGETABLE MILKS (1 cup)**	
Grape-Nuts (1/4 cup)	0.42	Edensoy	0.06
Nutri-Grain (3/4 cup)	0.40	Edensoy Extra	0.10
Pasta, enriched (1/2 cup)	0.18	Sno-E	0.17
Pasta, whole wheat (1/2 cup)	0.03	Soyagen	0.17
Rice Krispies (1 cup)	0.40	Take Care	0.42
Wheaties (1 cup)	0.42	Vegelicious	0.17
		Vitasoy Original	0.17
VEGETABLES (1/2 cup cooked)		Westsoy Plus	0.42
Alaria	2.73		
Asparagus	0.10	**NUTS AND SEEDS (2 tablespoons)**	
Beet greens	0.21	Almond butter	0.19
Collards	0.09	Almonds	0.25
Dulse	1.91	Peanuts	0.12
Kelp	2.48		
Mushrooms	0.14	**ANIMAL PRODUCTS**	
Nori	2.93	Egg (1 large)	0.25
Peas	0.12	Milk (1 cup)	0.40
Spinach	0.17	Yogurt, plain nonfat (1 cup)	0.59
Sweet potatoes	0.14		

milligram a day—or about half the adult RDA. Yet there were no outright symptoms of riboflavin deficiency. Campbell suggested that there was some danger in setting riboflavin requirements unnecessarily high, since this might encourage people to eat more animal foods—the primary source of riboflavin in the Western diet—which could lead to an increased risk of chronic disease.[20] There are other studies that support the idea that U.S. riboflavin requirements are too high. People who consume riboflavin at levels well below the RDA rarely if ever develop clinical signs of deficiency.[21]

Other researchers point out that in some parts of the world low riboflavin intake does, in fact, lead to true deficiency symptoms. Infants seem to be particularly vulnerable.[22] Also, even when true symptoms of riboflavin deficiency are absent, it is possible that low levels of the vitamin can result in impaired function.[23]

So it seems that, as is true with so many nutrients, the jury is still out on our requirement for riboflavin. Until we know for certain, it is best to strive to meet the RDA.

Food Sources of Riboflavin

Few plant foods are rich in this nutrient, but many contain moderate amounts. It is just a matter of including enough of these foods in your meals. Whole grains provide riboflavin. Enriched, refined grains are higher in riboflavin. Rice is an exception, however; because riboflavin gives white rice an undesirable yellow color, enrichment of this grain doesn't usually include riboflavin.

Green leafy vegetables, broccoli, mushrooms, avocados, and peas all contain substantial amounts of riboflavin. Legumes are even better sources, particularly soybeans and soyfoods. Of all the plant foods, sea vegetables appear to be the richest in riboflavin, so it is a good idea to try to make these a part of your diet.

Riboflavin Status in Vegetarians

Because milk and other dairy products are quite high in this vitamin, lacto-ovo vegetarians tend to meet their needs for riboflavin, and they have about the same intake as omnivores.[24] Vegans generally consume less riboflavin than omnivores but most come close to meeting the RDA.[25]

NIACIN

Niacin Requirements

Niacin is somewhat unique because we actually meet part of our needs for this nutrient through protein intake. One of the essential amino acids, called tryptophan, can be converted to niacin. Our bodies convert about sixty milligrams of tryptophan to one milligram of niacin. For this reason, the niacin RDA is expressed as niacin equivalents. One niacin equivalent is equal to a milligram of niacin, or sixty milligrams of tryptophan. The RDA for men is nineteen, and for women it is fifteen milligrams of niacin equivalents.

Pellagra is the disease that results when niacin intake is deficient. It is characterized by skin disorders, intestinal problems, and dementia and is still a common disease in some parts of Africa and Asia today.

Food Sources of Niacin

Grains are the main dietary source of niacin for vegetarians. Whole grains are rich in this vitamin, although it isn't very well absorbed. However, the niacin in enriched, refined grains is absorbed very well. It is interesting to note an example of how longstanding cultural practices sometimes serve to improve nutrition. Diets that make substantial use of cornmeal can be deficient in niacin because the niacin in corn is not very well absorbed. But in Latin America, where cornmeal is central to the diet, cooks traditionally use

TABLE 8.5 NIACIN CONTENT OF FOODS

Food and Serving Size	Niacin (milligrams)	Food and Serving Size	Niacin (milligrams)
BREADS, CEREALS, GRAINS		**VEGETABLES (½ cup cooked unless otherwise indicated)**	
Barley, pearled, cooked (½ cup)	1.6	Avocado (½, raw)	1.6
Barley, whole, cooked (½ cup)	2.1	Corn	1.0
Bran flakes (1 cup)	5.0	Mushrooms	2.1
Bread, white (1 slice)	0.9	Peas	1.6
Bread, whole wheat (1 slice)	1.0	Potatoes	1.7
Bulgur, cooked (½ cup)	1.6		
Cheerios (1¼ cups)	5.0	**LEGUMES (½ cup)**	
Corn flakes (1 cup)	5.0	Soybeans, green immature	1.1
Corn tortillas, enriched (1)	1.5	Tempeh	3.8
Granola (¼ cup)	4.9		
Grape-Nuts (¼ cup)	4.9	**NUTS AND SEEDS (2 tablespoons)**	
Millet, cooked (½ cup)	1.5	Peanut butter	4.6
Pasta, whole wheat, cooked (½ cup)	0.5	Peanuts	3.3
Rice, brown (½ cup cooked)	1.3	Tahini	1.5
Rice, white (½ cup cooked)	1.8		
Rice Krispies (1 cup)	5.0	**OTHER FOODS**	
Shredded Wheat (1 biscuit)	1.1	Brewer's yeast (1 tablespoon)	2.9

limewater to prepare tortillas. Lime frees the niacin so that it is readily absorbed. (It also happens to increase the calcium content of the tortillas.)

The niacin intake of vegetarians is consistently good.[26]

VITAMIN B6 (PYRIDOXINE)

It's rare to see vitamin B6 deficiency by itself. It usually occurs when the diet is generally poor, and it is usually one of multiple deficiencies. The clinical signs of this deficiency are anemia and skin problems.

Vitamin B6 Requirements

Vitamin B6 is used in more than sixty different enzyme systems, most of which are involved in protein metabolism. Therefore needs for this vitamin are directly proportional to protein intake. That is, the more protein you consume, the more B6 you need. Generally, we need 0.016 milligrams of B6 for every gram of protein consumed. The RDA for B6 is 2 milligrams for men and 1.6 milligrams for women.

Food Sources of Vitamin B6

Whole grains are especially rich in vitamin

B_6, but it is lost when the grains are refined. And since B_6 is not added back, refined grains tend to be a poor source of this nutrient.

There is some controversy over how well the B_6 in plant foods is absorbed. This may be one reason that a group of vegetarian African women had lower blood levels of B_6 than omnivore American women, even though the vegetarian women ate more

Food and Serving Size	Vitamin B_6 (milligrams)	Food and Serving Size	Vitamin B_6 (milligrams)
BREADS, CEREALS, GRAINS		Orange juice (1 cup)	0.22
Bran flakes (1 cup)	0.70	Prune juice (½ cup)	0.28
Cheerios (1¼ cups)	0.50	Raisins (⅔ cup)	0.32
Corn flakes (1¼ cups)	0.50	Watermelon (1 cup cubes)	0.23
Cream of Wheat, instant (1 packet)	0.50		
Granola (¼ cup)	0.50	**LEGUMES (½ cup cooked)**	
Grape-Nuts (¼ cup)	0.50	Chickpeas	0.57
Oatmeal, instant (1 packet)	0.70	Kidney beans	0.10
Rice, brown, cooked (½ cup)	0.15	Lentils	0.17
		Lima beans	0.11
VEGETABLES (½ cup cooked unless otherwise indicated)		Meat analogues (3 to 4 ounces)	0.30–0.70
Asparagus	0.12	Navy beans	0.15
Avocado (½, raw)	0.24	Pinto beans	0.15
Nori	0.16	Soybeans	0.20
Okra	0.15	Soy nuts	0.19
Peas	0.17	Tempeh	0.25
Plantain	0.18	Vegetarian baked beans	0.17
Potatoes	0.38		
Spinach	0.14	**NUTS AND SEEDS (2 tablespoons)**	
Squash, winter	0.14–0.20	Sunflower seeds	0.22
Sweet potato (1 medium)	0.28		
Tomato juice (1 cup)	0.26	**SOY AND VEGETABLE MILKS (1 cup)**	
		Soymilk, plain	0.12
FRUITS		**ANIMAL PRODUCTS**	
Banana (1 medium)	0.66	Egg (1 large)	0.06
Elderberries (1 cup)	0.33	**OTHER FOODS**	
Figs (10)	0.42	Brewer's yeast (1 tablespoon)	0.20

TABLE 8.7 FOLIC ACID CONTENT OF FOODS

Food and Serving Size	Folic Acid (micrograms)	Food and Serving Size	Folic Acid (micrograms)
BREADS, CEREALS, GRAINS		**FRUITS**	
Bran flakes (¾ cup)	100	Banana (1 medium)	21
Corn flakes (1¼ cups)	100	Cantaloupe (1 cup chunks)	27
Granola (¼ cup)	99	Grapefruit pink or red (½)	15
Most (⅔ cup)	400	Orange (1 medium)	39
Nutri-Grain (¾ cup)	100	Orange juice (1 cup)	109
Oatmeal, instant (1 package)	150	Strawberries (½ cup sliced)	20
Oatmeal, quick or regular, cooked (⅔ cup)	29	**LEGUMES (½ cup cooked)**	
Rice Krispies (1 cup)	100	Black beans	128
Wheat germ (2 tablespoons)	49	Black-eyed peas	86
		Kidney beans	63
VEGETABLES (½ cup cooked unless otherwise indicated)		Lentils	179
		Lima beans	78
Asparagus	88	Pinto beans	147
Avocado (½ medium)	56	Soybeans	46
Beets	45	Split peas	64
Broccoli	38	Tempeh	43
Brussels sprouts	46		
Cauliflower	32	**NUTS AND SEEDS (2 tablespoons)**	
Collards	64	Peanut butter	25
Endive (½ cup raw)	36	Peanuts	35
Mustard greens	51	Sunflower seeds	40
Parsnips	45	Tahini	27
Spinach	110		
Squash, acorn	11	**ANIMAL PRODUCTS**	
Sweet potatoes	25	Yogurt (1 cup)	27
Tomato juice (1 cup)	47		
Turnip greens	32		

vitamin B₆.[27] Fiber is thought to be one factor that hinders absorption.[28]

But other evidence shows that B₆ from plant foods is actually absorbed quite well.[29]

At any rate, foods high in fiber tend to be high in B₆, so that any negative effects of fiber intake would be offset by the high content of vitamin B₆.

Vegetarians and Vitamin B_6

Although vitamin B_6 was once targeted as a nutrient of concern for vegetarians, we think the evidence suggests otherwise. Most studies show the B_6 intake and status of vegetarians to be good.[30]

Vegetarians may have some advantages when it comes to B_6 needs. The RDA for vitamin B_6 is based on the assumption that men consume 126 grams of protein a day and women consume 100 grams. Clearly vegetarians, who consume less protein than omnivores, need less vitamin B_6. In fact, the ratio of B_6 to protein in your diet is much more important than meeting the B_6 RDA. Plant foods generally contain more B_6 relative to their protein content than animal foods.[31] And vegans have a better B_6-to-protein ratio in their diets than nonvegetarians.[32]

There may be another advantage to getting B_6 from plant foods. Animal protein in particular may raise B_6 needs. In one study women who ate diets based on plant protein needed 25 percent less B_6 to maintain normal body levels than when they ate diets based on animal protein.[33] Studies with men showed similar results.[34]

Vegetarians seem to have the advantage in meeting B_6 needs. And there is one more advantage to getting B_6 from plant foods. The B vitamins are fragile and are easily destroyed during the cooking process. But the type of B_6 found in plant foods is less vulnerable to destruction by cooking.

FOLIC ACID

You'll see this B vitamin referred to as "folic acid," "folate," and "folacin." These are different names for the same vitamin. Folic acid is needed for the metabolism of proteins and for cell division. Deficiency results in the same type of anemia that is seen in B_{12} deficiency. In fact, these two vitamins work together to help synthesize the new genetic material that is needed for cell division. As we noted earlier, large amounts of folic acid can prevent anemia even when B_{12} is deficient. So, in essence, it masks B_{12}-deficiency anemia and hides the fact that B_{12} is deficient. There is a certain danger in this situation, because it means that the B_{12} deficiency won't become noticeable until it affects the nervous system, causing problems that may be irreversible.

Folic Acid Requirements

The RDA for folic acid was significantly lowered when the latest set of RDAs were issued. The reason was that most people did not come close to meeting the former RDA for folic acid, but they also didn't seem to suffer from any deficiency problems. As a result, it was reasoned that folic acid requirements must be much lower than previously thought. The current RDA of 200 micrograms for men and 180 micrograms for women is much closer to the World Health Organization's recommendations.

Food Sources of Folic Acid

Foods that are especially rich in folic acid include vegetables (especially greens, broccoli, asparagus), orange juice, brewer's yeast, and legumes (especially soybeans and black-eyed peas). Not surprisingly, vegetarians have very high intakes of folic acid—higher than omnivores.[35] Blood levels of folic acid for vegans and lacto-ovo vegetari-

TABLE 8.8 BIOTIN CONTENT OF FOODS

Food and Serving Size	Biotin (micrograms)	Food and Serving Size	Biotin (micrograms)
BREADS, CEREALS, GRAINS		**LEGUMES (½ cup cooked)**	
Barley, pearled (½ cup cooked)	3.0	Black-eyed peas	10.7
Oat bran (½ cup cooked)	7.0	Lentils	13.0
Oatmeal, instant (1 packet)	7.0	Textured vegetable protein	17.5
VEGETABLES (½ cup cooked)		**NUTS AND SEEDS (2 tablespoons)**	
Corn	4.9	Almonds	23.0
Mushrooms	7.6	Peanut butter	12.8
Spinach	7.2	**ANIMAL PRODUCTS**	
		Egg (1 medium)	11.0

ans can be as much as three times higher than those for meat eaters.[36]

BIOTIN

We don't have much information about biotin, especially with respect to vegetarians. Although it is an essential nutrient, no RDA is established for it. We do, however, have what is known as an estimated safe and adequate daily dietary intake, which is thirty to one hundred micrograms per day. Biotin deficiency is rare.

Food Sources of Biotin

Biotin can be synthesized by bacteria in the large intestine, although it isn't certain that very much of it is absorbed into the blood. Soy flour, brewer's yeast, and grains are good sources of this vitamin, although the amount in grains is quite variable. Fruit and meat are low in this vitamin.

The little bit of information we have about biotin status in vegetarians suggests that their intake is higher than that of omnivores and that vegans consume more than lacto-ovo vegetarians.[37]

PANTOTHENIC ACID

The name "pantothenic acid" comes from the Greek *pantos*, which means "everywhere." It is widely distributed in foods and may also be synthesized by bacteria in the intestines. It's used by a wide variety of enzymes for metabolism of carbohydrates and fat. The only time a deficiency of pantothenic acid has been noted is in prisoners of war who complained of "burning feet" syndrome. The symptoms went away when the men were given pantothenic acid, so the symptoms were attributed to a deficiency of this vitamin.[38] There is no information about vegetarians and pantothenic acid, but because it is so abun-

TABLE 8.9 VITAMIN C CONTENT OF FOODS

Food and Serving Size	Vitamin C (milligrams)	Food and Serving Size	Vitamin C (milligrams)
BREADS, CEREALS, GRAINS		Squash, Hubbard	10
Cheerios (1¼ cups)	15	Sweet potatoes	28
Corn flakes (1 cup)	15	Swiss chard	15
Most (⅔ cup)	60	Tomato (raw, 1 medium)	22
Nutri-Grain (¾ cup)	15	Tomato juice (6 ounces)	30
Rice Krispies (1 cup)	15	Turnip greens	17
Special K (1⅓ cups)	15	Turnips	9
Wheaties (1 cup)	15		
		FRUITS	
VEGETABLES (½ cup cooked unless otherwise indicated)		Banana (1 medium)	10
		Blackberries (½ cup)	15
Asparagus	24	Blueberries (½ cup)	19
Beet greens	18	Cantaloupe (1 cup chunks)	68
Broccoli	58	Elderberries (½ cup)	26
Brussels sprouts	48	Grapefruit (½ medium)	47
Cabbage	17	Grapefruit juice (6 ounces)	70
Cauliflower	36	Guava (1 medium)	165
Collards	22	Honeydew melon (1 cup chunks)	92
Kale	27	Kiwifruit (1 medium)	75
Kohlrabi	44	Lychees (10 medium)	72
Mustard greens	18	Mango (1 medium)	57
Okra	13	Orange (1 medium)	69
Nori	39	Orange juice (6 ounces)	62
Parsnips	10	Papaya (1 medium)	188
Peas	11	Persimmon (1 medium)	17
Peppers, sweet bell	76	Pineapple (1 cup chunks)	24
Potatoes	16	Raspberries (½ cup)	15
Rutabagas	19	Strawberries (½ cup sliced)	42
Spinach	12	Tangerine (1 medium)	26
Squash, acorn	11	Watermelon (1 cup chunks)	15
Squash, butternut	15		

Table 8.10 Vitamin D Content of Foods

Food and Serving Size	Vitamin D (micrograms)	Food and Serving Size	Vitamin D (micrograms)
BREADS, CEREALS, GRAINS		Vegelicious	1.00
Bran flakes (1 cup)	1.83	Vitamite*	2.50
Corn flakes (1 cup)	1.83	Westsoy Plus	2.50
Granola (¼ cup)	1.83		
Grape-Nuts (¼ cup)	2.40	ANIMAL PRODUCTS	
		Milk (1 cup)	2.50
FORTIFIED SOY AND VEGETABLE MILKS (1 cup)		Egg (1 large)	0.67
Edensoy Extra	1.00	FATS (1 teaspoon)	
Rice Dream	2.50	Margarine	0.50
Soyagen	2.50		
Take Care	2.50	*Contains milk protein	

dant in plant foods, we can assume that vegetarians get plenty of it. The safe and estimated daily dietary intake is four to seven milligrams.

VITAMIN C

After years of research, there is still much debate about the role of vitamin C in curing the common cold. Two-time Nobel prize winner Linus Pauling was a great believer in the curative powers of this vitamin. He held that doses of vitamin C that were many times greater than the RDA could prevent or cure colds. Current thinking is that large doses of vitamin C won't prevent colds, but they do reduce the length and severity of the average cold.[39] If this is true, then we should see many fewer vegetarians sneezing and coughing, since plant diets provide much more vitamin C than omnivore diets.

Vitamin C Requirements

Vitamin C deficiency leads to scurvy, a serious disorder that was once the scourge of sailors—or anyone else who went without fresh fruit and vegetables for a long time. Because vitamin C is needed to maintain the connective tissues of the body, its lack causes a breakdown of these tissues and widespread bleeding. Vitamin C is also a powerful antioxidant, and it seems to be involved in maintaining a strong immune system.

It takes only about ten milligrams per day of vitamin C to prevent scurvy, but needs of individuals vary quite a bit. The RDA is set at sixty milligrams.

Food Sources of Vitamin C

Many fruits and vegetables are especially rich in vitamin C, especially citrus fruits, strawberries, pineapples, watermelons, peppers, potatoes, and broccoli. Grains and beans contain little, milk contains none, and the only meat with appreciable amounts is liver.

Vegetarians and Vitamin C

Vegetarians consume much more vitamin C than omnivores and considerably more than the RDA.[40] In nearly all cases, vegans have the highest vitamin C intakes of all.[41]

VITAMIN D

Is it a vitamin or a hormone? Nutritionists agree that it is both. It fits the classic definition of a hormone—a compound made in one part of the body (the skin, in this case) that travels to another part of the body (the bones, kidney, and intestines) to exert its effects. But vitamin D has some special features. One is that we can make it only when our skin is exposed to sunlight. And it is one of the few hormones that we can get from our diet.

Food Sources of Vitamin D

Historically, sun exposure has been by far our most important source of vitamin D. Depending on the natural food supply for vitamin D would put us in big trouble. It is found in a very few foods, including eggs and some fish oils. Many Americans erroneously believe that milk is a natural source of vitamin D. But milk contains vitamin D only because it is fortified. Several brands of soymilk and rice milk are also fortified, and so are many commercial breakfast cereals.

Vitamin D Requirements

Vitamin D is measured in two ways—as micrograms and as international units (IU). ("International unit" is the older terminol-ogy, and it isn't used much anymore.) One microgram equals forty international units. For adults, the RDA is five micrograms, or two hundred international units. But vitamin D requirements are actually quite hard to determine, since the amount needed from the diet is completely dependent on how much we make from sun exposure.

The primary function of vitamin D is to maintain normal blood levels of calcium. Vitamin D affects the amount of calcium absorbed from the intestines, the amount lost in the urine, and the amount released from the bones. The overall effect is to maintain normal blood levels of calcium and to increase the amount of calcium in the bones. But vitamin D seems to have other functions as well. It appears to have effects on the immune system, the skin, and the pancreas, and it might play a role in preventing cancer.[42]

In children, inadequate vitamin D leads to rickets, a disease of deformed bones, stunted growth, and swollen joints. Childhood rickets was the scourge of urban areas in northern Europe and the United States. It came to be called the English disease because, around the turn of the century, nearly 80 percent of London children suffered from rickets. The reason was that many northern European children worked long hours in factories and had little sun exposure in these cloudy, smoggy urban areas. Rickets was rare or even nonexistent in southern Europe.

In adults, the deficiency disease is osteomalacia, which is excessive bone loss. This is somewhat different from osteoporosis, in which bones are weak and porous. In osteomalacia, bones are actually smaller. But in both cases, bones are easily fractured.

Vitamin D and Sun Exposure

We can make *all* the vitamin D we need through adequate sun exposure. However, conditions that block sunlight, such as cloudiness and smog, increase the amount of exposure needed to make vitamin D. Using a sunscreen with a sun protection factor (SPF) of 8 can completely block vitamin D synthesis.[43] Aging also decreases the ability of the body to make vitamin D.

The darker your skin, the more sun exposure you need. It takes as much as six times more sun exposure to make the same amount of vitamin D in some African Americans as it does in Caucasians.[44] At one time, it was believed that this phenomenon protected people who evolved in sunny climates from making too much vitamin D, which could be toxic. This theory has been refuted, however, since scientists have found that the skin has built-in mechanisms to protect it from making too much vitamin D regardless of sun exposure.

Studies indicate that the average light-skinned adult can make adequate vitamin D with ten to fifteen minutes of sun exposure on the hands and face two or three times per week during the summer.[45] Because we store vitamin D, the vitamin we make during the summer can last us through the winter months. This is fortunate, since it appears that people don't make much vitamin D during the winter—at least in northern climates. Boston researchers found that in northern areas, exposing the skin to sunlight for three hours, just one day a month, resulted in significant vitamin D synthesis from April to October. But vitamin D wasn't synthesized during November and February.[46] Vitamin D was, however, made by the skin during winter months in Puerto Rico (and to a lesser degree in Los Angeles). However, despite these study findings—which used skin samples—the evidence in human populations is that some vitamin D is actually made during the winter months.[47]

Vegetarians and Vitamin D

There is very little information about blood levels of vitamin D in Western vegans. Also, it is difficult to determine whether low blood levels are due to inadequate intake or poor sun exposure. For example, Asian vegans living in England have low blood levels.[48] But most have a high vitamin D intake, which suggests that their reduced levels are most likely caused by inadequate sun exposure.[49] Conversely, American omnivores tend to have low dietary intakes of vitamin D but rarely suffer from deficiency, suggesting that they make up the difference from sun exposure. In the 1970s, vitamin D deficiency was somewhat common in macrobiotic children in the northern United States, England, Ireland, and the Netherlands.[50] Note that these are all northern areas where sun exposure is somewhat limited.

Studies of vitamin D status indicate that sun exposure is the most important factor affecting blood levels of this vitamin. In most people, blood levels of vitamin D (even during the winter) are more closely linked to summertime sun exposure than to diet.[51]

If you do rely on sunshine for most or all of your vitamin D, be sure to spend some time outdoors without using a sunscreen (but do use a sunscreen *most* of the time you are outdoors to protect against premature aging and skin cancer). Those people who have darker skin, live in northern or smoggy urban areas, or don't have much sun exposure may need to include some sources of vitamin D in their diet.

Vitamin D Toxicity

Like all of the fat-soluble vitamins, vitamin D is stored in the body, and excessive amounts are toxic. Too much vitamin D can lead to deposits of calcium in the soft tissues of the body and can therefore irreversibly damage the kidneys and heart. It may also increase absorption of aluminum and might be a risk factor for Alzheimer's disease.[52]

For most nutrients, you need to consume many times the RDA to have any adverse reactions. But this isn't so with vitamin D. In children, as little as four or five times the RDA could produce toxicity symptoms. In fact, in Great Britain, milk is no longer fortified with vitamin D because of such problems.[53] In the United States, there may also be problems with vitamin D fortification. Recently, scientists reported that eight people developed vitamin D toxicity from drinking fortified milk. The milk was found to contain five hundred times more vitamin D than federal regulations permit![54]

According to these regulations, milk must contain ten micrograms (four hundred international units) of vitamin D per quart.

However, surveys of the U.S. milk supply show that some samples of milk have very little vitamin D in them, while others have amounts many times what is allowed by the government.[55] This is because vitamin D is added to such huge volumes of milk at one time that it may not be dispersed throughout the milk properly.

Soymilks and other vegan milks that are fortified with vitamin D are likely to be more reliable (and safer), since these products are produced and fortified in much smaller quantities.

Clearly, the best way to get enough vitamin D is to get plenty of sunshine. Throughout human history—before people started working indoors—this probably provided plenty of vitamin D while protecting against too much. Vegetarians who use a vitamin supplement should be sure that it doesn't contain more than five micrograms of vitamin D. Vitamin D supplements are available from both plant and animal sources. Some evidence indicates that the plant form is used by the body in a more efficient manner.

VITAMIN A AND THE CAROTENES

Vitamin A is actually a group of three compounds (retinol, retinaldehyde, and retinoic acid) that are essential for vision, growth, reproduction, and protecting the integrity of the immune system. Vitamin A deficiency is rare in the United States and other Western countries. But elsewhere, a lack of this vitamin is widespread and serious. It is the leading cause of childhood blindness in the world. Every year, a half-million children develop eye problems due to vitamin A deficiency.[56]

TABLE 8.11 VITAMIN A CONTENT OF FOODS

Food and Serving Size	Vitamin A (micrograms)	Food and Serving Size	Vitamin A (micrograms)
VEGETABLES (½ cup cooked unless otherwise indicated)		Swiss chard	276
		Tomato (1 medium)	1,399
Beet greens	367	Tomato juice (6 ounces)	101
Bok choy	218	Tomato puree (½ cup)	170
Broccoli	110	Turnips	396
Carrots	1,915	Vegetable juice cocktail (6 ounces)	213
Carrots (1 raw)	2,025		
Chicory green (½ cup raw)	360	FRUITS	
Collards	422	Apricots (3)	277
Dandelion greens	608	Cantaloupe (1 cup chunks)	516
Kale	481	Mango (1 medium)	806
Mustard greens	212	Nectarine (1 medium)	100
Nori	520	Papaya (1 medium)	612
Plantain (1 cup cooked)	140	Persimmons (1 medium)	364
Pumpkin	2,691	Prunes (10 medium)	167
Spinach	737	ANIMAL PRODUCTS	
Squash, butternut	714	Cheese, cheddar (1 ounce)	86
Squash, Hubbard	616	Milk, skim (1 cup)	149
Sweet potatoes	2,797	Milk, whole (1 cup)	76

Vitamin A Requirements

Vitamin A is found only in animal products. Fortunately for vegetarians, humans can make their own vitamin A when they consume plants containing compounds called carotenoids. These are pigments in fruits and vegetables; they give these foods their bright colors. There are as many as six hundred carotenoids in plants, and fifty of these can be converted into vitamin A. The most commonly consumed of these is beta-carotene. In fact, nutritionists often speak of beta-carotene and vitamin A as though they were the same thing.

The RDA for vitamin A is expressed in *retinol equivalents* (RE). Recommended intakes are 1,000 RE for men and 800 RE for women. One retinol equivalent is equal to one microgram of preformed vitamin A, or six micrograms of beta-carotene, or twelve micrograms of any of the other carotenoids. The old unit of measure for vitamin A was international units, just as it was for vitamin D. One international unit equals about one-third retinol equivalents.

Theoretically, beta-carotene should be equal to preformed vitamin A. However, it is less well absorbed than vitamin A, and only half of it is converted to vitamin A. Beta-carotene is absorbed better from cooked foods than from raw ones. It also requires small amounts of fat in the diet for absorption.

Food Sources of Vitamin A

Most people in the United States consume only 25 percent of their vitamin A as carotenoids.[57] The rest is preformed vitamin A from animal foods. Lacto-ovo vegetarians get about half their vitamin A as preformed vitamin A and the other half from carotenoids.[58] Vegans meet their vitamin A requirements completely from beta-carotene and other carotenoids in plant foods. Foods that are especially rich in these vitamin A precursors are brightly colored vegetables and fruits such as broccoli, peppers, dark-green leafy vegetables (kale, collards, and so on), carrots, sweet potatoes, pumpkins, tomatoes, mangoes, cantaloupes, and papayas.

Vitamin A in Vegetarian Diets

When we measure total vitamin A retinol equivalents in the diet, which includes beta-carotene, vegetarians have a much higher intake than nonvegetarians.[59] In addition, there is an advantage to meeting vitamin A needs with beta-carotene and other carotenoids.

First, beta-carotene, as well as some of the other carotenoids that have vitamin A activity, act as antioxidants.[60] For this reason, the carotenoids are thought to reduce cancer risk, to prevent cataracts, and to reduce heart disease risk.[61] Carotenoids may also enhance the immune system.[62] Vitamin A from animal foods, on the other hand, does not have any antioxidant properties.

Another small advantage is that the carotenoids are not toxic, no matter how much you consume. Like all of the fat-soluble vitamins, vitamin A can be toxic, although it takes amounts that are many times the RDA to cause any problems. But the worst that will happen with big doses of beta-carotene is that your skin will turn orange. This condition, called hypercarotenosis, usually occurs when people drink large amounts of carotenoid-rich juices, such as carrot juice or tomato juice.[63] It isn't permanent or harmful, and skin returns to its normal color when the juices are discontinued.

VITAMIN E

Vitamin E is another nutrient that functions as an antioxidant. It is found in the membranes of cells along with the polyunsaturated fats that are a normal part of cells. Vitamin E "traps" free radicals and prevents them from damaging the fats in cell membranes. Because of its role as an antioxidant, vitamin E might help to prevent cancer, heart disease, cataracts, and may even slow the aging process. Two large studies—one involving eighty-seven thousand female nurses and one involving forty thousand male health professionals—found that people with the most vitamin E in their diet had a one-third reduced risk for heart disease.[64]

Vitamin E Requirements

Vitamin E is actually a group of eight compounds, all of which have some vitamin E activity—although the amount of activity varies for these compounds. So, as for vitamin A, this vitamin is measured in terms of equivalents—in this case, tocopherol equivalents (TE), since a compound called alpha-tocopherol is the form of vitamin E with the most activity. The adult RDA for vitamin E is ten milligrams of tocopherol equivalents for men and eight milligrams for women.

A deficiency of this nutrient is very rare. The most evident symptom of acute vitamin E deficiency is a type of anemia due to destruction of red-blood-cell membranes. It tends to occur only in premature infants or in people who have absorption problems. In adults, a deficiency can lead to neurological problems, but it can take as long as five to ten years for the deficiency to develop.[65]

Since vitamin E protects polyunsaturated fats from oxidation, our requirement for this

TABLE 8.12 VITAMIN E CONTENT OF FOODS

Food and Serving Size	Vitamin E (milligrams)	Food and Serving Size	Vitamin E (milligrams)
BREADS, CEREALS, GRAINS		**NUTS AND SEEDS (2 tablespoons)**	
Wheat germ (2 tablespoons)	1.90	Almond butter	2.90
		Almonds	1.50
VEGETABLES (½ cup cooked unless otherwise indicated)		Brazil nuts	2.10
		Hazelnuts	6.70
Asparagus	1.70	Peanut butter	6.00
Avocado (½, raw)	1.80	Peanuts	2.10
Cabbage	1.20	Sunflower seeds	8.90
Kelp	0.87		
Kohlrabi	1.30	**FATS (1 tablespoon unless otherwise indicated)**	
Mustard greens	1.40	Corn oil	1.90
Parsnips	0.77	Margarine (1 teaspoon) (varies by brand)	0.10–8.00
Pumpkin	1.20		
Stewed tomatoes	0.92	Mayonnaise (varies by brand)	3.00–11.00
Sweet potatoes	5.20		
Swiss chard	1.30	Olive oil	1.60
		Peanut oil	1.60
FRUITS (1 medium)		Safflower oil	4.60
Apple	0.80	Sesame oil	0.20
Mango	2.30	Soybean oil	1.50
Pear	0.80	Sunflower oil	6.10
Pomegranate	0.84	Wheat germ oil	20.30
LEGUMES (½ cup)			
Soybeans	1.60		

TABLE 8.13 VITAMIN K CONTENT OF FOODS

Food and Serving Size	Vitamin K (micrograms)	Food and Serving Size	Vitamin K (micrograms)
VEGETABLES (½ cup cooked unless otherwise indicated)		LEGUMES (½ cup cooked)	
		Black-eyed peas	23.0
Asparagus	35.0	Lentils	261.0
Broccoli	119.0	Split peas	81.0
Cabbage	90.0	ANIMAL PRODUCTS	
Kale	179.0	Egg (1 large)	25.0
Lettuce (1 cup raw)	56.0	Milk (1 cup)	10.0
Pumpkin	18.0		
Spinach	141.0	FATS (1 tablespoon)	
Turnip greens	53.0	Soybean oil	77.0

vitamin is directly related to our intake of these fats. Vegetarians may need more vitamin E because much of the fat in their diet is polyunsaturated. But foods high in unsaturated fats tend to also be high in vitamin E.

Food Sources of Vitamin E

The richest source of vitamin E in the diet is vegetable oil, particularly sunflower and wheat-germ oil. In other vegetable oils, the ratio of vitamin E to polyunsaturated fat is lower than ideal. Animal fats, like beef tallow, tend to be very low in vitamin E. It is important to include vitamin E–rich foods other than vegetable oils in the diet. Foods that are rich in vitamin E are sweet potatoes, cabbage, greens, parsnips, and other vegetables.

Vegetarians and Vitamin E

Vegetarians consume more vitamin E than nonvegetarians.[66] They also have a better ratio of vitamin E to cholesterol in their blood.[67] This is important because it means that LDL cholesterol, the "bad cholesterol," is more likely to be protected from oxidation, a process that promotes heart disease. Vitamin E might also inhibit the formation of blood clots in the arteries; this could be another way that this vitamin reduces the risk for heart disease.

Vitamin E also works closely with beta-carotene to protect cells from oxidation, so the high intake of both beta-carotene and vitamin E among vegetarians may give them an especially powerful edge against heart disease.[68]

VITAMIN K

Vitamin K Requirements

The vitamin K RDA for adult males is eighty micrograms per day, and for females it is sixty-five micrograms per day. The average American intake of vitamin K is more than

Carnitine is a compound that is necessary to transport certain fats into the interior parts of cells so that the fats can be metabolized for energy. At one time, carnitine was dubbed "vitamin B$_T$." In the past, concern was raised about carnitine in the diets of vegetarians. It is abundant in meat, but is negligible in plant foods. However, it isn't a vitamin and isn't even an essential nutrient for humans. Our liver can synthesize all of the carnitine our body needs from two amino acids.

Some people do have a genetic carnitine deficiency. They lack the ability to make this compound in sufficient amounts.[73] Although this is a rare occurrence, a vegan diet could exacerbate the problem.[74] In normal, healthy adult vegetarians—both lacto-ovo and vegan—blood levels of carnitine are adequate.[75]

four times the RDA—although there is some indication that this is an overestimate.[69]

Vitamin K is essential for blood clotting and for the manufacture of proteins that are found in the bones and in the kidneys. Vitamin K might play an important role in the health of bones. Elderly women with hip fractures have lower levels of vitamin K in their blood than women who don't get hip fractures.[70] People with low levels of this vitamin might not make enough of the proteins that are needed for optimal bone health.[71]

However, the most evident symptom of vitamin K deficiency is prolonged bleeding because blood doesn't coagulate. An acute deficiency of this vitamin is rare because it is widely available in foods, the body conserves it very carefully, and bacteria in the intestines make vitamin K. Usually, deficiency occurs only in people who undergo long-term antibiotic treatment (which can kill intestinal bacteria) or who have problems with absorption. Worldwide, newborn infants are also subject to vitamin K deficiency, which can cause hemorrhaging and death. This is because vitamin K doesn't reach the fetus very well and is low in breast milk. Most important, newborn babies have "clean intestines." This means that for the first few days of life, they don't have any bacteria in their intestines. In the United States, it is common practice for all infants to receive a vitamin K injection at birth.

Food Sources of Vitamin K

Determining the intake of vitamin K has been difficult because there has been very little information about the vitamin K content of foods. The USDA has released a provisional table of vitamin K in foods, and it is clear from this information that leafy green vegetables are by far the best sources of this nutrient. One serving of kale provides more than five times the RDA for vitamin K.[72]

Unlike the other fat-soluble vitamins, vitamin K is not toxic, even at very high doses. However, synthetic forms of the vitamin, which might be found in vitamin supplements, *can* be toxic at very high intakes.

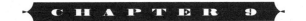

CHAPTER 9

MINERALS IN VEGETARIAN DIETS

It is now known that such inexpensive foodstuffs as greens and fresh vegetables not only contain more iron than does the finest beefsteak, but better food iron than is found in meats of any sort.

—JOHN HARVEY KELLOGG,
The Natural Diet of Man, 1923

◆

Most of the nutrients are large, complex molecules, but not so minerals. They are simple chemical elements that are integral parts of the earth and of all plant and animal life. They are also indestructible. If you burn any food to cinders, what is left in the ashes will be the perfectly intact minerals that were in that food.

Minerals perform a myriad of functions in the body. Like many of the vitamins, they can be a part of enzyme systems. But, as in the case of calcium, they can also be important components of the body's structures and cells.

Our body contains about sixty minerals, and many of these must be supplied by the diet. Recommended intake levels are established for fourteen minerals. Other minerals are required in the diet, but nutritionists have very little information about dietary needs and food sources.

We looked at the mineral calcium in chapter 7. In this chapter we will look first at the minerals that are of special interest in vegetarian diets—iron, zinc, and iodine. Then we'll touch briefly on the rest.

IRON

Iron is the substance that gives blood its red color. As long ago as the mid-1800s scientists demonstrated that blood contains iron by picking up dried blood particles with a magnet.[1]

One reason that iron gets so much attention is that its lack is one of the most common nutritional deficiencies in the world. More than 500 million people are believed to be iron deficient.[2] This problem is much more common in developing countries, where parasitic infections that can lead to iron loss are more widespread. But iron deficiency is also the most common nutritional deficiency in the United States, and 6 percent of the population might suffer from it. Four groups of people are most susceptible to poor iron status: infants and toddlers, teenagers, pregnant women, and premenopausal women.

Iron Requirements

Iron is primarily found in *hemoglobin*, the portion of the red blood cells that carries

TABLE 9.1 RECOMMENDATIONS FOR IRON INTAKE (IN MILLIGRAMS)

	United States	Canada	United Kingdom	Japan	Korea
Children	10	6–8	8.7	8–10	10–15
Adolescents	12–15	10–13	11–15	10–12	18
Adults	10–15	9–13	8.7–14.8	12	10–18
Pregnant Women	30	18–23	14.8	–	20

oxygen to all the cells of the body. It is also found in *myoglobin*, which provides a fast source of oxygen for muscles. About 25 percent of the body's iron is stored in the liver.

Of the body's 25 trillion red blood cells, about 25 billion are destroyed every day and need to be replaced. But even with that astounding number of lost red blood cells, we only need about one milligram of iron a day, since much of the iron in the body is recycled. We do lose iron every day via small amounts of intestinal blood loss and from sloughing off and excretion of cells lining the intestines.

We need to consume much more iron than what is lost because iron is poorly absorbed. The RDA for both men and post-menopausal women is ten milligrams, even though the actual biological need is just one milligram per day. Premenopausal women lose additional iron during menstrual bleeding, so their iron needs are 50 percent higher, at fifteen milligrams per day. Also, men tend to have enough stored iron to last them three years, whereas women have enough to last only six months.[3] When iron intake is too low, iron stores will eventually be depleted. Without enough iron to produce new red blood cells, a type of anemia develops in which red blood cells are tiny and pale. Fatigue is one symptom of anemia, as the tissues aren't receiving enough oxygen.

There is a strong agreement among scientists worldwide that vegetarians need more iron than omnivores. Much of the concern over iron in vegetarian diets is due to the fact that plant and animal foods contain different types of iron. The iron in animal foods, called *heme* iron, is better absorbed than that in plant foods, called *nonheme* iron. We'll see in a moment that this doesn't pose much of a problem, however.

Food Sources of Iron

Iron is widely distributed in plant foods. Both whole and enriched grains are good sources. So are legumes, nuts and seeds, many vegetables, and dried fruits.

Iron Absorption

The amount of iron that is absorbed from foods varies, depending on many factors. One major factor is iron need. Iron-deficient people absorb twice as much heme iron as people in good iron status. But they can absorb ten times as much nonheme iron when iron status is poor—an indication that

TABLE 9.2 IRON CONTENT OF FOODS

Food and Serving Size	Iron (milligrams)	Food and Serving Size	Iron (milligrams)
BREADS, CEREALS, GRAINS		**FRUITS**	
Barley, whole (½ cup cooked)	1.6	Apricots, dried (¼ cup)	1.5
Bran flakes (1 cup)	11.0	Prune juice (½ cup)	1.5
Bread, white (1 slice)	0.7	Prunes (¼ cup)	0.9
Bread, whole wheat (1 slice)	0.9	Raisins (¼ cup)	1.1
Cream of Wheat (½ cup cooked)	5.5		
Oatmeal, instant (1 packet cooked)	6.3	**LEGUMES (½ cup cooked)**	
Pasta, enriched (½ cup cooked)	1.2	Black beans	1.8
Rice, brown (½ cup cooked)	0.5	Chickpeas	3.4
Wheat germ (2 tablespoons)	1.2	Kidney beans	1.5
		Lentils	3.2
VEGETABLES (½ cup cooked unless otherwise indicated)		Lima beans	2.2
Alaria	18.1	Navy beans	2.5
Avocado (½, raw)	1.0	Pinto beans	2.2
Beet greens	1.4	Soybeans	4.4
Brussels sprouts	0.9	Split peas	1.7
Collards	0.9	Tempeh	1.8
Dulse	33.1	Textured vegetable protein	2.0
Kelp	42.0	Tofu	6.6
Nori	20.9	Vegetarian baked beans	0.7
Peas	1.2	**SOY AND VEGETABLE MILKS (1 cup)**	
Pumpkin	1.7	Soymilk	1.8
Spinach	1.5	**NUTS AND SEEDS (2 tablespoons)**	
Squash, acorn	0.9	Cashews	1.0
Swiss chard	1.9	Pumpkin seeds	2.5
Tomato juice (1 cup)	1.3	Sunflower seeds	1.2
Turnip greens	1.5	Tahini	1.2
		OTHER FOODS	
		Blackstrap molasses (1 tablespoon)	3.3

TABLE 9.3 FACTORS AFFECTING IRON ABSORPTION

Enhances Iron Absorption	Reduces Iron Absorption
Increased iron need	High levels of dietary iron
Vitamin C (affects only nonheme iron)	Tannins (in tea)
Other organic acids in fruits and vegetables	Coffee
	Calcium/milk
	Some Indian spices
	Fiber
	Phytates (in whole grains and legumes)

the iron in plant foods is much more sensitive to iron need.[4]

The total amount of iron ingested at any one time also affects absorption; as the amount of iron in a meal increases, the percentage absorbed drops. But, again, this seems to affect nonheme iron much more than heme iron.[5] Iron absorption is so closely tied to dietary factors that it can vary as much as twentyfold, depending on what else is in your diet. Vitamin C greatly enhances the absorption of nonheme iron—though not of heme iron. A cup of orange juice with seventy-five milligrams of vitamin C can boost the absorption of nonheme iron fourfold.[6] For this to be effective, though, the iron and vitamin C have to be consumed at the same time. It's easy to pair iron-rich foods with vitamin C sources. Here are a few examples of meals and snacks that take advantage of this combination:

- Sandwiches on whole wheat or iron-enriched bread with tomato slices

- Hot cereal with orange juice

- Cereal with sliced strawberries

- Pasta with tomato sauce

- Beans cooked in tomato sauce

- Soymilk shake with strawberries

- Green peppers stuffed with grain-and-nut mixture

Some foods are rich in both iron and vitamin C, including broccoli, spinach, Swiss chard, other dark-green leafy vegetables, and vitamin C–fortified breakfast cereals.

Substances in tea called tannins can reduce the absorption of nonheme iron by half. However, vitamin C can completely overcome this effect.[7] Coffee also inhibits iron absorption, and coffee with milk does so to an even greater degree.[8] Calcium is a potent inhibitor of iron, so that consuming dairy products with a meal can greatly reduce the amount of iron absorbed from that meal. Some spices commonly used in Indian cooking, such as turmeric and coriander, also reduce iron absorption.[9]

A high intake of dietary fiber also hinders iron absorption.[10] So do phytates. These phosphorus-containing compounds can lower iron absorption by as much as 90 percent.[11] But generally, people whose diets are high in fiber and phytate *don't* have poor iron status. One reason is that diets high in these two components tend to also be high in iron, which compensates for the poor absorption.[12] Also, vitamin C and other acids found in fruits and vegetables can overcome the effects of phytate.[13]

The high vitamin C content of vegetarian diets may help to make up for any potential problems with iron absorption. However, iron absorption is generally thought to be somewhat lower among vegetarians. While omnivores absorb about 10 to 15 percent of the iron in their diet, vegetarians may absorb only 5 to 10 percent.[14] In developing countries, absorption may be even lower, because of very high intakes of phytate and tannins and low intake of vitamin C. This is one reason that the World Health Organization recommendations for iron are very high compared with the RDA. But in many countries, including Western countries, it is common to recommend a higher iron intake for vegetarians.[15] So, with their greater iron needs, how do vegetarians fare when it comes to getting enough iron?

Iron Intake and Status in Vegetarians

Typical eating patterns of vegetarians show that vegetarian diets contain more iron than meat-containing diets and that vegans have the highest intakes of all. Studies suggest that this is also true for children. In one study of British vegan children, their iron intake was twice as high as that of omnivore children.[16]

Their higher intake probably makes up for the poorer iron absorption in vegetarian diets. Iron status bears this out, since vegetarians are no more likely to be iron deficient than omnivores.[17]

However, vegetarians do tend to have much smaller iron stores than meat eaters.[18] Although the smaller stores don't seem to result in any problems, vegetarians could be at greater risk for anemia if iron losses increased dramatically or iron needs increased. The dramatic rise in iron absorption when needs increase may help to protect against anemia, though. Because vegetarians have such high iron intakes, there is really no reason to give any special attention to iron in the diet. It's a good idea, however, to consume a source of vitamin C at most meals to make sure that iron is absorbed well. Some foods, like broccoli and spinach, have the double advantage of being high in both iron and vitamin C.

Iron and Plant-Based Diets: A Vegetarian Advantage

We noted earlier that absorption of nonheme iron—the kind found in plant foods—is much more subject to dietary factors than heme iron is. In the past, nonheme iron was considered to be inferior to heme iron for that reason. But now it seems as though there is a special advantage to consuming nonheme iron.

Too much iron in the body might raise the risk for chronic diseases like cancer and

TABLE 9.4 RECOMMENDATIONS FOR ZINC INTAKE (IN MILLIGRAMS)

	United States	Canada	United Kingdom	WHO
Children	10	4–7	5–7	4
Adolescents	12–15	9–12	7–9.5	5.5–7
Adults	12–15	9–12	7–9.5	5.5
Pregnant Women	15	15	7	7.5

heart disease. Iron can promote the process of oxidation, which results in formation of free radicals. These reactive substances wreak havoc on cells and may be involved in both cancer and heart disease.[19]

We are very limited in the ways we can get rid of excess iron. We don't simply excrete it in the urine as we do many of the vitamins. Instead, iron levels are regulated by absorption. But absorption of heme iron is very poorly regulated. We absorb pretty much the same amount of heme iron regardless of needs.

On the other hand, because nonheme iron is very sensitive to iron status and to dietary factors, its absorption is more tightly controlled. It may be safer to get iron from plant foods for this reason. What was considered a disadvantage—that nonheme iron is not always absorbed as well as heme iron—is now recognized as a possible advantage.

One Harvard University study has found that total iron in the diet isn't the critical factor that raises heart disease risk; rather it is the amount of *heme* iron in the diet.[20] That is, only iron from meat raises risk. So iron from meat may pose a double hazard, first because its absorption is poorly regulated and second because it may contribute to disease risk.

Many people—as many as 1 out of every 250—may be genetically susceptible to *iron overload*.[21] This is excessive iron storage, and it is a dangerous condition. For people with this condition, which can be diagnosed only through a blood test, it is especially important to guard against too much iron in the diet.

ZINC

Zinc Requirements

The RDA for zinc is fifteen milligrams for men and twelve for women. Outright deficiency of zinc is rather rare in Western countries, although it is sometimes seen in other parts of the world. A lack of this mineral can affect sexual maturation and growth in young people. The first documented case was seen in Middle Eastern men who suffered from hypogonadism (underdeveloped testicles) and also dwarfism.[22] In Turkey, children who indulge in a common practice called geophagy, or clay eating, also suffer from poor growth due to zinc deficiency, since clay interferes with the absorption of zinc.[23] Scientists in China note that as many as 30 percent of Chinese children might suffer stunted growth from zinc deficiency.[24]

For North Americans, marginal zinc defi-

TABLE 9.5 ZINC CONTENT OF FOODS

Food and Serving Size	Zinc (milligrams)	Food and Serving Size	Zinc (milligrams)
BREADS, CEREALS, GRAINS		Chickpeas	1.30
Barley, whole (½ cup cooked)	1.20	Cranberry beans	1.00
Bran flakes (1 cup)	5.00	Hyacinth beans	2.70
Granola (¼ cup)	0.71	Kidney beans	0.95
Grape-Nuts (¼ cup)	1.20	Lentils	1.20
Millet (½ cup cooked)	0.42	Lima beans	0.95
Nutri-Grain (¾ cup)	3.70	Navy beans	0.90
Oatmeal, instant (1 packet)	1.00	Pinto beans	0.90
Shredded Wheat (1 biscuit)	0.93	Soybeans	1.00
Special K (1⅓ cups)	3.70	Split peas	1.00
Wheat germ (2 tablespoons)	2.30	Tempeh	1.50
		Textured vegetable protein	1.37
VEGETABLES (½ cup cooked)		Tofu	1.00
Asparagus	0.43		
Collards	0.61	**NUTS AND SEEDS (2 tablespoons)**	
Corn	0.87	Brazil nuts	1.30
Irish moss	1.95	Cashews	0.96
Kelp	1.23	Peanut butter	1.00
Mushrooms	0.68	Peanuts	1.80
Nori	1.05	Pumpkin or squash seeds	1.20
Okra	0.57	Sunflower seeds	0.90
Peas	0.95	Tahini	1.30
Potatoes	0.44		
Spinach	0.69	**ANIMAL PRODUCTS**	
		Cheese, cheddar (1 ounce)	0.88
LEGUMES (½ cup cooked)		Cheese, Swiss (1 ounce)	1.10
Adzuki beans	2.00	Milk (1 cup)	0.95
Black-eyed peas	1.10	Yogurt (1 cup)	1.80

ciency may be more relevant than outright deficiency. A zinc intake that is chronically low might not lead to acute deficiency symptoms, but it could result in some chronic problems. The most common ones that have been seen in Western children are poor appetite, suboptimal growth, and impaired taste sensations.[25] Low-income children in the United States tend to have a poor zinc intake.[26]

One problem is that we really don't store any zinc in our bodies. So once zinc intake gets too low, deficiency symptoms can appear quite quickly. The effects of this deficiency can be widespread, since zinc has so many functions. It is involved in more than sixty different enzyme systems and is needed for optimal cell growth. It also is needed to make new proteins in the body and to aid blood formation, and it is involved in the immune system. One consequence of low zinc intake is that when people are injured, their wounds heal more slowly.

Many healthy people—both omnivores and vegetarians—don't meet the RDA for zinc.[27] However, in this case, as in others, we view the RDA with a bit of skepticism. The fact that in healthy American populations only a small percentage of people meet the RDA could mean that the zinc RDAs are too high. Canada, the United Kingdom, and the World Health Organization all recommend intakes that are quite a bit lower than the RDA (see table 9.4). This is largely due to a difference in opinion on how well zinc is absorbed.

One reason that people may do just fine with lower zinc consumption is that absorption increases with low zinc intakes. Also, the amount of zinc that is excreted from the body goes down dramatically.[28] So the body works in two ways to ensure that it is getting and keeping more zinc when intake is low.

Food Sources of Zinc

Zinc is fairly widespread in plant foods, although most of these foods supply only moderate amounts. Legumes, nuts, sea vegetables, and some breakfast cereals are among the best sources. Dairy products are also fairly high in zinc.

Zinc in Vegetarian Diets

A number of factors in vegetarian diets affect zinc absorption. Phytate is a potent inhibitor of zinc absorption.[29] As little as 5 percent of the zinc is absorbed from meals that are high in whole grains.[30] Since vegetarians consume about two or three times as much phytate as omnivores, this could have a significant impact on their zinc status.

Fiber also impairs zinc absorption.[31] Because of these two factors, refined grains may be as good a source of zinc as whole grains.[32] Processing removes much of the zinc from grains, but it also removes fiber and phytate, so that more of this zinc is available for absorption. In one study, when subjects switched from a diet containing white bread to one that used whole wheat bread, they consumed more zinc, but their zinc blood levels didn't change.[33]

But other factors in vegetarian diets tend to favor zinc status. Calcium reduces zinc absorption, especially when phytate is present.[34] This may work against lacto-ovo vegetarians, since they tend to have a high calcium intake, but it is to the advantage of vegans, who consume less calcium than either lacto-ovo vegetarians or omnivores.

Protein may directly raise zinc needs, so vegetarians may have lower needs due to their lower protein intake. In fact, in a typical American diet with about one hundred grams of protein and a moderate amount of phosphorus, zinc needs are estimated to be twice as high as they are for a vegetarian diet.[35] Vegetarians consume about the same amount of phosphorus as omnivores, but much of their phosphorus, particularly in the case of vegans, is not absorbed, so it won't increase zinc needs.

Zinc Intake of Vegetarians

Vegetarians generally consume less zinc than omnivores, and neither group tends to meet the RDA.[36] Studies of British vegan preschoolers show that their diet is also low in zinc but is about the same as nonvegetarian children.[37] A few studies have found very low intakes of zinc in vegetarians, particularly in vegetarian women.[38]

However, vegetarians have blood levels of zinc in the normal range.[39] In some cases, though, they are on the low end of normal, and some subjects have zinc levels that are generally too low, although not quite low enough to be outright zinc deficiency. Two recent studies put zinc in perspective: one found that zinc absorption was about 25 percent lower on a lacto-vegetarian diet, but the other found that the zinc status of vegetarians was normal on a diet that contained only five milligrams of zinc, because they became more efficient at conserving zinc.[40]

We noted that the RDA for zinc may be too high. Also, vegetarians may have lower zinc requirements than meat eaters because they consume less protein. On the other hand, absorption of zinc from plant foods can be quite poor.

At any rate, we recommend that vegetarians include several sources of zinc-rich foods in their diets every day and strive to meet the RDA for zinc.

IODINE

Iodine Requirements

Most Americans never give a second thought to the iodine content of their diet. But throughout much of the world, getting enough iodine is a serious problem. Iodine is a part of two hormones produced by a small gland in the neck called the thyroid gland. These thyroid hormones are needed for normal energy production and growth. When iodine is in short supply, the thyroid gland becomes enlarged, producing a goiter. In severe deficiency, goiters can become as large as grapefruits and are plainly visible at the front of the neck.

Worldwide, more than 500 million people are iodine deficient. When pregnant women become iodine deficient, their infants can suffer from cretinism, a disease of growth problems and mental deficiencies. In some parts of India, China, and Indonesia, as many as 10 percent of children are affected by cretinism.[41]

The RDA for adults is 150 micrograms. However, the RDA may be twice as high as what is actually needed.

Food Sources of Iodine

In the United States, iodine deficiency disappeared rapidly after 1924, when iodine was added to salt.[42] Common, iodized table salt contains about 400 micrograms of iodine in a teaspoon. In other parts of the world, iodized salt is also available and so are iodine injections. In China, iodine is sometimes added to soy oil.[43] The content of iodine in plant foods varies considerably, depending on where the food is grown. The amount of iodine in a region is a matter of geography. Both very

TABLE 9.6 SELENIUM CONTENT OF FOODS

Food and Serving Size	Selenium (micrograms)	Food and Serving Size	Selenium (micrograms)
BREADS, CEREALS, GRAINS		**LEGUMES (½ cup cooked)**	
Barley, pearled (½ cup cooked)	5	Lentils	10
Barley, whole (½ cup cooked)	.03	Navy beans	10
Bran flakes (1 cup)	4	**NUTS AND SEEDS (2 tablespoons)**	
Bread, white (1 slice)	7	Brazil nuts	10
Bread, whole wheat (1 slice)	11	**ANIMAL PRODUCTS**	
English muffin (½)	8	Egg (1 large)	12
Oatmeal (½ cup cooked)	10		
Rice, white (½ cup cooked)	5		

mountainous areas—like the Himalayas and the Andes—and areas that are subject to flooding, like the Ganges Valley in India and all of Bangladesh, tend to be iodine poor.

Although the iodine content of many plant foods is variable, sea vegetables are reliably rich in this mineral. Some brands of nutritional yeast provide iodine as well.

Vegetarians and Iodine

Even without the use of iodized salt, most Westerners consume plenty of iodine. However, vegetarians may be the exception. There is very little information about the iodine intake of vegetarians, but two studies show it to be quite a bit below the RDA.[44] Since milk is quite high in iodine (because it is in the solution used to disinfect milk storage tanks), vegans may have lower intakes than lacto-ovo vegetarians. However, neither study considered whether vegetarians used iodized salt. And one study took place in Sweden, which is a low-iodine area.[45]

However, we would recommend that vegans choose iodized salt whenever they salt foods (as little as a quarter teaspoon a day provides nearly three-quarters of the RDA for iodine, so don't overdo your salt intake).

SELENIUM

Although we've had RDAs for many of the vitamins and minerals since the 1940s, the first RDA for selenium was established in 1989. Prior to that, there just wasn't enough information to say how much people needed of this mineral. Also, selenium deficiency is extremely rare. When it does occur, it results in diseases that can cause damage to the heart.

Selenium Requirements

Selenium is an antioxidant that protects cells against damage caused by free radicals. It works very closely with vitamin E, another antioxidant. There is some evidence that it might play a role in preventing

TABLE 9.7 COPPER CONTENT OF FOODS

Food and Serving Size	Copper (micrograms)	Food and Serving Size	Copper (micrograms)
BREADS, CEREALS, GRAINS		LEGUMES (½ cup cooked)	
Barley, whole (½ cup cooked)	0.22	Lentils	0.24
Bran flakes (1 cup)	0.29	Navy beans	0.24
Bread, whole wheat (1 slice)	0.09	Soybeans	0.35
Graham crackers (2 whole)	0.14	Split peas	0.25
Millet (½ cup cooked)	0.19	Tempeh	0.55
		Textured vegetable protein	0.33
VEGETABLES (½ cup cooked unless otherwise indicated)		Tofu	0.23
Avocado (½, raw)	0.23	NUTS AND SEEDS (2 tablespoons)	
Mushrooms	0.24	Almond butter	0.28
Peas	0.13	Almonds	0.29
Potatoes	0.27	Brazil nuts	0.50
Sweet potatoes	0.23	Cashews	0.38
Tomato juice (1 cup)	0.23	Peanuts	0.37
		Pumpkin or squash seeds	0.23
		Sunflower seeds	0.30
		Tahini	0.45

breast cancer, possibly by participating in reactions that detoxify carcinogens.[46] It may help to prevent heart disease, which makes sense, since it is an antioxidant. However, this role for selenium is somewhat controversial right now.[47] The RDA for selenium is seventy micrograms for men and fifty-five micrograms for women.

Food Sources of Selenium

The selenium content of foods varies widely because it depends on the selenium in the soil in which the food was grown. For example, grains and other crops grown in one area of China are a thousand times higher in selenium than those grown in a selenium-poor area of China. The selenium content of animal foods is fairly stable, because animals absorb more or excrete more depending on their needs.

Selenium Intake in Vegetarians

Not surprisingly, the selenium intake of vegetarians varies quite a bit according to where they live. In northern European countries such as Sweden and Finland, soil is low in selenium and so are vegetarian diets.[48] In the United States, selenium intake of vegetarians is comparable to that of nonvegetarians.[49] The levels of selenium in the body are also similar between vegetarians and omnivores.[50]

COPPER

Copper has been used therapeutically since at least 400 B.C., when Hippocrates prescribed it to treat lung disease and other conditions.[51]

Copper Requirements
There is no RDA established for copper. However, we do have an estimated safe and adequate daily dietary intake, which is between 1.5 and 3.0 micrograms. Outright copper deficiency is quite rare in humans and seems to occur only when a person is severely malnourished or has a serious problem in absorbing nutrients.

Food Sources of Copper
Vegetarians tend to have high copper intakes, since it is found in many plant foods. Good sources of copper for vegetarians include whole grains, nuts, seeds, and legumes.

Vegetarians and Copper
There is some concern about copper absorption in vegetarians because both vitamin C and fiber can reduce the amount that gets into the blood. Also, a lower protein intake may raise copper needs. However, all of these effects might be negated by the fact that vegetarians consume more copper than omnivores, and their intake exceeds the RDA. Lacto-ovo vegetarians eat slightly more copper than meat eaters, and vegans eat about twice as much as either of those groups.[52]

The higher copper intake of vegetarians could have some real advantages, as a high copper-to-zinc ratio might decrease the risk for heart disease.[53]

MAGNESIUM

Magnesium is responsible for a lot of activity in the body. It is involved in more than three hundred different enzyme systems. It's also very important for bone structure.

Magnesium Requirements
The RDA for magnesium is 350 milligrams for men and 280 milligrams for women. Americans tend not to meet the RDA for magnesium, and a substantial number of people may have low levels of this mineral in their blood. While true magnesium deficiency doesn't seem to be a problem, it is possible that lower-than-normal levels could cause problems. Vegetarian diets contain more magnesium than omnivore diets.[54] Vegan diets seem to be even higher in this nutrient than lacto-ovo-vegetarian diets.[55]

Food Sources of Magnesium
Whole grains are extremely rich in magnesium. Most of it gets lost when grains are processed, and the magnesium isn't added back, so processed grains are generally low in this nutrient. Also, meat and milk are very poor sources of this mineral.

PHOSPHORUS

Phosphorus Requirements
Most of the phosphorus in the body is found in the skeleton, where it works hand in hand with calcium to form the bone structure. Phosphorus is also crucial in the process by which cells release energy from

TABLE 9.8 MAGNESIUM CONTENT OF FOODS

Food and Serving Size	Magnesium (milligrams)	Food and Serving Size	Magnesium (milligrams)
BREADS, CEREALS, GRAINS		**LEGUMES (½ cup cooked)**	
Barley, whole (½ cup cooked)	61	Black-eyed peas	41
Bran flakes (1 cup)	71	Kidney beans	40
Bread, whole wheat (1 slice)	26	Lima beans	41
Millet (½ cup cooked)	52	Navy beans	48
Oatmeal (½ cup cooked)	28	Pinto beans	47
Pasta, whole wheat (½ cup cooked)	21	Soybeans	74
Rice, brown (½ cup cooked)	43	Split peas	35
Wheat germ (2 tablespoons)	45	Tempeh	52
		Tofu	127
VEGETABLES (½ cup cooked unless otherwise indicated)		**NUTS AND SEEDS (2 tablespoons)**	
Avocado (½, raw)	35	Almond butter	96
Beet greens	49	Almonds	79
Beets	31	Brazil nuts	64
Okra	45	Cashews	44
Peas	31	Peanut butter	60
Potatoes	32	Peanuts	52
Pumpkin	27	Pumpkin or squash seeds	92
Spinach	70	Sunflower seeds	63
Squash, winter	43		
Swiss chard	75	**ANIMAL PRODUCTS**	
		Milk (1 cup)	34
FRUITS		Yogurt (1 cup)	43
Banana (1 medium)	33		
Orange juice (1 cup)	24		

food. Ideally, the ratio of calcium to phosphorus in the diet should be 1:1. The RDA for adults is 800 milligrams.

Food Sources of Phosphorus

Foods that are especially high in phosphorus are meats, processed foods that contain food additives, and soft drinks. Omnivores tend to consume too much phosphorus relative to calcium, and this may adversely affect bone health.[56] The dietary phosphorus-to-calcium ratio may be especially problematic in teenage girls, who have a low calcium intake but drink a lot of soft drinks that are high in phosphorus.

Vegetarians consume about the same or

TABLE 9.9 POTASSIUM CONTENT OF FOODS

Food and Serving Size	Potassium (milligrams)	Food and Serving Size	Potassium (milligrams)
BREADS, CEREALS, GRAINS (1 cup)		Honeydew melon (1 cup chunks)	461
Bran flakes	248	Kiwifruit (1 medium)	252
		Mango (1 medium)	322
VEGETABLES (½ cup cooked unless otherwise indicated)		Nectarine (1 medium)	288
Asparagus	279	Orange (1 medium)	250
Avocado (½, raw)	548	Orange juice (6 ounces)	350
Beet greens	659	Papaya (1 medium)	780
Beets	265	Pear (1 medium)	208
Parsnips	287	Pineapple juice (6 ounces)	250
Peas	217	Prune juice (6 ounces)	528
Plantain	358	Prunes (5 dried)	313
Potatoes	498	Strawberries (1 cup whole)	247
Pumpkin	252		
Spinach	305	**LEGUMES (½ cup cooked)**	
Squash, acorn	448	Black-eyed peas	346
Sweet potatoes	397	Chickpeas	398
Swiss chard	480	Kidney beans	329
Tomatoes, stewed	304	Lentils	365
Tomato juice	521	Navy beans	395
		Pinto beans	400
FRUITS		Soybeans	443
Apple juice (6 ounces)	225	Split peas	296
Apricots (3 medium)	313		
Cantaloupe (1 cup chunks)	494	**NUTS AND SEEDS (2 tablespoons)**	
Dates (10)	541	Almond butter	242
Figs (5 dried)	666		
Grapefruit juice (6 ounces)	283	**ANIMAL PRODUCTS**	
		Milk (1 cup)	381
		Yogurt (1 cup)	590

somewhat less phosphorus than meat eaters, and vegans consume a bit less than lacto-ovo vegetarians. More important, the phosphorus in plant foods is not absorbed as well as that in animal foods.

SODIUM AND CHLORIDE

Sodium and chloride usually occur together in the diet because they are the two elements that make up common table salt—also called sodium chloride. Along with potassium, they are crucial for maintaining fluid balance in the body.

Sodium Requirements

The last thing that most Westerners need to worry about is a deficiency of sodium. Most of us eat too much of this mineral. In some individuals, it is linked to high blood pressure. Between 30 and 50 percent of people with hypertension are sensitive to sodium.[57] Although too much sodium is a problem in Western diets, it is an essential nutrient. We need about 500 milligrams of sodium a day; however, most Americans consume four to ten times that amount.[58] They also have chloride intakes that are well above the estimated 750 milligrams that are needed daily.

Food Sources of Sodium

Most foods contain small amounts of sodium and chloride, but only about 10 percent of what we consume comes from these natural sources. Some sodium chloride is added during cooking (as table salt), but most is added during processing.[59] Like everyone else, vegetarians need to decrease their sodium intake by using less salt, since their diets tend to be just about as high in sodium as omnivore diets.[60]

POTASSIUM

Potassium Requirements

High levels of potassium in the diet may improve bone health and may also help to lower blood pressure. There is no RDA for potassium, but the minimum recommended daily amount is 1,600 to 2,000 milligrams. Most Americans eat slightly more than this,

but people who consume generous amounts of fruits and vegetables can eat as much as eight to eleven grams of potassium every day—or four or five times the minimum recommendations.[61] Vegetarian diets contain more potassium than omnivore diets, which may partly explain vegetarians' lower blood pressure.[62]

FLUORIDE

Fluoride helps to protect tooth enamel and can reduce dental decay. It's widely present in Western countries, primarily because it is added to water. This widespread use of fluoride since the 1950s has resulted in a decline in cavities. There is also evidence that fluoride promotes bone health, as it is part of the skeletal structure.[63]

Fluoride Requirements

Although fluoride has been proven to improve dental health, there is no real, life-threatening deficiency disease associated with it, so it isn't classified as an essential nutrient. However, it is recommended that adults consume between 1.5 and 4 milligrams of fluoride a day.

Excessive fluoride can be toxic and damage kidneys and possibly muscles and nerves. But this occurs only after years of consuming twenty to eighty milligrams a day.[64] The average intake in the United States is less than two milligrams a day.

Food Sources of Fluoride

Water, either naturally containing fluoride or with fluoride added to it, is the best source of this mineral. Foods can take up fluoride from water used for cooking,[65] as

TABLE 9.10 MANGANESE CONTENT OF FOODS

Food and Serving Size	Manganese (milligrams)	Food and Serving Size	Manganese (milligrams)
BREADS, CEREALS, GRAINS		**FRUITS**	
Barley, whole (½ cup cooked)	0.89	Pineapple (½ cup)	0.82
Bran flakes (1 cup)	1.70	Strawberries (½ cup sliced)	0.32
Oatmeal (½ cup cooked)	0.68	**LEGUMES (½ cup cooked)**	
Pasta, whole wheat (½ cup cooked)	0.96	Black-eyed peas	0.36
Rice, brown (½ cup cooked)	1.00	Lentils	0.48
Rice, white (½ cup cooked)	0.38	Pinto beans	0.47
Shredded Wheat (1 biscuit)	0.75	Soybeans	0.71
Wheat germ (2 tablespoons)	2.80	Tempeh	1.10
VEGETABLES (½ cup cooked)		Textured vegetable protein	0.65
Beet greens	0.37	Tofu	0.75
Carrots	0.33	**NUTS AND SEEDS (2 tablespoons)**	
Collards	0.56	Almond butter	0.75
Lima beans	0.48	Pumpkin or squash seeds	0.52
Peas	0.42	Sunflower seeds	0.36
Spinach	0.96		
Sweet potatoes	0.63		
Turnip greens	0.39		

can foods that are cooked in Teflon-coated pans, which also contain fluoride.[66]

CHROMIUM

Chromium Requirements

Although nutritionists don't have a completely clear picture of how chromium works, it is believed to be important in order for the hormone insulin to do its job. It appears to be part of a complex called glucose tolerance factor, which might also include niacin and several amino acids.[67] Some people suffer from glucose intolerance, which is an inability to properly regulate the levels of glucose in their blood. This can be a sort of mild diabetes. Giving supplements of chromium often helps to improve this condition.[68] Chromium also might help to lower blood cholesterol levels.[69]

Adults need somewhere between fifty and two hundred micrograms of chromium per day, and there is evidence that many Westerners don't get enough of this essential nutrient.[70]

Food Sources of Chromium

Whole grains are rich in chromium, although most of the chromium is lost when grains are refined. Beer can also be a good source, but the chromium content varies quite a bit from brand to brand.[71] Fruits, vegetables, and dairy products are all low in chromium. Stainless-steel containers that hold processed foods can actually add chromium to food.[72]

There isn't much information on the chromium intake of vegetarians. However, a study of Indian vegetarians showed chromium intake to be adequate.[73]

MANGANESE

Manganese is involved in enzyme systems that produce energy in the cells. It is abundant in plant foods, and deficiency is extremely rare.

Vegetarians consume much more manganese than nonvegetarians.[74] Humans appear to have very low requirements for this mineral. The estimated safe and adequate daily dietary intake is two to five milligrams.

MOLYBDENUM

Molybdenum is involved in several enzyme systems, including those that help to detoxify foreign compounds that enter the body. The recommended daily intake is 75 to 250 micrograms, and most Americans seem to get enough molybdenum. This includes vegetarians and vegans, because legumes, bread, grains, and milk are all rich in molybdenum.

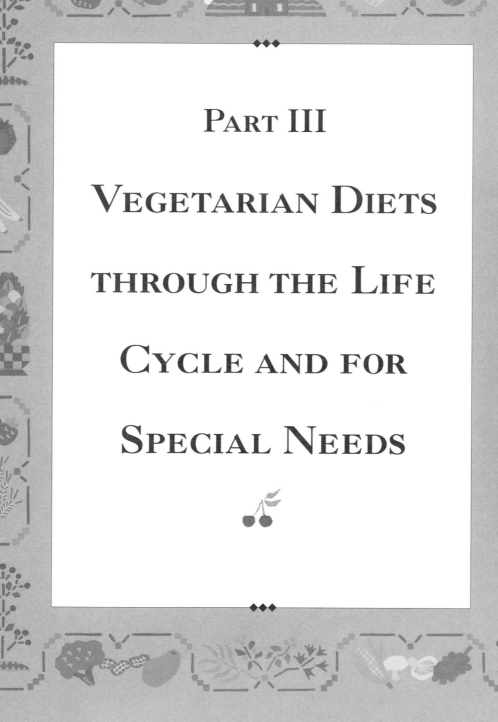

PART III

VEGETARIAN DIETS

THROUGH THE LIFE

CYCLE AND FOR

SPECIAL NEEDS

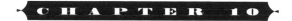

CHAPTER 10

GUIDELINES FOR MEAL PLANNING

There is no single pattern of diet which must be followed to ensure good nutrition.

—ROBERT S. GOODHART, M.D.,
Modern Nutrition in Health and Disease, 1980

◆

There are many ways to plan healthy diets for vegetarians. In fact, chances are, if you were simply to make whole grains the center of your meals and add plenty of legumes, vegetables, and fruits, keeping the diet low in fat and consuming adequate calories, you would likely meet nutrient needs. After all, most people in the world who have enough food meet dietary needs by consuming plenty of whatever is at hand. They don't consult meal-planning tools or draw up menu plans.

Westerners are at somewhat of a disadvantage, however. Many are not frequent consumers of some of the more nutritious plant foods that are commonly consumed in other parts of the world. So eating a healthy, plant-based diet doesn't necessarily come naturally to us. Some structured guidelines can help.

The guidelines in table 10.1 are a fairly simple approach to planning healthy menus. They should not be taken as the final word in menu planning, but they should work for a wide variety of vegetarians with different food preferences. The guidelines can be used by either lacto-ovo vegetarians or vegans. Macrobiotic vegetarians can use this guide also; they will find that some of the foods in the groups are not suitable for them, but each of the groups should contain enough choices to make the guide usable.

The food guide in table 10.1 can be used to plan meals for anyone over the age of one year. The numbers of servings listed here are for adults. (See chapters 13 and 14 for guidelines for meal planning for children and teens.) They represent minimum amounts of food for a healthy adult and provide about 1,600 calories. People who need more calories can increase their servings.

Depending on your food choices in each of these groups, this food guide describes a diet that gets about 15 to 20 percent of its calories from fat. You can reduce the calories by omitting the servings of added fats. They certainly aren't required for healthy eating. On the other hand, avoidance of all added fats isn't required for good health either. For normal, healthy vegetarians whose diets are low in saturated fat and cholesterol, and who are at a desirable weight, there is no evidence that a fat intake below 15 to 20 percent of calories provides any advantage.

TABLE 10.1 VEGETARIAN FOOD GUIDE

Food Group	Foods Included	Serving Size	Number of Servings Suggested
GRAINS	Breads, muffins, crackers, cereals, pasta, *tortillas,* and whole grains such as amaranth, barley, bulgur, kamut, kasha, oats, popcorn, quinoa, rice, wheat berries	1 slice breads, 1 small muffin, ½ cup cereal, ½ cup pasta, 1 6-inch tortilla, 1 pancake, ½ cup grain, 2 cups popcorn	8 or more
VEGETABLES	Asparagus, beets, *bok choy, broccoli,* Brussels sprouts, cabbage, carrots, cauliflower, chard, *collards,* corn, eggplant, *greens,* jicama, *kale,* leeks, lettuce, mushrooms, okra, peas, peppers, potatoes, rutabagas, *sea vegetables (dulse, kelp, nori, wakame),* spinach, squash, sweet potatoes, tomatoes, turnips, or any other vegetable	½ cup cooked or 1 cup raw vegetable	4 or more (include at least 1 serving a day of broccoli, kale, collards, or other dark-green leafy vegetables)
FRUITS	Apples, apricots, bananas, berries, cantaloupe, dates, *figs,* grapefruit, grapes, honeydew, kiwifruit, oranges, papaya, peaches, pears, persimmons, pineapple, plums, prunes, raisins, strawberries, watermelon, all fruit juices	1 piece fresh fruit, 1 wedge melon, ½ cup cooked or canned fruit, ¾ cup fruit juice, ¼ cup dried fruit	3 or more

Foods printed in italic type are good sources of calcium.

TABLE 10.1 VEGETARIAN FOOD GUIDE (cont.)

Food Group	Foods Included	Serving Size	Number of Servings Suggested
LEGUMES, NUTS, SEEDS, MILK			5 or more
Legumes	Adzuki beans, *black beans,* black-eyed peas, *chickpeas, great northern beans,* kidney beans, lentils, limas, mung beans, *navy beans, pintos, soybeans,* split peas, *vegetarian baked beans, tempeh, textured vegetable protein, tofu,* meat analogues	½ cup cooked beans, tempeh, tofu, vegetable protein; 3 ounces meat analogue	
Nuts/Seeds	*Almonds,* cashews, Brazil nuts, pecans, pine nuts, pistachios, walnuts, coconut, *almond butter,* peanut butter, *tahini,* pumpkin seeds, *sesame seeds,* sunflower seeds	2 tablespoons nuts, nut butter, seeds	
Milks	*Soymilk, fortified soymilk, Vegelicious, Take Care, 2% or nonfat cow's milk, soy yogurt,* cow's milk yogurt	1 cup fluid milk or yogurt	
FATS	Vegetable oils, margarine, butter, salad dressing	1 teaspoon oil, margarine, butter; 2 teaspoons salad dressing	2 or 3
OTHER FOODS	Soy cheese, *cow's-milk cheese,* eggs, baked sweets, snack chips	1 ounce cheese, 1 egg, 1 ounce snack chips, 2 ounces cookies or baked goods	Limit these foods

Foods printed in italic type are good sources of calcium.

Where's the Milk Group?

U.S. diet-planning guidelines have devoted a whole food group to dairy products since the first food guide was published in 1916. Even many food guides devised specifically for vegetarians include a milk group. You'll notice that our guide doesn't. While dairy products are present in this guide, they are simply one choice in a larger group of foods that includes a variety of legumes, nuts, seeds, and milks.

There are two reasons for this. The first is that we wanted our guide to be usable by both lacto-ovo vegetarians and vegans. This way, the guide is also useful to people who are moving from a lacto-ovo eating pattern to a vegan diet or for any vegetarian who simply wants to experiment with a variety of foods. If you are a vegan, you can ignore the dairy choices in that food group. If you are a lacto-ovo vegetarian, instead of looking toward cow's milk to meet all of your calcium needs, you can sometimes choose soymilks or other sources of calcium.

Second, it is faulty nutritional advice to devote a whole food group to dairy products with the idea that healthy diets must include choices from that group. The concept that diets must include dairy foods is an erroneous one. Unfortunately, even modern meal-planning guidelines, like the USDA's food guide pyramid, promote that false information.

Of course, dairy foods are not essential in the diet. We know this because of the adequate health of vegans and of people throughout the world who don't use these products. We placed cow's milk where it belongs—as one choice in a group of foods that all contribute generous amounts of protein and calcium to the diet.

Planning Meals with the Food Guide

Grains

It is often said that bread is the staff of life. A more accurate rendering would be that grains are the staff of life. Most of the people in the world make grains the center of their diet. Often they rely on just two or three grains that are locally grown and readily available. Thus in Africa, millet and corn are common parts of meals. In China, dishes are based on rice and millet, and in Central and South America, rice and corn are the center of meals. In North America, wheat is the most commonly consumed grain, though most of what we eat is made from processed, refined wheat flour.

Grain-based diets represent the healthiest way of eating. Grains are rich in protein, B vitamins, iron, and other minerals. Whole grains are more nutritious than refined grains; they are higher in fiber and in some B vitamins and minerals than processed grains. Even when refined grains are enriched and have some nutrients added back, they are less nutritious than whole grains. However, processed grains are still healthful foods. Do focus on including whole grains in your diet. But vegetarians have fairly high fiber intakes, so it is fine to include a few servings a day of processed grains in your meals. There is nothing wrong with eating these foods.

Making grains the center of your diet

means planning all of your meals around these foods. We suggest that adults consume eight or more servings of grains a day. That may seem like a lot, but it really isn't that difficult. For one thing, a serving of grains is just a half cup or a slice of bread.

To get more grains into your diet, it helps to think along the lines of ethnic cuisine. Since most international menus make good use of grains, this is a great way to have fun exploring these healthy foods. After all, when you think of Italian food, doesn't pasta come to mind? Latin American cuisine brings images of corn tortillas and rice. Rice and noodles are also the foundation of many Asian dishes.

It's easy to make all of your meals and snacks grain based. Build breakfasts around toasted whole-grain breads, satisfying stick-to-your-ribs cereals like oatmeal, Cream of Wheat, or multigrain cereals. Cold cereals tend to be highly processed and are always long on packaging and short on value. But there are good choices, and many of the available cereals are nutritious, at least through fortification. Some of the old-fashioned classics are among the best, including Grape-Nuts and Shredded Wheat.

Whole-grain muffins, made with bran flakes or rolled oats, for example, are also good for starters in the morning. So are pancakes or waffles made with whole wheat flour. We even offer an eggless French toast recipe in the recipe section of this book.

The all-American favorite lunch—a sandwich—is a great way to go, especially if you choose whole-grain bread and stuff the sandwich with something low fat and fiber rich. Good sandwich stuffers are bean spreads, sautéed vegetable mixes, or vegetarian burgers. Look for mixes in natural foods stores or check our recipe section in the back of the book for ideas.

If you get tired of sandwiches, try pasta or rice salads with beans, chopped vegetables, and vinaigrette dressing for a nice portable lunch. Or carry a thermos to work or school that is filled with soups thick with rice, barley, or pasta.

Start every dinner by filling your plate with a mound of hearty, whole grains, like brown rice, wheat berries, quinoa, or barley. Cook the grains in vegetable stock to make them more flavorful. You can also create lovely sweet-tasting grain dishes by replacing up to half the cooking water with apple juice or by adding raisins or other dried fruits to grains. Team these sweeter dishes with hot and spicy curries for a nice flavor contrast.

Don't shy away from trying new grains because you think you need to wade through cookbooks or go through elaborate preparation. Keep it simple. Toss hot grains with garlic and ginger or with fresh herbs and sautéed onions.

Think grains when choosing snacks, also. Bagels, graham crackers, popcorn, toasted bread, and whole-grain muffins are all good ways to boost your intake of whole grains throughout the day.

Vegetables

Working four servings of vegetables into your diet may take some effort at first, especially if the extent of your relationship with these foods is an occasional oil-drenched salad. Again, remember that a serving of vegetables is just one-half cup cooked vegetable or one cup raw.

A little bit of planning helps. Include one to two servings of vegetables at both lunch and dinner. But don't let traditional meal-planning guidelines interfere with your attempts to eat a healthier diet. Very few people in this country eat vegetables for breakfast, but who says you can't?

Remember to include vegetables in snacks, also. Munch on raw carrots or enjoy other raw vegetables with dips made from nonfat yogurt or from tofu.

Everyone, but vegans in particular, should include one to two servings of dark green leafy vegetables in their diet every day. These foods, which include kale, mustard greens, turnip greens, collards, spinach, Swiss chard, beet greens, dandelion greens, and some of the new Asian greens that are appearing in many grocery stores, are rich in beta-carotene, iron, riboflavin, and other nutrients. With the exception of Swiss chard, beet greens, and spinach, they are super sources of calcium.

Cruciferous vegetables also deserve a prominent role in your diet. These include broccoli, Brussels sprouts, cabbage, cauliflower, kale, rutabagas, and turnips. Besides being great sources of many nutrients, they are thought to help protect against cancer, especially colon cancer. Try to consume these foods several times a week. Many children will shun these stronger-tasting vegetables. Try raw broccoli or cauliflower, the mildest-tasting of the group, and serve these foods in very small quantities to acclimate children's taste buds.

Make every attempt to buy vegetables in season. They are cheaper, and they taste better. They are also likely to be more nutritious. Vegetables that are shipped from great distances can spend more than a week on the road from the time they are harvested until they land in the produce bin at the grocery store. And then they can sit there for another week. While some vegetables store very well, many lose much nutritional value over a relatively short time. In fact, in the winter, frozen and canned vegetables are likely to be more nutritious than fresh ones, since they are processed immediately after harvest. They lose some nutritional value in processing, but not as much as is lost when vegetables sit for a week or two.

Many vegetables grow well in colder weather and are a good bet for fresh choices in the wintertime. These include some of the cruciferous vegetables, many of the dark leafy greens, winter squash, and potatoes. Your best guide to what is in season is price. When the price goes down, that food is likely to be in season and becomes a good choice for meals.

Legumes, Nuts, Seeds, Milks

This is a large group that includes a variety of different types of foods. While grains, vegetables, and fruit play central roles in the diet, legumes, nuts, seeds, and milks have supporting roles. The exception is for children. Milks—either soymilk, vegetable milk, or cow's milk—can be one important way to boost calories and nutrients in a child's diet, especially for young children who may express strong food dislikes.

We suggest five or more servings a day of

LEARNING TO LOVE VEGETABLES

If you are not a vegetable lover, it may be that you were raised—as many of us were—on mushy canned green beans. Some people never had a chance to taste actual vegetables because they grew up on ones that were smothered in butter and salt or that only appeared in casseroles buried under layers of sour cream, bread crumbs, and cheese.

A first step in learning to love vegetables is to learn to cook them properly. Gently steamed vegetables tend to taste the most mild and have the most pleasant texture. Steam or sauté them just until they are slightly tender but still crisp. Of course, some of the starchy vegetables, like potatoes or winter squash, need to be cooked more thoroughly. And older people who have problems chewing may need to cook vegetables to a more easily chewed tenderness.

If you are used to drowning vegetables in butter, margarine, salt, and fatty sauces you might be surprised to find that when they are gently cooked, lighter treatments will enhance the flavor and allow you to enjoy many new vegetables. Try a dash of tamari (soy sauce) or a sprinkle of fresh or dried herbs. A pungent dressing of fresh lemon juice and Dijon mustard is wonderful on a variety of vegetables. A dash of herb-flavored vinegar dresses up steamed greens like kale or collards. Every vegetable has its own unique flavor. And that flavor varies depending on whether the vegetable is cooked or raw. So the person who doesn't care for cooked carrots may like them very well when they are shredded raw in a salad. Give yourself a chance to enjoy vegetables by trying a wide variety of them, prepared in different ways. You will probably find a good assortment of vegetables that you like.

these foods, which include all cooked beans, soyfoods like tofu and tempeh, nuts, seeds, nut and seed butters, and milks such as soymilk and cow's milk. Foods in this group fall into three categories: legumes, nuts and seeds, and milks. You can choose your five servings from among these categories in any way you wish, though we suggest including a variety of foods from this food group.

Legumes. These are dried beans, peas, and lentils. In the diets of most Americans, they are largely absent. An occasional bean burrito or a side of baked beans at a Fourth of July picnic describes the beginning and end of most people's relationship with legumes. In other cultures, beans play a supporting but ever-present role in the diet. Generally used as a sauce served over grains, beans are common fare in Latin America, Asia, Africa, and the Middle East. Where food tends to be scarce, beans are an important source of high-quality protein because they are so efficiently and inexpensively produced.

You can likely plan a healthy vegetarian diet without beans, but they are such a versatile food that most vegetarians feel they couldn't live without them. They are less popular with the rest of the population because of ideas that they are "poor people's food" and that they are bland. They *are* inexpensive and are a virtual must in the diet of anyone counting grocery pennies. But cheaper foods are often the most nutritious options. The foods we pay a premium for—meats, cheese, processed cereals, and packaged dinners—are also the foods that are most detrimental to our health. The basic stuff—whole grains, legumes, fresh greens—are the healthiest foods you can eat. This is one case where cheaper is nearly always better.

As far as their blandness is concerned, many beans don't have a lot of flavor right out of the pot. But because they are so central to different international cuisines, we have endless, delicious ways to prepare them. Some of the best vegetarian dishes include beans.

A pestier problem for some bean eaters is the gas that they produce. Beans contain small amounts of carbohydrates that our digestive enzymes can't break down. These carbohydrates cause flatulence. People who are just getting acquainted with beans can take some solace in the fact that many people find these symptoms lessen the more frequently they eat beans. For people who really experience discomfort, there are products available made of natural compounds that help to digest the carbohydrates in beans. Put a few drops of one of these products on your first forkful of beans, and you should have no problems. One of these, called Beano, is sold in most drugstores.

Another solution to the problem of gas is to cook your beans according to our gas-reducing method (see pages 308–11).

People often don't realize that beans provide a wonderful opportunity to add variety to meals. Worldwide, people eat hundreds of different types of beans. Beans available in specialty grocery stores are heirloom varieties that are regaining popularity. Many are so pretty that you will want to display them in jars in your kitchen. For a treat for your eyes and palate, look for Christmas limas, Jacob's cattle beans, Anasazi, soldier beans, yellow eyes, and calypso beans. But your local grocery store carries a good selection of beans as well. You'll find chickpeas, black beans, kidney beans, navy beans, great northerns, pintos, yellow and green split peas, lentils, and limas.

A special category in the bean group is soyfoods. These include soybeans and a host of products made from them. Many foods made from soybeans mimic meat and dairy products for those who find meal planning difficult without those foods. The best known of the soyfoods is probably tofu, a fantastically versatile food. Chapter 24 includes some ideas for using tofu in your meals.

New vegetarians may find it daunting to include several servings of beans in their diet each day. But again, serving sizes are modest—just a half cup of beans. Try some dishes that are familiar and easy, like canned vegetarian baked beans or lentil soup. Then try a few new bean dishes from our recipes or from some of the recommended cookbooks in the resource section at the back of this book.

A good way to increase your intake of beans is to add them to dishes that you already enjoy. Add beans to soups, stews, pasta primavera, or salads. Some of the best dishes are the simplest. Pasta, great northern beans (or any white beans), and tomatoes cooked in vegetable broth generously flavored with garlic and onions is a very traditional Italian soup. Serve it with bread and a salad for a taste of the Mediterranean that is healthy and delicious.

Beans can be a simple but delicious dinner. Make a sauce of your favorite beans sauteed with chopped onion, garlic, and herbs and served over grains. Add chopped tomatoes, peppers, or salsa if you like.

Beans are also a good sandwich stuffer. Mash your favorite beans with chopped onions and herbs and spread on whole wheat bread or stuff into a pita pocket.

How about beans for breakfast? While that seems a little unusual to many of us, it is standard fare in many countries. In some Latin American countries, black beans on bread or a tortilla with an eye-opening dash of salsa is a common breakfast. At British bed-and-breakfasts, vegetarian guests are likely to be served baked beans on toast instead of eggs for breakfast.

Nuts and seeds. Nuts and seeds are rich in protein, calcium, and minerals and earn a place in this food group for that reason. However, they are also extremely high in fat. A serving of nuts or seeds each day is a super way to boost nutritional intake, but don't overdo it with these high-calorie foods. An exception might be a vegan child who is a picky eater and is having trouble meeting calorie needs.

A serving of nuts or seeds consists of two tablespoons of chopped nuts, seeds, or nut or seed butter. Make this amount go a little further by mixing nut butters with fruits— such as peanut butter and mashed banana spread—or by tossing a few tablespoons of

seeds into a salad or casserole for some extra flavor or crunch.

Milks. To many people, milk means one thing: milk from a cow. But many vegetarians enjoy a much wider range of milks in their diet. Soymilk has been a staple in many vegan households for years. Plain soymilk contains eighty milligrams of calcium in an eight-ounce serving. Over the past few years, a number of fortified soymilk products have become available. Most of these have upward of 240 milligrams of calcium, making them comparable to cow's milk as far as nutrition is concerned.

More recently, a whole new generation of vegetable-based milks have made their way onto the market. Milks made from rice or almonds are becoming popular. A new product, called Vegelicious, is made from potatoes and other ingredients. It's a nutritious product, and it doesn't taste anything like potatoes; it tastes like milk! Use vegetable-based milk just as you would cow's milk. Try it on morning cereal, in shakes, for French toast, in baked goods, or plain, as a beverage.

For our purposes, milk includes fortified soymilk and rice milk, Vegelicious, cow's milk, and, for babies and toddlers, human milk. Unfortified rice and almond milks are less nutritious. They are fine for occasional use, but they don't count toward servings from this food group.

There are a number of fortified soymilks on the market, and they vary considerably in their nutrient makeup. We recommend using a soymilk that provides at least 25 percent of the RDI for calcium in one cup and at least 10 percent of vitamin D, riboflavin, and vitamin B$_{12}$. A new product called Take Care is not a true soymilk but is manufactured from protein that has been isolated from the soybean. However, it is a vegan product and is well fortified, so it is comparable to milk in its nutritional quality. In fact, since it contains no animal protein or animal fat and is free of lactose, we would consider it nutritionally superior to cow's milk.

Use any of the milks in this group interchangeably. Lacto-ovo vegetarians might sometimes want to choose some of the vegan milks to explore new foods, add variety, and reduce their intake of animal protein. These milks are also free of lactose, making them a great choice for anyone with problems digesting this milk sugar. Whichever milk you choose, adults can use low-fat or nonfat versions to lower the fat content of their diet.

There is no dietary requirement for any type of milk. However, we are recommending that vegetarian children consume *two or three cups* of some type of milk every day. This is an especially easy way to boost the calorie and nutrient intake of children. But as with any food plan, there is some room for flexibility. If your child doesn't like milk of any kind, you can omit this food. Just be sure that you are supplying additional servings from the other food groups and that your child is eating plenty of calcium-rich foods. One good way to encourage children to drink milk is to make fruit-flavored shakes using soymilk, Vegelicious, Take Care, or cow's milk with frozen fruit, whirred together in a blender.

While milks are good sources of nutrition, it is also wise not to overdo it. All of the milks are low in fiber (cow's milk contains no fiber). Children or adults who drink too much milk may not have room for other foods. Also, cow's milk is extremely low in iron. Children who fill up on this milk may not have room for iron-rich foods and can become anemic. Breast milk is a nutritious choice for babies and toddlers, but, in toddlers, it should be a supplemental food, not the center of the diet.

Fats and Oils

Historically, added fats have played an important role in human nutrition. Where food is scarce and people perform a great deal of physical labor, fat provides additional calories. But most Americans get more than enough fat. People who eat diets based on meat and dairy foods are likely to get too much. And even a vegan diet is apt to provide plenty of fat.

There is much debate over how much fat people need in their diet. While fat is an essential nutrient, our dietary requirement is really just for two types of fat, linoleic acid and linolenic acid, which are both found in plant foods. A mixed diet that includes whole grains and beans will easily provide plenty of these fatty acids, since they are found in small amounts in these low-fat foods.

Adults probably don't need more than 10 percent of their calories to come from fat. Children may need a bit more fat to help them meet calorie needs. We get fat from foods that are inherently rich in fat, such as nuts, seeds, soybeans and soybean products, avocados, and olives; from foods

TABLE 10.2 THREE DAYS OF MEALS FOR A VEGAN ADULT

Day 1

BREAKFAST

Strawberry-banana shake (½ banana, ¼ cup strawberries, 1 cup soymilk)

English muffin, with 2 tablespoons peanut butter

LUNCH

Large whole wheat pita, stuffed with ½ cup curried tofu chunks, chopped peppers, tomatoes, and celery

Salad (lettuce, mushrooms, avocado, 2 tablespoons tahini dressing)

Orange

DINNER

1 cup vegetarian baked beans

1 cup mixed quinoa and amaranth

1 cup collard greens, braised in 1 teaspoon olive oil

SNACK

2 small oat-bran muffins, with 1 teaspoon margarine

Day 2

BREAKFAST

½ cup scrambled tofu in 1 teaspoon oil

2 slices rye toast

6 ounces calcium-fortified orange juice

LUNCH

1½ cups pasta-and-bean soup

Pumpernickel roll

Salad (¾ cup lettuce, ¾ cup raw broccoli, 2 tablespoons shredded carrots, 1 tablespoon oil-and-vinegar dressing)

DINNER

Bean burrito, with chopped tomatoes and lettuce

1 cup Spanish rice

½ cup steamed turnip greens

½ cup carrots

SNACKS

1 cup vanilla soymilk

4 graham crackers

½ cup watermelon chunks

Day 3

BREAKFAST

2 slices French toast

½ cup applesauce

Coffee, with nondairy creamer

LUNCH

Large whole wheat pita, stuffed with ½ cup hummus and chopped tomato

Carrot sticks

Oatmeal cookie

DINNER

1½ cups lentil soup, with sliced tofu hot dogs

2 whole wheat dinner rolls

1 cup steamed broccoli

Lettuce, tomato, and mushroom salad, with 1 tablespoon oil-and-vinegar dressing

SNACKS

5 figs

1 cup vanilla soymilk

2 slices raisin bread, with 1 teaspoon margarine

TABLE 10.3 THREE DAYS OF MEALS FOR A LACTO-OVO VEGETARIAN ADULT

Day 1

BREAKFAST
1 cup 7-grain cereal, with 1 cup skim milk
½ cup sliced peaches
Slice whole wheat bread, with 1 teaspoon margarine

LUNCH
1 cup vegetable soup
Bean-spread sandwich (½ cup great-northern-bean spread, with lemon and garlic, 2 slices whole wheat bread)
Sliced tomatoes
Bean sprouts

DINNER
1 cup curried chickpeas
1 cup rice
½ cup broccoli
½ cup cauliflower
1 teaspoon butter

SNACKS
Bran muffin, with 2 tablespoons almond butter
Orange

Day 2

BREAKFAST
1 cup Shredded Wheat, with 1 cup skim milk
2 slices rye bread, with 1 teaspoon margarine
½ cup strawberries

LUNCH
1½ cups vegetable chili, with ½ cup textured vegetable protein (½ cup tomato sauce, ¼ cup chopped green peppers, ¼ cup chopped carrots)
1 cup brown rice
½ cup coleslaw
Corn muffin

DINNER
1 slice chickpea nut loaf
1 cup mashed potatoes, with ¼ cup mushroom gravy
½ cup steamed carrots
1 tablespoon diet margarine

SNACKS
6 ounces apple juice
1 bagel, with 2 tablespoons almond butter

Day 3

BREAKFAST
English muffin, with 2 tablespoons peanut butter
6 ounces orange juice
Coffee

LUNCH
½ cup curried tofu spread, with 2 slices whole wheat bread
1 cup nonfat yogurt, with ½ cup blueberries
1 cup vegetable soup

DINNER
2 green peppers, stuffed with lentil-rice-walnut mixture, topped with 2 tablespoons shredded cheddar cheese
½ cup cauliflower, sautéed in 1 teaspoon olive oil

SNACKS
2 cups popcorn

like muffins or cookies that are prepared with added fats; and from small amounts of processed fats like margarine and vegetable oils that are added to foods. Adults and children who use few high-fat foods might include up to two or three servings of added fat in their diet each day. Added fat really isn't necessary to meet nutrient needs, but it can help some vegetarians to maintain adequate calorie intake. But remember to be conscious of all the fat in your diet or in a child's diet. A serving of French fries or potato chips contains a lot of added fat. Loading up on foods like peanut butter and trail mix will also increase your fat intake.

A serving of fat is small: just one teaspoon. Try to use vegetable oils rather than margarine or butter as much as possible. Where possible, opt for olive oil.

Other Foods

Cheese, eggs, baked products, and snack items can contribute calories and some nutrition to the diet, but they don't earn a place in one of the essential groups of foods. Eat these foods only occasionally. Most of them contribute artery-clogging saturated fat and cholesterol. No more than one serving per day is a good guideline. Adults or teens who are aiming for weight loss might start by eliminating these foods completely.

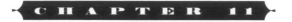
PREGNANCY AND BREAST-FEEDING

*If ever there is a need for simplicity
of diet and special care as to quality, it is
in the prenatal period.*

—ELLEN WHITE, *Counsels on Diet and Foods,* 1926

◆

*Green vegetables, fruits, fresh and
dried and whole grain cereals such as
rolled oats, wheatena, etc should be
liberally used.*

—ALIDA FRANCES PATTEE,
"Diet in Pregnancy" IN *Practical Dietetics,* 1923

◆

Good nutrition is a crucial part of the total health package that will ensure your baby the best start in life. And you'll see here that planning a vegetarian diet for a healthy pregnancy is easy.

FINDING A HEALTH CARE PROVIDER

The most important step you can make for a healthy pregnancy is to see a health care provider right away. It can be a family practice physician, an obstetrician, or a nurse-midwife, as long as he or she is a medical expert in pregnancy. Women who have regular health care visits during pregnancy have the best chance of giving birth to a healthy baby.

But if you are a vegetarian, and especially if you are a vegan, you may run into problems with the very first visit. Your doctor or midwife will probably give you nutrition information about diet during pregnancy, and there is a good chance that the information will center on conventional beliefs about maternal nutrition. That is, you may be told to eat plenty of high-protein meats and to drink as many as four glasses of milk a day. Your health care provider may not be familiar with vegetarian diets.

The material in this chapter can help you get started in planning a healthy vegetarian diet for your pregnancy. In order to address your own specific concerns and questions, you might enlist the help of a registered dietitian (RD). Check the resources section in the back of this book for groups that can refer you to a nutrition professional.

HOW YOUR BABY GROWS

During the 266 days of the average human pregnancy, a single fertilized cell grows into a complex and organized human being consisting of about 200 million cells. It also increases in weight by about a billionfold. Understanding just a little of what takes place during those 9 months can help you to see the crucial role that good nutrition plays in human development.

Pregnancy is usually divided into three trimesters, each of which is three months long. At the very beginning of the first trimester, the fertilized egg begins to divide rapidly, forming a round mass of cells. As the cells divide they travel down one of the Fallopian tubes—the tubes leading from the ovary to the uterus. It takes about two weeks for the cell mass to reach the uterus, where it firmly attaches to the uterine wall.

Beginning with the third week of pregnancy, this mass of cells is called an embryo, from the Greek word for "to swell." At this stage, the cells begin to differentiate—or become different from one another. Cells on the outer part of the mass will become the baby. The inner cells become the placenta. The placenta is central to the well-being of the baby throughout pregnancy because it extracts oxygen and nutrients from the mother's blood and delivers waste products back to the mother's blood for disposal. Nutritionists once believed that the placenta formed a protective layer around the growing baby, guarding it from all harmful substances while letting only oxygen and nutrients through. Now we know that many harmful substances can pass through the placenta to the baby, including alcohol, drugs, nicotine, and caffeine.

By the twentieth day after conception, the embryo is just one-tenth of an inch long and doesn't look even remotely like a baby, but it has a weakly beating heart and is beginning to develop eyes, a spinal cord, a nervous system, lungs, and intestines.

By the third week, the neural tube, which will become the brain and spinal cord, has formed. This is of great significance: failure of the neural tube to close properly can result in a host of common birth defects, including spina bifida. Researchers think that neural-tube defects may be the result of nutrient deficiencies. A lack of the B vitamin folic acid is thought to lead to neural-tube defects.[1] Your health care provider will most likely recommend that you use a folic acid supplement throughout pregnancy. Vegetarian women may have the edge with folic acid intake, since it is abundant in fruits, vegetables, and whole grains.

These important events—formation of the heart and closing of the neural tube—take place before a woman might even know that she is pregnant. Also, at this early stage of pregnancy, some women suffer from nausea that makes it difficult to follow a good diet. For this reason, a woman's prepregnancy diet and her stores of nutrients can be just as important as her diet during pregnancy.

The fourth through eighth weeks of pregnancy are the most critical in all human development. Drugs, alcohol, or extreme malnutrition can disturb the process of development at this point. By the end of eight weeks, the growing baby is no longer an embryo but is called a fetus, a Latin word meaning "young one."

By the end of the first trimester, the fetus has all of its working body systems. Nerves, muscles, and the newly developing bones are coordinated so that the fetus can move its arms and legs even though the whole body is only two and a half inches long.

During the second trimester, the fetus grows rapidly, the skeleton hardens, and some of the finer features like hair and fingernails appear. At the end of sixteen weeks, the fetus is easily recognizable as a human baby, with well-developed facial features, although it is still fewer than five inches long. During this time, most women find that any nausea of early pregnancy begins to ease. They also might notice an increase in appetite, accompanied by some slow but steady weight gain. Increased calorie and nutrient needs become especially important. The growing fetus needs a good supply of all nutrients, especially protein and calcium.

During the last trimester of pregnancy the fetus grows and deposits body fat fairly rapidly. Both poor nutrition and cigarette smoking during the last part of pregnancy can interfere with growth of the fetus. The number of brain cells also is increasing during the third trimester and, in fact, will continue to increase well past birth, until the baby is about eighteen months old. Therefore, adequate protein and generous amounts of all the essential nutrients are important to the baby's future well-being. The lungs mature during this period so that a baby born at the end of the seventh month of pregnancy has a fair chance of survival. By the end of the eighth month, the chance of survival is very good. Generally, the closer to full term the baby is carried, the better.

The growth of the fetus is the exciting part of pregnancy. But many changes take place in the mother's body during pregnancy as well. All of these changes are important for a healthy pregnancy and are supported by good nutrition. For example, the uterus, the organ that houses the fetus, is about the size of a grapefruit at the onset of pregnancy. By the end of the ninth month, of course, it is big enough to hold a seven-pound baby.

The amount of blood circulating in the mother's body increases by about 50 percent. This increased blood volume requires more protein, iron, folic acid, and vitamin B_{12}. Pregnant women also deposit about four to eight extra pounds of fat throughout pregnancy. This is a storage form of calories that will provide energy for labor and delivery and then for breast-feeding.

NUTRITIONAL NEEDS FOR A HEALTHY PREGNANCY

Vegetarian diets can easily meet the needs of pregnant women. Table 11.1 compares the amounts of nutrients needed by pregnant women with the needs of nonpregnant women. It is clear that pregnant women require more of almost all of the essential nutrients. In some cases the needs are just slightly higher, whereas in others they are several times higher. For example, protein needs are only about 20 percent higher, while the need for iron doubles.

While it would seem obvious that a woman needs to eat healthfully in order to produce a healthy baby, people didn't always understand this. For a long time, medical science considered the growing fetus to be a "perfect parasite." That is, it was believed that the fetus would take whatever nutrition it needed from the mother; if any nutritional shortages occurred, the mother was the one who would suffer, not the baby. We know now

PREGNANCY WEIGHT GAIN

• For healthy women over the age of eighteen, ideal weight gain will fall somewhere between twenty-five and thirty-five pounds, although many women have weight gains greater than thirty-five pounds.

• Women who are underweight at the start of their pregnancy should try to gain a little extra, with a recommended range being between twenty-eight and forty pounds.

• Overweight women may need to gain a little less. For some overweight women, a weight gain of fifteen pounds may be enough. Women who are not near their ideal weight at the beginning of pregnancy should consult with their health care provider about a weight gain goal.

• Pregnant teens are still growing themselves, so they need to gain enough weight to support their pregnancy *and* their own growth. A pregnant adolescent might need to gain anywhere from thirty to forty or even forty-five pounds during pregnancy. Again, the teen's health care provider can help to set an appropriate weight gain goal.

• Finally, women who are carrying twins will need to gain extra weight, as much as thirty-five to forty-five pounds, to support the growth of two babies.

that this isn't entirely true. In many cases, nature protects the mother at the expense of the fetus. From a practical standpoint, this makes sense—or at least it did in earlier times of human history. The healthiest baby in the world didn't stand much of a chance if its mother was too sick to take care of it.

Poor nutrition during pregnancy raises the risk of problems in the infant. For example, if a woman restricts her intake of calories during pregnancy, the growth of the fetus will suffer. On the other hand, for some nutrients, the fetus does act a bit like a parasite. If iron intake is low, the mother might show signs of iron-deficiency anemia, but the infant will rarely be anemic at birth.

The goal, of course, is to provide plenty of good nutrition to produce a healthy baby *and* to protect the health of the mother as well. Table 11.2 lists some of the most

important functions of the nutrients during pregnancy. A few of the nutrients deserve special attention in the diets of pregnant women.

Calories

Believe it or not, a pregnant woman needs to consume a total of about eighty thousand extra calories to produce a baby. If that seems a little overwhelming, don't worry. Over the 266 days of pregnancy, that works out to just about three hundred extra calories a day. Eating for two doesn't mean a woman should double her food intake. After all, the second person being fed is a little one. The most important point to remember about the extra three hundred calories is that they should be nutrient dense. Given the small caloric increase and the rather significant increase in nutrients needed during pregnancy, it is important to make sure those calories are packed with good nutrition.

The extra calories a woman eats during pregnancy directly affect weight gain. Weight gain during pregnancy is more closely associated with the chance of having a healthy baby than any other dietary factor.[2] As recently as thirty years ago, women who gained substantial amounts of weight were scolded by their doctors. A healthy weight gain was considered to be about fifteen to eighteen pounds total, or no more than two pounds a month. Health experts now stress that normal-weight women should gain a *minimum* of twenty-five pounds. Actually a woman's weight-gain goal will vary a little, depending on how old she is and how close she is to her ideal weight at the beginning of pregnancy.[3]

All women need to gain weight during pregnancy. No matter what, a net weight loss during pregnancy is taboo. Inadequate weight gain can result in a low-birth-weight baby, which is defined as a baby who weighs less than five and a half pounds. Low birth weight is the single most important cause of illness and death in babies during the first year of life. Statistically, the more weight a woman gains during pregnancy, the larger her baby will be.[4]

The *pattern* of weight gain is just as important as the total amount of weight gained. Most women gain very little weight during the first part of pregnancy. During the first trimester, average weight gain isn't usually much more than two to four pounds over the entire three months of this period. In fact, women who suffer from nausea dur-

ing the first part of the pregnancy might even lose one or two pounds during this time. Beginning with the second trimester, recommended weight gain is about one to one and a half pounds per week.

Although plant-based diets tend to be lower in calories, vegetarian women give birth to normal-weight babies.[5]

Protein

Every cell of the growing fetus contains protein. At birth, the fetus will contain about one pound of protein, and the mother will have deposited another extra pound of protein in her own tissues. But despite the importance of this nutrient, rarely do American women get too little protein. The protein RDA for pregnancy is sixty grams, which is just ten grams more than that for nonpregnant women. Since the average American woman consumes about seventy-five grams of protein a day, most nonpregnant women are consuming more than enough protein to support a pregnancy.[6] Vegetarian women, particularly vegans, eat less protein than omnivores, but most easily consume enough to meet the needs of pregnancy. One study showed that the average vegan woman consumes about sixty-five grams of protein a day.[7]

The food guides in tables 11.3 and 11.4 ensure that pregnant vegetarians consume enough protein. Remember that grains, legumes, soy products, nuts, seeds, and many vegetables are rich in protein.

Vitamin D

Vitamin D helps the body to absorb and use calcium. It's essential for the development of the fetus's bones. Vitamin D recommendations double during pregnancy, increasing from five to ten micrograms a day. Although vegan women typically have low intakes of vitamin D, pregnant vegans can make all the vitamin D they need if they get adequate exposure to sunshine.[8] However, dark-skinned women or those who live in cloudy or smoggy areas or at northern latitudes need extra exposure. A little extra insurance doesn't hurt where vitamin D is concerned. Pregnant vegans can include foods in their diet that are fortified with vitamin D, such as many brands of soymilk or other milk substitutes and some commercial cereals. Check labels to see whether a particular brand is fortified with vitamin D. For women who don't use these products and who are at risk for vitamin D deficiency a supplement might be a good idea. Use supplements only under the supervision of your health care provider, because high doses of vitamin D can be toxic.

Vitamin B12

Many vegans have stores of vitamin B_{12} adequate enough to last for many years. But a couple of studies showed that a fetus may not have access to the vitamin B_{12} stored in the mother's body. The fetus may depend entirely on its mother's intake *during* pregnancy.[9] More recent evidence suggests that this isn't true, at least for breast-feeding.[10] But to be on the safe side, it is important to include a source of vitamin B_{12} in your diet throughout pregnancy.

Pregnant women who eat a lacto-ovo vegetarian diet have no trouble getting plenty of vitamin B_{12}. A cup of milk contains about one microgram of vitamin B_{12}. Vegans who use fortified foods on a regular basis will get plenty of B_{12}. Those who don't use fortified foods need to use a supplement during pregnancy.

Calcium

About thirty grams—or one ounce—of calcium are deposited in a fetus's bones during pregnancy, most of it during the third trimester. A high calcium intake seems to be most important for pregnant women who are under the age of thirty, since the bones of these woman are still growing and depositing calcium.[11] After age twenty-five low calcium intake during pregnancy doesn't seem to affect a woman's risk of eventual osteoporosis.[12]

Pregnant women absorb calcium especially well, and absorption is probably even higher when their calcium intake is low. And, of course, calcium needs may be lower in vegetarians because of their lower protein intake. This is one reason that the recommended calcium intake for pregnant women varies so much from country to country. The amount of calcium needed really depends to a great extent on a woman's overall lifestyle. In some parts of the world six hundred milligrams per day, or just half of the RDA for calcium, are considered enough for a healthy pregnancy.[13]

Vegan women generally have a lower intake of calcium than women who use dairy products.[14] But the relationship of bone health to diet is a complex one, involving protein, calcium, vitamin D, phosphorus, and other nutrients, as well as genetics and exercise. Right now, we really don't know what the exact calcium needs of a pregnant vegan are. Most will probably do well on fewer than the 1,200 milligrams per day specified by the recommended dietary allowance. Until we can say with certainty how much calcium a pregnant vegan needs, we recommend striving for 1,000 to 1,200 milligrams a day by including at least five or six servings of calcium-rich plant foods in the diet. The food guides in tables 11.3 and 11.4 can help pregnant women get plenty of calcium in their diet with or without dairy products.

Iron

Iron needs increase dramatically during pregnancy, since a woman's blood volume increases by about 50 percent. In addition, the fetal blood requires iron, and so does the placenta. The RDA for pregnant women is thirty milligrams a day. Iron supplements are almost always prescribed for pregnant women because it is somewhat difficult to meet needs through diet alone, regardless of the type of diet followed. Recently, however, the belief that *all* women need iron supplements has been questioned, as there is no indication that pregnant women who use supplements are any healthier than those who don't, when the overall diet is healthy.[15]

When iron supplements are used they usually provide between thirty and sixty milligrams of iron a day, with higher doses for women who are already anemic. However, very high doses of iron are not recommended. Iron can interfere with the absorption of other nutrients, most notably zinc. If your health care provider recommends iron supplements, take them between meals with liquids other than milk, tea, or coffee.

It is important to eat an iron-rich diet during pregnancy whether or not you use supplements. Pregnant vegetarian women should try to include an iron-rich food *and* a vitamin C–rich food at every meal.

Women with low blood levels of iron are more likely to give birth to low-birth-weight babies; the babies of these women have a higher rate of infant death. Low iron levels are most often seen in low-income populations. These women are at generally high risk for pregnancy problems for a whole host of reasons. It's difficult to say that the iron deficiency itself is the cause of low birth weight.

However, iron is a concern for all pregnant women. Iron-deficiency anemia is fairly common among pregnant women, although pregnant vegetarians are no more likely to suffer from this deficiency than pregnant women who eat meat.[16]

Zinc

Zinc is important for the formation and growth of all cells in the fetus. The zinc intake of pregnant vegetarians is about equal to that of pregnant meat eaters.[17] But all pregnant women—including meat eaters—may not get enough zinc.[18] Dairy foods can be a significant source of zinc for lacto-ovo vegetarians, although vegetarians may actually get much of their zinc from plant foods. Because zinc from plant foods is less easily absorbed, pregnant women should make an additional effort to include

TABLE 11.1 RDAs for Pregnant Women and Nonpregnant Women

Nutrient	Pregnant	Nonpregnant
Protein	60 grams	50 grams
Vitamin A	800 micrograms	800 micrograms
Vitamin D	10 micrograms	5 micrograms
Vitamin E	10 milligrams	8 milligrams
Vitamin K	65 micrograms	65 micrograms
Vitamin C	70 milligrams	60 milligrams
Thiamine (B_1)	1.5 milligrams	1.1 milligrams
Riboflavin (B_2)	1.6 milligrams	1.3 milligrams
Niacin	17 milligrams	15 milligrams
Vitamin B_6	2.2 milligrams	1.6 milligrams
Folic acid	400 micrograms	180 micrograms
Vitamin B_{12}	2.2 micrograms	2.0 micrograms
Calcium	1,200 milligrams	800 milligrams
Phosphorus	1,200 milligrams	800 milligrams
Magnesium	320 milligrams	280 milligrams
Iron	30 milligrams	15 milligrams
Zinc	15 milligrams	12 milligrams
Iodine	175 micrograms	150 micrograms
Selenium	65 micrograms	55 micrograms

plenty of zinc-rich foods in their diet. Whole grains, legumes, and nuts are good choices.

PREECLAMPSIA

One of the most serious problems of pregnancy is called pregnancy-induced hypertension (PIH), also sometimes referred to as preeclampsia. PIH is actually a set of symptoms that include high blood pressure and the loss of protein in the urine. An early sign of this disease is very rapid weight gain, which is generally due to edema, or excessive water retention. Untreated PIH can lead to convulsions and coma, a condition called toxemia or eclampsia. Low-income women, teenagers, and older mothers-to-be are all at higher risk of developing PIH.

Although the exact cause of PIH isn't understood, there are some interesting observations about its relationship to diet. Some studies show that vegetarians may actually have a lower risk of developing these problems.[19] In a study of women who were strict vegans, only one case of PIH out

Table 11.2 Functions of Nutrients during Pregnancy

Nutrient	Function	Nutrient	Function
Protein	Development of all new tissue in the fetus, formation of the placenta, growth of the uterus, increase in mother's blood volume	Vitamin E	Development of new blood cells
		Vitamin C	Part of cells that hold tissues together, iron absorption
Calcium	Formation of fetal skeleton and teeth	Folic acid	Development of red blood cells, part of enzymes involved in energy production and protein use, crucial role in formation of spinal cord
Phosphorus	Formation of fetal skeleton and teeth		
Iron	Formation of hemoglobin for mother's increased blood volume, formation of fetal blood (Extra iron is stored in the fetus's liver for the first several months of life.)		
		Niacin and riboflavin	Part of enzymes involved in energy production and protein use
Iodine	Formation of hormones for mother's increased metabolic rate	Thiamine	Part of enzymes involved in energy production
Magnesium	Part of enzymes involved in energy production and protein use	Vitamin B_6	Assistance in body's use of protein to build new tissues
Vitamin A	Development of teeth and new cells in the fetus's body	Vitamin B_{12}	Assistance in body's use of protein to build new tissues, formation of new red blood cells
Vitamin D	Formation of skeleton and teeth		

of 775 pregnancies was noted.[20] In the average American population, PIH occurs in about 10 percent of pregnancies.[21]

It is possible that antioxidants in the diet reduce the risk of PIH.[22] Because antioxidants, such as vitamin C and beta-carotene, are found only in plant foods (except for some vitamin C in liver) and are especially high in fruits and vegetables, vegetarians generally have a higher intake of these protective compounds.

MEETING THE NUTRIENT NEEDS OF PREGNANCY ON A VEGETARIAN DIET

We've seen that pregnancy is a time of greatly increased nutritional needs. All pregnant women need to pay attention to their diet in order to make sure they are meeting those needs. Weight gain is especially important, too.

But remember that nutritional science is young. The first vitamins weren't even discovered until this century. While the chance of having a healthy baby is vastly greater today than it was a hundred years ago, the fact is that women have been having healthy babies since the beginning of time. One reason might be that a lot of things work in favor of a healthy pregnancy. Appetite increases during pregnancy. Nutrients are more readily absorbed because the movement of the intestines, which pushes food through, slows down during pregnancy. This gives the body more time to absorb nutrients.

We've provided two sets of guidelines for meeting nutrient needs during pregnancy. The first plan, table 11.3, can be used by either lacto-ovo vegetarians or vegans, though it specifies that vegans should consume four servings a day of a vegetable milk, like fortified soymilk, Vegelicious, or Take Care. This represents a very easy way to meet the elevated calcium needs of pregnancy as well as other nutrient needs. The second guide, table 11.4, is a vegan plan that does not have a milk or milk-alternatives group. Calcium is supplied from a variety of foods in all of the groups. Those who choose to use this guide should be certain that they include five or six good sources of calcium throughout the day. (Remember that calcium-rich foods are printed in italic in the food guide in chapter 10.) This plan requires a bit more attention to food choices, but it may be easier for women who don't use dairy products or dairy substitutes or who find it difficult to drink four glasses of either of these beverages every day. Soymilk, Vegelicious, and Take Care are still options in this plan, but they represent one choice from the legume group and aren't required every day.

These food guides are fairly conventional approaches to planning vegetarian diets, and they are based on foods that vegetarians are likely to enjoy. Bear in mind, however, that they are not the final word in menu planning. There are any number of vegetarian eating patterns that can provide adequate nutrition for pregnancy.

If you find that neither of these eating plans is right for you, and that you have trouble planning meals that you enjoy by using them, you may wish to contact a professional nutritionist to help you plan a healthy diet.

Some guidelines *are* more or less written in stone, however. It is pretty much a given that a healthy diet for pregnancy is going to include generous amounts of vegetables. If you are not a vegetable lover you may want to reread chapter 10 on meal planning for some hints on how to sneak vegetables into your diet. If the four servings of vegetables a day recommended in the food guides seem overwhelming, remember that a serving is just a half cup of cooked vegetables or one cup of raw. Take a look at your half-cup measure, and you'll be reassured that this is not a large amount. A little planning will help, also. Munch on some raw vegetables with lunch every day and then again for an evening snack. For dinner, have a salad and a serving of steamed greens.

Pregnant women who have small children will likely find that they don't have much leisure time to prepare elaborate meals. If morning sickness is a problem, you may not feel like spending much time in the kitchen. The sample menus in this chapter can be adapted to take advantage of fast-food preparation and the use of convenience foods. Use canned beans, prepared soups, mixes for chili, tacos, or vegetarian burgers, and frozen vegetables. Although our menus provide ideas for a wide variety of meals, you can save a lot of cooking time by making use of leftovers as often as possible. Many of the tips for fast meals in chapter 22 will also help pregnant women plan healthy and easy meals.

What about Sweets, Chips, and Treats?

The fact that pregnant women have significantly increased nutrient needs but need only about three hundred extra calories a day means that it is important to choose nutrient-dense foods. These are foods that have lots of good nutrition packed into a moderate number of calories. The problem with foods like sweets and snack chips is not so much that they are unhealthy— although they do tend to be too high in fat—but that they are skimpy on nutrients and can displace other, more nutritious foods in the diet.

But pregnant women can certainly enjoy some special treats. Whenever possible, it is a great idea to make the treats those that just happen to provide some good nutrition. For example, choose roasted soy nuts over potato chips, since the soy nuts provide some calcium. Peach crisp made with fresh peaches and an oatmeal topping, baked

apples stuffed with raisins, walnuts, and cinnamon, and peanut-butter cookies are all good choices.

BREAST-FEEDING

Breast-feeding is a wonderful choice for your newborn infant. The nutrient makeup of breast milk is a close match to the nutrient needs of a baby. Although infant formulas come close to matching those needs, there are some important advantages to breast-feeding. Breast milk contains factors that enhance the baby's immune system so that breast-fed infants are less likely to get illnesses, and breast milk is also very unlikely to cause allergies in babies.

Since breast milk contains all of the nutrients needed to support a rapidly growing infant, the mother's nutritional needs are quite high during the time she is breast-feeding. As during pregnancy, you will need to consume a diet that supports your own nutritional needs as well as those of the rapidly growing infant. Nutritional needs are similar to those for pregnancy. In some cases they are a bit higher. Breast-feeding mothers need an additional five hundred calories per day over their own calorie needs. Calorie needs are high because milk needs to contain enough energy for the infant's growth, and the physiological process of producing milk takes quite a bit of energy.

Breast-feeding mothers also need more vitamin B_{12} and protein than pregnant women, and they need plenty of fluids. Iron needs go down quite a bit, however.

Some women prefer to cut back on calories during breast-feeding so that they can lose any weight they gained during pregnancy. A slightly reduced calorie intake and a *very* gradual weight loss are fine during breast-feeding. However, a significant reduction in calories can reduce the production of milk, so fast weight loss is never recommended for breast-feeding mothers.

Although nutrient needs are high during breast-feeding, studies of women throughout the world show that even when women are malnourished, the quality of their breast milk is quite good.[23] In fact, the levels of some nutrients in breast milk aren't at all affected by the mother's diet.

Other nutrients do reflect the mother's diet, however. They include most of the B vitamins, vitamin D, vitamin C, and vitamin A. Vegetarian mothers generally have breast milk that is nutritionally adequate, and their infants grow normally.[24] Some studies of macrobiotics have found that the breast milk of these women is low in vitamin B_{12}. We mentioned earlier that there is some concern about whether vitamin B_{12} from a woman's stores can reach the fetus. The same may true of breast-feeding. It may be that only the vitamin B_{12} in the mother's diet while she is breast-feeding is available to her infant.[25] Until we know otherwise, it is important that breast-feeding vegan women include a source of vitamin B_{12} in their diet.

Interestingly, the milk of vegan mothers is about 50 percent higher in the mineral selenium than the milk of omnivores.[26] We don't know whether this has any significance or not, but it might give infants added protection against cell damage from oxidation.

Environmental Contaminants in Breast Milk

People living in industrial countries are exposed to a variety of environmental contaminants, including many pesticides and industrial compounds. Because these are fat soluble, the body is very limited in its ability to get rid of them. One of the most significant routes of excretion is through a woman's breast milk. In some cases, breast milk is a very concentrated source of these compounds, and infants are exposed to fairly high levels. The level of contamination varies depending on diet and geography. But the levels in breast milk are commonly high enough that federal law would prohibit its sale as a food for infants.[27] It is estimated that 30 percent of breast milk samples have higher levels of PCBs (toxic industrial by-products) than are considered safe according to the World Health Organization and the Food and Drug Administration. Wisconsin, New York, and the Canadian government have recommended that women have their milk tested for safety.[28]

One of the best ways to protect against contaminants in milk appears to be to eat a vegetarian diet. In a study of twelve women living in a vegan community in Tennessee, all but one had lower levels of seventeen chemicals in their milk compared with the general population. In fact, the highest value seen among these women was still lower than the lowest value seen in the milk of nonvegetarian mothers.[29] In most cases, vegetarian mothers had levels of contaminants that were just 1 to 2 percent of the values seen in nonvegetarians.

TABLE 11.3 FOOD GUIDE 1		
Minimum Daily Servings for Pregnant and Breast-Feeding Lacto-Ovo and Vegan Women		
Food Group	Pregnant	Breast-Feeding
Grains	6	7
Vegetables	4	5
Fruits	4	4
Legumes, nuts, seeds	3	4
Milk or milk alternatives	4	4

See Table 10.1 for serving sizes.

Note: These are minimum numbers of servings. Many women will need to add more servings and/or include some added fats in their diet to meet calorie needs and to support adequate weight gain.

TABLE 11.4 FOOD GUIDE 2		
Minimum Daily Servings for Pregnant and Breast-Feeding Vegan Women		
Food Group	Pregnant	Breast-Feeding
Grains	7	8
Vegetables	4	5
Fruits	4	4
Legumes, nuts, seeds, milks	5	6

See Table 10.1 for serving sizes.

Note: These are minimum numbers of servings. Many women will need to add more servings and/or include some added fats in their diet to meet calorie needs and to support adequate weight gain.

In a study of macrobiotic women, pesticide and PCB levels were lower than in nonvegetarians, even though the macrobiotics lived in an area of high PCB contamination.[30] In this study, the frequency of consumption of meat, dairy products, and fish was directly proportional to milk contamination. Women who had a high consumption of meat and animal fat had more contaminants in their milk.[31]

Some mothers might choose not to breast-feed because of the fear of passing contaminants to their baby. In some cases, when breast milk tests very high for contaminants, this might be the best decision. For most women, however, breast-feeding is always the best choice. But it is clear that babies of vegetarian mothers have a considerable advantage. All women who are pregnant or thinking of becoming pregnant should consider reducing the meat in their diet, especially the use of fatty meats and fatty fish, which are very high in contaminants. We think that there is a clear advantage to following a vegetarian diet if you plan to breast-feed.

TABLE 11.5 SAMPLE MENUS FOR PREGNANT WOMEN

Menus Based on Food Guide 1

Day 1	Day 2	Day 3
BREAKFAST	**BREAKFAST**	**BREAKFAST**
1 cup bran flakes, with 1 cup fortified soy or cow's milk	Fruit shake (1 cup fortified soy or cow's milk, strawberries, banana)	1 cup oatmeal, with chopped apple
½ cup orange juice		½ cup orange juice
Slice toast, with 1 teaspoon margarine	Bran muffin, with 1 tablespoon tahini	Slice toast
		1 cup fortified soy or cow's milk
LUNCH	**LUNCH**	**LUNCH**
1 cup vegetarian chili	Peanut-butter-and-banana sandwich	Whole wheat pita bread, stuffed with ½ cup hummus
1 cup steamed broccoli	1 cup fortified soy or cow's milk	
2 slices whole wheat bread		Tossed salad
Raw carrot sticks	Carrot sticks	1 cup yogurt, with ½ cup fruit
Peach	Apple	
1 cup fortified soy or cow's milk		
DINNER	**DINNER**	**DINNER**
1 cup vegetable soup	1 cup baby lima beans	2 cups pasta primavera, with steamed broccoli and mushrooms
Baked potato	1 cup wheat berries	
1 cup steamed kale	1 cup steamed broccoli	½ cup steamed collards
Slice whole-grain bread	Sliced tomatoes	Slice bread
1 cup fortified soy or cow's milk	Slice bread	1 cup fortified soy or cow's milk
	1 cup fortified soy or cow's milk	½ cup fruit cocktail
SNACKS	**SNACKS**	**SNACKS**
1 cup soy- or cow's-milk yogurt, with ½ cup strawberries	Raw vegetables, with yogurt dip	Orange
Slice bread, with 2 tablespoons tahini	Graham crackers	Milk shake (1 cup fortified soy or cow's milk, flavored with fruit)
Banana	Nectarine	Crackers and peanut butter

TABLE 11.5 SAMPLE MENUS FOR PREGNANT WOMEN (cont.)

Menus Based on Food Guide 2

Day 1

BREAKFAST

1 cup bran flakes, with 1 cup fortified soymilk

½ cup strawberries

Slice toast, with marmalade

LUNCH

2 tomatoes, stuffed with missing-egg salad

Spinach salad

Roll

½ cup fresh fruit cocktail

DINNER

2 slices lentil-tomato loaf

1 cup roasted red potatoes

1 cup steamed collards, sprinkled with wine vinegar

Slice whole wheat bread

SNACKS

Cantaloupe wedge

1 cup soy yogurt, with ¼ cup dates, ¼ cup granola

½ bagel, with 1 tablespoon peanut butter

1 cup fortified soymilk

Day 2

BREAKFAST

1 cup 7-grain cereal

1 cup fortified soymilk

Banana

½ cup orange juice

Slice toast

LUNCH

1 cup bean soup

½ cup steamed asparagus, with herbs

Endive-and-romaine-lettuce salad

Orange wedges

DINNER

1 cup vegetable curry

1 cup brown rice

1 cup steamed kale

½ cup fruit salad

Slice bread

SNACKS

Bran muffin, with 2 tablespoons almond butter

1 cup fortified soymilk shake, flavored with banana

½ cup soynuts

Day 3

BREAKFAST

½ cup scrambled tofu in 1 teaspoon oil

2 slices toast

½ cup fortified orange juice

LUNCH

Peanut butter–sliced apple–raisin sandwich

Carrot sticks

DINNER

1 cup baked beans

Baked sweet potato

Corn bread

1 cup steamed kale

Baked apple

SNACKS

Raw vegetables

Bagel, with 2 tablespoons almond butter

Fresh fruit salad

1 cup fortified soymilk

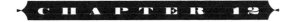
RIGHT FROM THE START: FEEDING VEGETARIAN INFANTS

◆◆◆

*I had the good sense to be born
in a vegetarian family.*

—HELEN NEARING,
Good Food for the Simple Life, 1980

◆

Growth is faster during the first six months of life than during any other period of the life cycle. During that time, an infant's weight more than doubles, and a baby can add as much as eight inches to his or her length. It is interesting to note that the pre-scribed diet for this time of speedy growth is a lacto-vegetarian one. All young infants consume only milk for the first few months of their lives, and their first solid foods are always grains, fruits, and vegetables. So until higher-protein foods are introduced at around eight months, all babies are normally vegetarians.

As we will show you, it is easy enough to keep your baby on a healthy vegetarian diet beyond the first eight months. When it is time to introduce protein-rich foods, you can feed your vegetarian infant mashed beans or tofu, and, if you are a lacto-ovo-vegetarian family, you can also use cottage cheese and egg yolks instead of meat. Otherwise, the rules for feeding vegetarian infants are the same as for feeding omnivore infants. As long as appropriate guidelines are followed—and they are simple ones—vegetarian and vegan infants grow normally.

GROWTH AND DEVELOPMENT OF VEGETARIAN INFANTS

Breast-fed infants of both lacto-ovo-vegetarian and vegan mothers thrive in early infancy.[1] After the age of six months, they continue to grow well as long as they receive adequate breast milk and good sources of iron, vitamin B_{12}, and vitamin D.[2] Infants who are fed either cow's-milk formula or soy formula also grow and develop normally.[3] Infants in vegetarian families may grow at a slightly slower rate, since vegetarian mothers are more likely to breast-feed and breast-fed infants grow more slowly than formula-fed infants.[4] Because breast milk is the preferred food for infants, a slower rate of growth may actually be the natural, healthier growth rate.

Findings from a few studies demonstrate how deficient growth may occur when diets are very restrictive.[5] Rickets, due to lack of vitamin D, and vitamin B_{12} deficiency have been seen in some vegan babies.[6] However, these studies, done in the 1970s, looked at infants on very restrictive macrobiotic diets. These were poorly planned diets that didn't conform to guidelines for healthy vegetarian infant diets. Since that time, macrobiotic teachers have liberalized their diet guidelines for children.[7]

Unfortunately, very few recent studies examine growth and nutrient intake in non-macrobiotic vegan infants. The older studies of infants who were fed very poor diets cannot be used as an argument against well-balanced vegan diets. However, they do indicate that some planning is required so that diets for vegetarian infants include enough calories and protein for growth as well as appropriate amounts of vitamins and minerals. Vegan infants may have slightly higher protein needs than omnivore infants because plant protein is less digestible than animal protein.[8] But, regardless of those needs, it is easy for all vegetarian infants to meet protein needs by adhering to the basic principles of infant feeding.

FEEDING VEGETARIAN INFANTS

The first food for all infants is either breast milk or infant formula. Infant formula is a relatively new option for parents, but it has become a popular one. Today, about 50 percent of all infants are formula fed. Although breast-feeding was on the rise a couple of decades ago, the number of breast-fed infants has fallen off a bit in recent years.[9]

While both breast-feeding and formula feeding are fine for infants, parents should know that there are some clear advantages to breast-feeding. Breast milk contains immunologic factors that help to protect newborns against illness. Breast-fed infants are less likely to have respiratory and gastrointestinal infections, and they also have fewer allergies.[10] Breast-feeding is also a much more economical choice.

Unless the mother is ill, breast-feeding is nearly always possible. It is a good choice for premature babies—although sometimes the breast milk must be pumped and fed to the infant in a bottle. Breast-feeding is also a wonderful option for babies with developmental disabilities, such as Down syndrome. Mothers can breast-feed after a cesarean delivery or if they have had a mastectomy.

For mothers who wish to breast-feed but who must spend time away from their infants, there are several options. Even a month or so of breast-feeding before the mother returns to work offers advantages to a newborn infant, providing some of the immunologic factors in breast milk. Or a mother can pump her breasts and leave refrigerated milk for a baby-sitter to feed to the baby. She can also breast-feed in the morning and evening and offer formula the rest of the day.

Of course, sometimes breast-feeding is not an option. A mother may be on medication that could be passed on to her baby, for example. Adopted babies can't be breast-fed except in very rare instances. In other cases, women are simply not comfortable with breast-feeding. Fortunately, commercial infant formulas are good, nutritious options for babies. Contrary to popular opinion, babies who are formula fed bond perfectly well with their mothers and are not at any psychological disadvantage. In fact, it is probably more important that the feeding experience be a positive one. For mothers who truly do not like the idea of breast-feeding, formula feeding may be the better choice.

Whole, low-fat, and skim cow's milk are *not* good options for infants. In fact, none of these should be fed to an infant during the first year of life. Cow's milk is too high in protein and minerals that can stress infant kidneys.[11] It is also difficult to digest. The protein in cow's milk may cause intestinal bleeding, which can lead to anemia.[12] Cow's milk is also too low in vitamin C, vitamin E, and essential fatty acids for infants. The American Academy of Pediatrics recommends that infants not receive cow's milk for the first year.[13] Goat's milk is also a poor choice. While the protein is more easily digested than that in cow's milk, it is too high in protein and minerals and is deficient in vitamins D, C, B$_{12}$, and folic acid.[14]

Commercial infant formula made from cow's milk is fine for most infants. The protein is treated to make it easier to digest, and the mineral levels are altered to be more appropriate for young babies. It is also fortified with the vitamins and minerals that are missing in plain cow's milk. Some of these formulas are also fortified with iron, since cow's milk is very low in this mineral. Generally, newborn infants don't need any additional iron in their diet until they are about four months old.[15] However, some health professionals recommend using iron-fortified formula right from the beginning.

For infants in vegan families, formulas based on soy protein are free of all animal products. Soy-based formulas can be good choices for infants who are allergic to cow's-milk protein or who are lactose intolerant. Also, there is some concern about the use of cow's-milk formula for infants; a few recent studies have shown that cow's-milk formula raises the risk for diabetes in some infants.[16]

If you choose to feed your baby soy formula, make sure you choose a product that is designed especially for babies. Brand names are Isomil, Prosobee, and Soyalac. (Another infant soy formula, Nursoy, contains some animal fat.) Regular soymilk is *not* an appropriate food for infants.

Some parents choose to make their own formula, since commercial formulas tend to be costly. Homemade formula can be prepared using whole evaporated cow's milk, water, and corn syrup, but we *do not* recommend this. Although the protein in evaporated milk is well digested by infants, the fat is difficult to digest. Homemade formula is also too high in sodium and phosphorus and is low in iron and vitamin C. Babies raised on this formula need special vitamin supplements that breast- or formula-fed infants don't require. Homemade soy preparations should *never* be used for babies. Nor should homemade or commercial nut milks or rice milk. Some parents are not comfortable with commercial formulas because they can't control what goes into these foods. But after breast milk, they really are the only healthy choice for infants.

The only foods that babies should receive in their bottles are infant formula, breast milk, or water. Never feed a baby diluted cereals in the bottle. Babies don't need juices either until they are ready to drink from a cup—around seven months of age. If you decide to discontinue breastfeeding before your baby is one year of age, it is best to switch to an infant formula. At around one year, your baby can start drinking fortified soymilk or whole cow's milk.

Nutrient Supplements

If the mother consumes a vegan diet, it is important to make sure that she is consuming enough vitamin B_{12}. As we noted in chapter 11, there is some evidence that the mother's B_{12} *stores* don't get into breast milk. This means that the mother can have significant B_{12} stores, but her baby can still become deficient. If there is any question about the B_{12} in a vegan mother's diet, then the infant should have B_{12} supplements.

Babies can make their own vitamin D if their hands and face are exposed to the sun for a total of two hours per week or if they are exposed to the sun for thirty minutes per week wearing only a diaper. Frequent exposure for short periods of time is best since this helps to prevent sunburn. However, dark-skinned babies and babies who live in cold climates, especially in urban areas, will need much more exposure to the sun to make adequate vitamin D. If sun exposure is limited, a breast-fed infant should receive supplements beginning at around three months.

Both breast- and formula-fed infants need iron supplements by the age of about four months. Formula-fed infants can be switched to an iron-fortified infant formula. Other ways to introduce more iron into your baby's diet are to begin feeding iron-fortified infant cereals or to provide supplemental iron drops.[17]

Fluoride is recommended for both breast-fed and bottle-fed babies if the water supply is not fluoridated.

Solid Foods for Vegetarian Infants

Parents are often eager to start a new baby on solid foods. First, solid feedings are seen as a happy milestone. Some parents worry that their baby is hungry and that early feeding of solids will help the baby sleep through the night. (It won't.) Also, solid foods seem like such a nice treat. Doesn't that diet of nothing but milk get boring for a baby?

Actually, babies are perfectly content to consume nothing but milk for the first months of their lives. Feeding solids before your baby needs them provides absolutely no advantage. Babies are rarely ready for solid foods before four months of age and often aren't ready until they are six months old. There are a few signs that tell you when a baby is ready for solid foods. Babies will have generally doubled their birth weight. And babies may be demanding more than eight feedings if they are breast-fed or may be drinking more than a quart of formula per day if they are bottle fed. Most infants need the additional calories that solid foods provide by the time they are six months old.[18]

Just as important are some developmental signs. Babies aren't ready for solids until they can hold their head up, sit upright without help, and reach and grab objects while sitting without assistance. They will have lost the extrusion reflex—a reflex to push things out of the mouth with the tongue. They must also be able to swallow diluted solid foods; younger infants can't do so. If an infant chokes or gags with solid foods, it is a clear sign that the baby isn't ready for solids yet.

TABLE 12.1 FOODS FOR YOUR BABY'S FIRST YEAR

There is some overlap in ages and much variation in amounts because babies develop at different rates.

1 to 4–6 months	4 to 6 months	6 to 7 months	7 to 8 months	8 to 9 months	10 to 12 months
Breast milk or infant formula	Breast milk or 3 to 4 cups infant formula 1 tablespoon to ¼ cup iron-fortified cereal	Breast milk or 3 to 4 cups infant formula 2 table-spoons to ½ cup iron-fortified infant cereal 1 to 3 tablespoons mashed or pureed fruits and vegetables	Breast milk or 3 to 4 cups infant formula ¼ to ½ cup iron-fortified infant cereal ¼ slice soft bread 3 table-spoons to ½ cup mashed or pureed fruits and vegetables 1 to 3 table-spoons pro-tein foods 3 ounces juice with vitamin C from a cup	Breast milk or 3 to 4 cups infant formula ¼ to ½ cup iron-fortified infant cereal ¼ to ½ cup mashed or pureed fruits and vegetables 1 to 3 table-spoons pro-tein foods 3 ounces juice with vitamin C from a cup Soft finger foods	Breast milk or 3 cups infant formula ¼ to ¾ cup iron-fortified infant cereal ¼ to ¾ cup soft chopped fruits and vegetables 2 table-spoons to ¼ cup protein foods Mealtime milk or juice in a cup Soft finger foods

There are no set rules about what to offer your baby as a first solid food, but an excellent choice is iron-fortified infant cereal. Nutritionists suggest rice cereal, as it doesn't cause allergies. Mix and dilute the cereal with formula or breast milk. Start with just a few teaspoons a day, and work up to two feedings a day. At that point, you can introduce other cereals, such as iron-fortified infant oat and barley cereals. Introduce one new food at a time, and always wait three days or so between foods. This way, if your baby has an allergic reaction, you'll know which food it is right away.

Once your baby is eating several types of cereal and is consuming a third to a half cup of cereal per day, offer cooked mashed fruits and vegetables, continuing with one new food at a time at three-day intervals. Good choices for infants are smooth applesauce, pureed canned peaches or pears (canned in their own juice without added sugar), potatoes, carrots, sweet potatoes, or green beans. Mashed bananas and avocados are also good early foods and are easy to prepare, since they don't need to be cooked. At seven to eight months, if your baby is learning to drink from a cup, offer fruit juices. Most babies are also ready to explore some higher-protein foods at this point. There are many excellent choices for vegetarian babies. Try thoroughly cooked and pureed legumes or mashed tofu. You can also offer

small amounts of smooth nut butters when your baby reaches his or her first birthday. Babies in lacto-ovo-vegetarian families can have plain yogurt mixed with mashed fruit or blended cottage cheese. You might also introduce your baby to some of the stronger-tasting vegetables at this point. Try mixing steamed, pureed kale with blander additions such as pureed tofu or mashed avocado. You can also use applesauce to sweeten these vegetables.

By ten months your baby will most likely be enjoying finger foods, such as small tofu chunks, crackers, and bread. Frozen bagels are a soothing food for babies to gnaw on when they are teething. Of course, infants need to continue to drink breast milk or infant formula as solid foods are being introduced.

Some parents prefer the convenience of using commercially prepared baby foods. However, these products are expensive and offer limited choices. You won't find jars of pureed tofu, lentils, or kale in the baby food aisle at your grocery store. We suggest making your own baby foods when possible. Begin by removing skins, seeds, and any stringy portions from fruits and vegetables. Cook the foods, then puree them in the blender, adding small amounts of cooking liquid to reach a smooth consistency. Be sure to cook beans very well—you may need to press the pureed beans through a sieve to remove the skins.

You can purchase a small, portable food mill, which is especially nice for travel or eating out. It allows you to prepare baby food right at the table in any restaurant that will provide you with a serving of steamed vegetables.

Baby foods can be frozen in two-tablespoon portions in ice-cube trays, or you can keep foods for up to two days in the refrigerator. Use only fresh or frozen vegetables, since canned foods are high in sodium. There is no need to add either salt or sugar to the baby foods you prepare. While plain, unflavored foods may seem bland to you, your baby will be perfectly happy with them.

You can also make your own baby cereals by grinding uncooked rice or oats to a fine powder and then cooking them well in plenty of water. If you aren't using iron-fortified commercial baby cereals, make sure that your baby is receiving another good source of iron—either iron-fortified formula or a supplement in the form of iron drops.

ALLERGIES

Between 4 and 6 percent of babies develop allergies to one or more foods.[20] Symptoms of allergies can include coughing, wheezing, runny noses, skin rashes, diarrhea, and vomiting.

About one or two out of every one hundred infants is allergic to cow's-milk protein (although some researchers have found that it could be as many seven out of every one hundred babies).[21] Allergic babies can be switched to either a soy-based formula or to a special formula with predigested cow's-milk protein. Since soy formulas can also cause allergies in sensitive babies, some physicians think that allergic babies should be switched right to the special predigested formulas.[22] However, the number of cow's-milk sensitive infants who are also allergic to soy protein is somewhere between 15 and 50 percent, so soy formula can still be a good option for many babies.[23] Trying soy formula is probably worthwhile because the special allergy formulas are very expensive. The special formulas for allergic babies are also not vegan. This is another reason that breast-feeding is the best choice in vegan families. If a formula-fed baby develops a sensitivity to soy formula, there are no other vegan formula options.

Infants who are allergic to cow's milk are often allergic to other foods. Vegetarian foods likely to cause problems include eggs, nuts, peas, chocolate, citrus fruit, corn products, soy products, and wheat.[24] If your baby is allergic to a food, keep that food out of the diet for at least a year. Food sensitivities often disappear by one or two years of age.

Breast-fed infants are much less likely to develop allergies. However, breast-fed infants can show adverse reactions to food components in the mother's diet that are passed on to the baby through the milk. For example, if a breast-feeding mother drinks cow's milk, the protein can cause symptoms in her baby.[25] Other foods that might cause discomfort or problems in breast-fed infants include coffee, chocolate, cabbage and other gas-producing vegetables, onions, beans, and chili. Of course, it is probably a minority of babies who react to foods in the mother's diet. Breast-feeding mothers don't need to be too particular about their diet unless there is a specific problem.

HEALTHY VEGETARIAN BABIES

You're likely to hear some criticism of your decision to feed your baby a meatless diet. Everyone loves to give advice about feeding and raising babies; unfortunately, most people don't know much about vegetarian diets for infants. Sometimes, even family doctors have concerns about vegetarianism for babies. But the growth and good health of vegetarian babies is good evidence that a meatless diet is a perfect choice for these youngest family members.

To ensure your baby the best start in life, a healthy vegetarian diet is easy to plan when you keep in mind the following simple guidelines:

• Choose either breast milk from a well-nourished mother or an infant formula.

• Use appropriate supplements (iron, vitamin D, and perhaps vitamin B_{12}) as prescribed by your pediatrician.

• Introduce iron-fortified infant cereal when your baby is developmentally ready, usually between four and six months.

• Gradually offer other solid foods, including pureed fruits, vegetables, beans, tofu, nut butters, and cottage cheese as tolerated and enjoyed by your baby.

It's as simple as that to give your baby a great start to a healthy life.

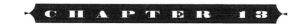

VEGETARIAN CHILDREN

Meats should be fed sparingly all the early years of childhood, not only on account of their over stimulation, but because they create a distaste for the cereals and vegetables which are essential for the child's growth.

—*The Ann Arbor Cookbook,* 1904

It would be wonderful if, left to their own devices, children always chose healthy foods—but they don't. Children do need some guidance from adults in making food choices. Guidance doesn't mean hovering, though. In fact, once your child gets to be about two years old, he or she will certainly have developed strong opinions about different foods and will want to have some say about food choices. We suggest the following approaches to developing good eating habits in children:

- Plan meals to include healthy foods that your child enjoys.

- Introduce new foods frequently, but casually, so that your child is exposed to a wide variety of foods without feeling threatened by strange and unappealing ones.

- Keep your kitchen well stocked with healthy foods. Turn your child loose for snacks so that he or she has some control over food choices, but in an environment that you create.

That's childhood-feeding theory in a nutshell. While these guidelines are certainly helpful, they won't solve all childhood eating problems. Children can be picky eaters, and parents sometimes have to do some pretty fancy footwork to get healthy foods into a preschooler.

Growth is fairly erratic during childhood, but, in general, it slows down quite a bit after the growth spurt of infancy. A child's eating behavior will mirror this to some extent. Parents who sometimes feel that their preschooler lives on next to nothing should find it reassuring that the very slow growth of these preschool years is generally accompanied by a decrease in appetite. This, along with a surge of independence that is so typical of preschoolers, can create real struggles at mealtime.

Parents can rest assured that no toddler or preschooler will willfully starve to death. Food jags—like the week your child wants only peanut-butter-and-jelly sandwiches for breakfast, lunch, and dinner—may be exasperating, but are essentially harmless. Eating behavior tends to improve with age.

So if you faithfully introduce a variety of healthy foods, your child should enjoy a good selection of vegetarian foods by the school years.

Vegetarian diets are great choices for children. Children who are raised in vegetarian homes are exposed to healthy foods and have a better chance of learning to enjoy meals that are low in fat and rich in fiber. While some people might challenge your decision to raise your child as a vegetarian, including such experts on child health as your pediatrician, vegetarian children who receive well-balanced diets do grow and develop normally.

Any diet carries its own risks of nutritional problems when it is thoughtlessly or poorly planned. When parents raise children on omnivore diets, they must take great care that the diet is not too high in fat, saturated fat, and cholesterol, since those are abundant in many animal foods. Too many fatty foods like meat, milk, eggs, and cheese can produce lifelong health problems. Omnivore children have low intakes of a number of nutrients, including calcium, iron, and vitamin B6.[1] Parents of vegetarian children also need to give extra attention to meeting some nutrient needs in the diet. This is easily accomplished by varying and expanding food choices.

Growth in Vegetarian Children

We run into the same problems in evaluating the impact of vegetarian diets on the growth of children that we noted in chapter 12. Many studies of vegan children are older studies and are based upon vegetarians who ate very restricted and unhealthy diets. Today's parent has access to a greater amount of information on planning vegetarian diets. And vegetarian children can include in their diets a wide array of nutrient-rich foods, such as fortified soymilk, fortified meat analogues, nut and seed butters, soy yogurt, and flavored tofu products. Achieving adequate nutrient intake for vegetarian children today is simply easier.

When poor growth is observed in vegan children, it is most often seen in macrobiotic populations.[2] Restrictions on the use of added fats, oils, and nut butters in some macrobiotic diets may impact the growth of very young children.[3] We consider moderate amounts of fats and nut or seed products to be important components of the diet for many vegetarian children. Eliminating these foods can reduce calorie intake and can jeopardize growth.

Several studies of both vegan and lacto-ovo-vegetarian children show that they grow at rates similar to nonvegetarian children.[4] In one study of Seventh-day Adventist school-age children, vegetarians were actually somewhat taller than their classmates.[5]

A study of British vegan toddlers and preschoolers showed that they were as tall as omnivores but were slightly lighter.[6] In a study of American vegans between the ages of four months and ten years, vegetarian children were slightly shorter than the average American child. However, this difference in heights decreased with age, and by age ten the vegetarians were only about one-third inch smaller than omnivores.[7] It is doubtful that small differences in height have any real meaning; they are certainly not harmful. Since taller adults are at higher risk for some cancers, there may even be an advantage to slightly smaller stature.[8]

Vegetarian children clearly enjoy some health benefits over their meat-eating counterparts. Vegetarian children consume less cholesterol and fat and more fiber than nonvegetarian children,[9] and they also eat more fruits and vegetables.[10] They are slimmer and have lower cholesterol levels than average nonvegetarian American children.[11] Some nutritionists have been concerned about the effects of reduced fat intake in children. However, as long as calories are sufficient, a lower fat intake doesn't affect growth. For instance, children consuming a 27-percent-fat diet grew just as well as those consuming a 38-percent-fat diet in one study.[12] The U.S. government's National Cholesterol Education Program recommends that all children over the age of two years should consume 30 percent or less of their calories as fat.[13] Since the development of atherosclerosis begins in childhood, the lower fat intake of vegetarian children is an important health advantage. Of course, some fat is important in children's diets to help ensure adequate calories. You'll see that our meal-planning guidelines for vegetarian children (table 13.2) include some fat-rich nuts or seeds and other foods that contain moderate amounts of fat.

Finally, for anyone who still believes that meat increases brain power, one comparison of vegetarian and nonvegetarian children showed the vegetarians to be above average in mental development.[14]

MEETING THE NUTRIENT NEEDS OF VEGETARIAN CHILDREN

Compared with adults, children have much higher nutrient needs on a body-weight basis. But an easier way to understand their nutrient needs is to compare them with their calorie needs. This is a concept called nutrient density. Nutrient density compares the amount of nutrients in a food with the number of calories in that food. A higher ratio of nutrients to calories is usually desirable. Toddlers, aged one to three years, need almost three times more *calories* for each pound of body weight than an adult, but they need only one and a half times more *protein* per pound. This means that they actually need a less protein-dense diet than adults do. On the other hand, they need six times more iron than adults. So a young child needs a diet that is very iron dense.

Children's nutrient needs are highest for vitamin D, iron, calcium, and zinc, when we look at those needs on a per calorie basis. Other nutrients of special interest in the diets of vegetarian children are protein, vitamin B_{12}, and riboflavin. We'll look briefly at how these nutrient needs are met by vegetarian children before discussing the specific guidelines and tips for feeding vegetarian children.

Protein

Lacto-ovo-vegetarian and vegan children have no problems meeting protein needs.[15] Protein needs go hand in hand with calorie intake. So make sure your child is eating enough food in general—not just enough high-protein food. When calories are inadequate, protein needs go up. Although you may think that we've put the protein-combining theory forever to rest, we have to bring it up again here. Some experts in protein nutrition believe that there may be some advantage to combining proteins for very young children.[16]

We noted previously that children need diets that are less protein dense than adults do. So why would children need to worry about protein combining when adults don't? The reason is that children have much higher needs for specific amino acids. We know that this can immediately raise a lot of concerns for parents. The idea of protein combining conjures up images of measuring foods and carefully following a chart of food combinations.

It doesn't have to be at all that complicated. It isn't necessary to measure foods and to analyze each meal to make sure it contains a protein combination. A basic rule is to serve several different foods at each meal. The chance that some of those foods are a good protein match is likely. Most children will consume some type of grain (bread, cereal, crackers, rice, or pasta) at most of their meals and snacks. If that meal also includes a legume, nut, seed, or dairy product, such as soymilk, beans, peanut butter, tahini, or cow's milk, then your child is receiving complementary proteins. Also, while a soy product in the diet (tofu, soymilk, tempeh, textured vegetable protein) will enhance the protein in other foods, soyfoods are very rich in high-quality protein even when consumed alone. Finally, any need to combine proteins may be somewhat diminished because young children eat so frequently. A child who eats three meals and two or three snacks per day will be eating every three hours or so. In that short time, foods eaten at one meal should easily combine with foods eaten at the next meal.

We think that most parents unconsciously serve complementary proteins to their toddlers and preschoolers throughout the day. It may not be true at every single meal, but it doesn't have to be. In fact, because protein combining just happens in the lives of most vegetarians, we don't think that parents should be at all concerned about this aspect of feeding vegetarian children. However, parents of vegetarian children should realize that children do utilize nutrients differently from adults. A variety of protein-rich foods is important in the diets of all vegetarians; it is even more so for vegetarian children.

While we encourage vegetarian parents to make sure their child is getting adequate protein, we also urge you to not be overly concerned about this. When children consume adequate calories, eat frequently throughout the day, and consume a variety of foods, protein deficiency is virtually nonexistent.

Calcium

Children have very high calcium needs relative to the calories they eat. Some studies show that vegan children consume less calcium than omnivores or lacto-ovo-vegetarian children.[17] Again, most of the studies that show this are twenty years old and limited to macrobiotic populations. Today's vegan child is likely to consume more calcium. Adequate calcium intake is very important for young children, since the heavier and denser that bones are to begin with, the less the risk of osteoporosis later in life.

Vegan children may, in fact, have better calcium utilization than omnivore children because their diet is free of animal protein. As we saw in chapter 7 animal protein can cause increased calcium loss. Although this effect has been documented only in adults, it is also likely to occur in children. However, we recommend that children consume the RDA of eight hundred milligrams until there is firm evidence that they need less. Calcium-rich foods that appeal to many children include figs, calcium-fortified orange juice, oranges, tofu, baked beans, raw broccoli, almond butter, tahini, fortified soymilk, Vegelicious, Take Care, and cow's milk. See chapter 7 for a more extensive list of foods that are high in calcium.

Vitamin D

Vitamin D is crucial for bone formation in children. Its lack produces rickets in young children, causing weak, stunted bone growth. Rickets has occurred in some macrobiotic children who weren't receiving supplements or using fortified foods.[18] Children should be able to make plenty of vitamin D in their skin from sun exposure.[19] For light-skinned children in relatively sunny climates, exposing the hands and face to the sun for twenty to thirty minutes, two or three times per week, should be enough. However, dietary sources of vitamin D are good insurance, especially for children who are dark skinned or who live in northern urban areas, where sun exposure is limited by geography and smog.

Cow's milk in the United States is fortified with vitamin D, so lacto-ovo vegetarians will usually consume considerable amounts of this nutrient. (See chapter 8 for a cautionary note about the vitamin D content of cow's milk, however.) Eggs also contain vitamin D. Vegans can consume plenty of this nutrient by using fortified soymilks, cereals, and meat analogues. Be sure to read labels, though, since fortification varies from product to product. If vegan children are not using any of these fortified products and if there is any question about whether they are getting enough sun exposure, a vitamin D supplement of five micrograms per day is a good idea.

Vitamin B12

Lacto-ovo-vegetarian children seem to get plenty of vitamin B_{12}.[20] However, adequate B_{12} is certainly an issue for vegan children. It's an easily resolved one, however, because a number of vegan foods that children enjoy are fortified with this nutrient. Some brands of fortified soymilk contain B_{12}—but not all of them, so be sure to read the label. Red Star nutritional yeast labeled T-6635+ is the only one that is a reliable source of B_{12}. Mix it into pasta and tomato sauce for children or sprinkle it on popcorn. Many commercial breakfast cereals and meat analogues are also B_{12} fortified. Children who follow strict vegan diets and who don't use fortified foods absolutely must have a B_{12} supplement.

Iron

Iron-deficiency anemia is the most common nutritional deficiency in the United States.[21]

It is most likely to occur between the ages of eighteen and twenty-four months, and it can affect children regardless of the kind of diet they eat—omnivore, lacto-ovo-vegetarian, or vegan. The iron content of vegetarian diets is typically high. Lacto-ovo-vegetarian children may have the disadvantage here, since milk contains no iron and often displaces other iron-rich foods. Soymilk, Vegelicious, and Take Care are all good sources of iron.

Iron is abundant in plant foods and is found in many foods that children enjoy. Toddlers should continue to eat iron-fortified infant cereals until they are eighteen months old. Make sure children eat plenty of whole or enriched grains, iron-fortified cereal, soy products, dried fruits, beans, and nuts. Serve good sources of vitamin C to your child frequently because vitamin C increases iron absorption. Good combinations of iron-rich and vitamin C–rich foods for children are spaghetti with tomato sauce, oatmeal and orange juice, fruit salad with raisins, soymilk-and-strawberry shake. Some foods, such as spinach, greens, broccoli, and watermelon, are high in both vitamin C and iron.

Zinc

There is very little information about zinc in the diets of vegetarian children. Vegetarian foods that contain zinc include dairy products—especially hard cheeses—whole grains, wheat germ, fortified cereals, nuts, and vegetables. However, phytate and fiber in some cereals may reduce zinc availability. Restricting the fiber somewhat in your child's diet can enhance zinc absorption.

You can do this by serving some refined grains like white rice, pearled barley, and muffins made with unbleached white flour.

Good sources of zinc for children include bran cereals, oatmeal, wheat germ, peas, legumes, tofu, textured vegetable protein, nuts, and seeds.

Riboflavin

Riboflavin is needed for the production of energy, so it is important for overall growth in children. Cow's milk is very high in riboflavin and usually provides enough of this vitamin for lacto-ovo-vegetarian children. Although fortified soymilk is generally low in riboflavin, other fortified milks like Take Care and Vegelicious are excellent sources. Other riboflavin-rich foods that may appeal to children are enriched and whole grains, almonds, almond butter, and avocados. Leafy green vegetables and mushrooms are good sources, although it may be difficult to get very young children to eat enough of these foods to contribute much riboflavin.

GUIDELINES FOR MEAL PLANNING FOR VEGETARIAN CHILDREN

Vegetarian children need the same foods that vegetarian adults do: grains, legumes, vegetables, and fruits. We also recommend that vegetarian children, toddlers through teens, consume a nutrient-rich "milk." For a variety of reasons, we think the best choice is a soymilk or other vegetable milk that is fortified with calcium, vitamin D, and vitamin B_{12}.

Some nutritionists recommend that a fortified infant soy formula be continued

TABLE 13.1 FORTIFIED SOY AND VEGETABLE MILKS

SOY AND VEGETABLE MILKS FORTIFIED WITH CALCIUM, VITAMIN D, AND VITAMIN B_{12}

Edensoy Extra (Eden Foods)
Sno-E soymilk (A and A Amazing Foods)
Soyagen (Loma Linda Foods)
Take Care (Nutritious Foods, Inc.)
Vegelicious (Abersold Foods)

SOY AND VEGETABLE MILKS FORTIFIED WITH CALCIUM AND VITAMIN B_{12}

Better Than Milk (Sovex Natural Foods)

SOY AND VEGETABLE MILKS FORTIFIED WITH CALCIUM AND VITAMIN D

Pacific Select and Pacific Rice Milk (Pacific Foods of Oregon)
Rice Dream, fortified (Imagine Foods)
Westsoy Plus (Westbrae)

---

until vegan children are two years old. Of course, breast milk is a good choice also. Many children receive breast milk well into their second year. Children in lacto-ovo-vegetarian families can begin consuming whole cow's milk after their first birthday. If your family drinks cow's-milk products, you might also introduce children to soymilk at a young age. This helps them expand their food preferences and provides additional iron in the diet. Nut milks and unfortified soymilks are fine for occasional use in children's diets, but they don't provide as much nutrition as fortified products.

Not only are milks good sources of many nutrients, but because they can be used in so many ways, they make it easy to get these nutrients into children. We don't mean to imply, however, that this is the only way for children to meet nutrient needs. In other cultures, children do well on diets that don't include substantial servings of milks. However, they are also likely to eat a greater variety of nutrient-rich plant foods that are less common in this country. If your family prefers not to use any of these milks, you can still plan healthy diets for children. Just make sure that they are getting plenty of calcium, vitamin D, and vitamin B_{12} from other foods. The food lists in chapters 7 and 8 can help.

As is true for adults, a child's diet should be based on grains. Try to include a few servings of whole grain or enriched bread as part of those grain servings. Children who eat bread tend to have good iron status—although many grains and other foods actually provide more iron than bread does.[22]

We also recommend a daily serving of nuts or seeds (or nut or seed butter) for children, as they are an appealing source of minerals such as zinc and manganese. Because children need slightly more fat in their diets

TABLE 13.2 MEAL-PLANNING GUIDELINES FOR CHILDREN

	1–4 years	5–6 years	7–12 years
Grains	4 servings	6 servings	7 servings
Leafy green vegetables	2–4 tablespoons	¼ cup	1 serving
Other vegetables	¼–½ cup	¼–½ cup	3 servings
Fruits	¾–1½ cups	1–2 cups	3 servings
Legumes	¼–½ cup	½–1 cup	2 servings
Nuts and Seeds	1–2 tablespoons	1–2 tablespoons	1 serving
Fortified soy or vegetable, cow's, or breast milk	3 cups	3 cups	3 cups
Fats	3 teaspoons	4 teaspoons	5 teaspoons
Nutritional yeast (Red Star T-6635+) and blackstrap molasses	Use frequently to flavor dishes		

than adults do, these higher fat foods can be used on a daily basis. To make sure that children are getting enough calories, you might include some added fat in the form of oil or margarine. Remember, though, that this fat can come from commercial baked goods like muffins as well as from fats used in cooking.

Finally, a few supplemental items can really boost the nutrient intake of children. Nutritional yeast is abundant in a host of nutrients. Choose Red Star brand T-6635+, which is rich in vitamin B_{12}. Other brands of nutritional yeast tend to be variable in the amount of B_{12} they contain. Blackstrap molasses is one of the few sweeteners that is also nutritious. One tablespoon provides nearly 140 milligrams of calcium and more than three milligrams of iron. Children don't need to have nutritional yeast and blackstrap molasses on a daily basis but do flavor

dishes with these items often to boost your child's intake of both calcium and iron.

The food guide in table 13.2 follows the meal-planning guidelines for adults that are found in chapter 10. Amounts for children are, of course, much smaller. For toddlers and preschoolers we've sometimes specified amounts of foods rather than number of servings, since some amounts are measured in tablespoons. For older children, serving sizes are identical to those noted in the meal-planning guidelines for adults in chapter 10.

Note that we often give a range of intake for younger children. Children grow at different rates, so that your two-year-old may eat less than your neighbor's two-year-old. In another couple of months, just the opposite may be true. Remember, too, that these are guidelines, not laws. Do strive for the minimum amounts we've suggested here.

But it isn't the end of the world if a child has only two cups of soymilk one day or turns down everything but spaghetti for a week. What counts is a variety of nutrient-rich foods most days over the long term.

A Word About Fat in the Diets of Children

Over the past several years there has been much legitimate concern about the fact that American children eat too much fat and have cholesterol levels that are too high. In response to this, among some health professionals there is a trend toward encouraging very low-fat diets for children. These diets are about 10 to 15 percent fat.

These low-fat diets are considerably more healthy than the diets consumed by the average American child. However, there is no evidence that they are any healthier than a vegan or lacto-ovo-vegetarian diet that derives 20 to 25 percent of calories from fat and that is very low in saturated fat and cholesterol. We don't think that there is any reason to recommend elimination of all high-fat foods and added fats from a vegetarian diet for children—or for adults for that matter. For children in the two-to-five-year-old age range, some higher-fat foods can provide an important way to meet calorie and nutrient needs. These include soymilk, tofu, nuts, seeds, and very small amounts of added fats.

But this doesn't mean we are encouraging a free-for-all with fatty foods for vegetarian children. The average vegan adult consumes a diet that is about 30 percent fat, and we can assume that vegan diets of children are comparable. This may very well be an acceptable amount of fat in a diet that contains no cholesterol and very little saturated fat, but we would still rather see adult vegans reduce their fat intake to 20 percent or so of calories. In our guidelines for children in table 13.2, we've aimed for diets that are 20 to 25 percent fat; the guidelines for preschoolers and toddlers are a bit higher. If your child grows well on a diet that is lower in fat than what we've specified and is eating enough food to meet nutrient needs, there is absolutely nothing wrong with a lower-fat menu. However, there is also no reason to recommend a lower fat intake for children than what we have recommended here.

Parents in lacto-ovo families should remember that eggs and dairy foods offer quite a bit of saturated fat. We recommend the use of nonfat or low-fat milk only for children over the age of two and suggest limiting cheese, other dairy foods, and eggs to very occasional use. In all vegetarian families, it is wise to limit the use of processed, prepared foods and baked goods, which can be very high in saturated fats and trans fatty acids.

Getting Children to Eat Healthy Vegetarian Foods

In writing this chapter, we asked for input from vegetarian parents about what their vegetarian kids like to eat or don't like to eat and what kinds of problems they've experienced. As we expected, there is simply no typical vegetarian child. Eating habits vary a lot from child to child. Since young children generally like blander-tasting foods, you might expect that tofu would be a hit with children. For the most part it isn't. At least plain tofu doesn't seem to appeal to many vegetarian children. However, studies at Southern Illinois University show that familiar dishes like macaroni and cheese, tuna casserole, and quiche with tofu blended in were very popular with preschoolers—even more popular than the original versions of these dishes.[23]

We did hear surprising accounts of children who thoroughly enjoy spicy bean burritos, steamed kale, and other stronger-tasting foods. It's a good idea to keep an open mind about foods for children. Perhaps your child will defy conventional wisdom by adoring all of the foods that other parents struggle to include in their child's diet. Children can be very surprising in their food likes and dislikes. The following sections offer some suggestions for encouraging children to eat healthy foods and to eat appropriate amounts of those foods. None will work for every child, but many might work for yours.

Getting Enough Calories

Small children have small stomachs, but they need a lot of nutrients and calories to grow. A pattern of three meals a day is not likely to satisfy a toddler's or preschooler's nutrient and calorie needs. Snacks are important for young children. People often have a negative image of snacking, since snack foods are often junk foods. Think of snacks as "mini-meals" that include smaller amounts of the same nutritious foods that you serve your child at mealtime. Some good snack ideas for vegetarian children include:

Apple muffin with soy or cow's milk

Fruit milk shake

Vegetable soup and crackers

Graham crackers with nut butter

Trail mix

Graham crackers with juice

Bananas rolled in chopped peanuts, raisins, or chocolate sprinkles and then frozen

Frozen juice bars

Dried fruits

Nonfat or low-fat soy- or cow's-milk yogurt mixed with fruit or applesauce

Celery sticks stuffed with peanut butter

Because fiber is so filling, a diet too high in roughage can fill a small child up before he or she has consumed enough calories. Consider peeling apples and other fruits to cut down on fiber and to make them more appealing to children. Don't be afraid to give your child some refined foods. Some hot and cold cereals, fruit juices, muffins made with white flour, applesauce, and white rice are all examples of refined products that are healthy and nutritious. A steady diet of these foods can make the diet too low in fiber, but for young children—and for all people—as long as whole foods play a central role in the diet, some refined products are perfectly acceptable. In the case of young children, these foods can help them meet calorie needs.

Include higher-calorie foods in your child's diet as often as possible. Some good choices are legume spreads, peanut butter–tofu spread, nut butters, avocado either in child-sized chunks or as a spread on bread, and dried-fruit spreads. To make dried-fruit spreads, blend ¼ cup of dried fruit with 1 to 1½ tablespoons of water in a blender. This makes a nice, sweet topping for toast or bread for a toddler or preschooler. To make peanut butter–tofu spread, put equal amounts of smooth peanut butter and soft tofu in a blender and blend until smooth. Don't overly restrict the fat in diets of toddlers and preschoolers. Higher-fat foods like nuts, seeds, and soy products can help a child to meet calorie needs.

Smaller serving sizes can also help to foster better appetites in small children. A plate piled high with food can be overwhelming and can blunt a child's appetite. A rule of thumb for toddlers and preschoolers is to serve one tablespoon of each food for each year of age. More is fine, of course, if your child is hungry.

Too Much of a Good Thing

Some children prefer a lactarian diet. That is, all they want is milk. For children who drink cow's milk, this can be a particular problem, since cow's milk contains virtually no iron. It can displace iron-rich foods from the diet. Overdependence on cow's milk is one reason for the iron deficiency that is so common between the ages of eighteen and twenty-four months. Soymilk is higher in iron, but, even so, children who drink too much of it can miss out on other nutritious foods and end up with a diet that is unbalanced.

If your child is drinking from a bottle, switching to a cup will certainly slow him down. If too much milk is a problem, offer soymilk or cow's milk with meals but offer only water or juice with snacks and only water for between meals if a child is thirsty.

Children love juice. While fruit juice is a nutritious beverage, it is extremely high in sugar. It can be very filling for a small child and can also feed a preference for sweets. Given a choice, most young children will nearly always choose juice to quench their thirst. Limit juice to a half to one cup per day for small children. Diluting it with extra water is also a good idea.

Getting Children to Eat Beans and Vegetables

Children really are natural vegetarians. Very young children often don't care for the tough (especially to them) texture of meat. Many parents in omnivore households complain that they can't get toddlers and preschoolers to eat meat.

But that doesn't mean that all children love all plant foods. Most children do well with a variety of grains and fruits. Nuts and nut butters are also pretty appealing. But getting children to eat and enjoy a wide variety of vegetables and legumes can be a challenge. It helps to serve these foods often, in a variety of guises, and to make them fun. Here are a few tips for getting young children to eat and enjoy new foods:

• Very young children like foods that are easy to eat. Finger foods are especially appealing. Cut vegetables into strips, steam them gently, and serve them as finger food.

• Make salads in the shape of animals and other favorite characters using raw vegetables and fruits. Try a Raggedy Ann salad using a pear half for the body, banana or zucchini slices for limbs, a mound of missing-egg salad or cottage cheese decorated with raisins for a face, and shredded carrots for hair.

• Raw vegetables are much milder than cooked ones. Preschoolers who reject cooked vegetables may be likely to accept a raw version of the very same vegetable. Offer small pieces of raw vegetables with dips made from tofu or cottage cheese.

• Experiment with "fun" vegetables. Some children will get a kick out of baby vegetables, like inch-long zucchini, baby carrots, and cherry tomatoes. Arrange these on a skewer and let older children roast them over the backyard grill (with supervision, of course).

• Introduce your child to new foods frequently. If a food is rejected, serve it again in a few weeks. Always serve new foods along with ones that are familiar and well liked. Don't make a big deal if your child doesn't want to try the new food or doesn't like it. Nagging, cajoling, and bribing will rarely help to change your child's mind and may discourage him or her from trying the food again in the future. Food dislikes and eating behavior problems are more likely to persist if a great deal of attention is paid to them.

• Add tofu or soymilk to puddings and milk shakes. Pancakes made with soymilk and shaped like animals are good snacks for children.

• When children really balk at vegetables, you might dress them up with a sauce of peanut butter diluted with water and perhaps flavored with some orange juice concentrate. Try diluting the strong taste of kale, collards, and other greens by blending them with a bland ingredient such as tofu, avocado, or ricotta cheese.

• Keep mealtime pleasant. Children eat best when they are well rested, undistracted, and happy.

• Let children participate in meal preparation. Younger children have limited culinary skills, but they can toss handfuls of chopped vegetables into a salad or raisins into muffin batter. As they get older, they can shell peas or tear up lettuce. Older school-age children can chop vegetables and follow a recipe. Children are likely to have more interest in eating a meal if they had a hand in making it.

• For children who are extremely picky about vegetables, sneak some into well-liked dishes. Greens can be very finely shredded and mixed into spaghetti sauce. Finely chopped vegetables can be added to nut or bean loaves or burgers. Shred carrots or zucchini into muffins, or make pumpkin or winter-squash muffins.

• Grow a garden for children. Let them have their own little patch of vegetables and strawberries. They'll feel pride and enjoy eating foods they grew themselves. Foods that are easy to grow and that children are likely to enjoy are strawberries, beans, lettuce, and carrots. Child-sized gardens can be planted in a sandbox, a plastic swimming pool, or even in pots on a balcony.

• Create interest in new foods by giving a child the facts behind the food. Older children may be intrigued by tofu if they know that it is a dietary staple of Chinese children. Plan special international nights to make new foods more fun. Serve a Chinese stir-fry with chopsticks to older children.

Setting Good Food Examples for Children

Parents and older siblings are the most important role models for children who are learning new food habits. On television and outside of the home they are likely to see adults enjoying Big Macs, fried chicken, and ice cream. It's important that they see you enjoying healthy and fun vegetarian foods. They won't like *everything* you like, but they will be positively influenced if they see you eating and enjoying healthy foods.

The same goes for the folks at day care or preschool. They have considerable influence on the children in their care and have an obligation to create positive attitudes toward healthy foods. You'll be very lucky if you can find a vegetarian day-care situation for your child. At the very least, look for one where healthy food is served and enjoyed, where some lunches and snacks are vegetarian, and where the provider has a thorough understanding of which foods you don't want your child to eat. People who are unfamiliar with vegetarian diets are more than likely to serve a tuna-fish sandwich to your vegetarian preschooler or egg salad to your vegan toddler. If you are unsure about what your child is getting to eat, it might be a good idea to pack lunches and snacks yourself.

Young children who watch television are an advertiser's dream. Very young children can't distinguish between regular programming and commercials and are fascinated by the upbeat, fast-paced nature of advertisements aimed at kids. They are sure to want all of the sugary cereals, fast-food meals (with toys), and frozen desserts shaped like cartoon characters that they see on television. Because young children are so impressionable, it is a good idea to guard them from as many commercials as possible. One way is to stick to videos during TV time for children.

Desserts

Humans have an inherent taste for sugar, so it is no surprise that children love sweets. In earliest times, this sweet tooth probably served an important nutritional purpose by attracting our ancestors to vitamin C–rich fruits. Today, sugar is abundant in our diet. Because it is added to so many foods and because we are exposed to so many highly sweetened foods, our sensitivity to sugar has probably decreased so that we like sweeter and sweeter foods. Many new products on the market boast "no sugar" on the label. That means they contain no white sugar. But they might be chock-full of honey, maple syrup, malted barley, or fruit juice concentrates—all of which are aliases for "sugar."

While sugar isn't exactly a health food, it probably gets a worse rap than it deserves. Contrary to popular opinion, it doesn't cause hyperactivity. The real health problem associated with sugar is that it leads to tooth decay. Another problem is that when kids fill up on sugar's empty calories, they may not have room for other more nutritious foods. And they may not appreciate the more subtle, pleasant tastes of other foods like whole fruits, lightly sweetened muffins, and unsweetened cereals.

Desserts and sweets can have a role in a healthy diet. Choose items that are lower in fat and sugar and that include healthy ingredients. Consider serving dessert as part of the main meal so that it doesn't earn a place as the special part of the meal. Good choices for desserts include apple crisp, pumpkin pie, rice pudding, bread pudding, zucchini bread, zucchini pancakes with applesauce, and frozen juice bars. A variety of vegan baked goods can be prepared from recipes that call for eggs and dairy. Use soymilk in place of the milk and one of the egg replacers (see page 313) in place of the eggs.

ON THEIR OWN

Most eating problems are resolved by the age of six or so. Quirky food jags have played out, and children are likely to have expanded their food likes and to be open to trying more new foods. It seems like it's time for the vegetarian parent to breathe a sigh of relief—just in time for your child to head out the door to the danger-ous world of school lunches, birthday parties at McDonald's and overnights at friends' homes with hot dogs, pepperoni pizza, and ice cream. Children who have gone to preschool may already be savvy to the ways of the meat-eating world. But for others, the school years may be their first exposure to the fact that most people eat meat.

Vegetarian parents have a few things to worry about when they send their children out the door. Will their vegetarian habits follow them? A hungry vegan child at a birthday party may be unwilling to pass up the ice-cream cake. A vegetarian toddler is unlikely to be too analytical about the tuna-fish sandwich served to him for lunch.

Second, how will your child feel about his or her different eating habits? Being singled out as different is not attractive to the average schoolchild.

For some children, this is simply not an issue. Children who live in urban areas or college towns may find that they are one of several vegetarians in their class. Also, a vegetarian diet is increasingly seen as "cool" among younger people. More and more, there is a sense of pride among even very young children about their vegetarian diet. Some parents say that their children have a strong sense of ethics regarding a vegetarian diet and the wrongness of killing animals. They won't consider eating meat. This may be more true when the child has been raised as a vegetarian or at least has been a vegetarian since a very young age and when parents talk to the child about the reasons their family doesn't eat meat.

But some parents find that there can still be problems. Children in strictly vegan families might receive "special foods" in the classroom when birthday treats are served or have to bring their own food to a birthday party. Some children don't mind. Others might feel uncomfortable.

Parents can take a variety of approaches. None is right or wrong. Some parents insist on vegetarianism for their young children 100 percent of the time—at least to the extent that they have control over this. There is some value to that kind of consistency. Children can be confused if they believe that things that are wrong inside the home are allowed outside the home. And for those who feel that this is too inflexible, it helps to remember that most families have inflexible rules about something, depending on their particular values.

Other parents feel that some circumstances are too difficult for children. Also, because vegan diets in particular are so far from the mainstream, some parents fear that a rigid approach can invite rebellion in children. This is probably more true when the children grew up on an omnivore diet and recently converted to vegetarianism or when the family is vegan and the child is faced with a party with nonvegan goodies. Families need to find their own comfort zone. You might send your child to a party with his or her own supply of vegetarian hot dogs and tofu ice cream, but let the birthday cake slide. Every parent has to decide where to set limits for his or her family.

Nearly all vegetarian parents agree that there comes a time when they simply don't have control over every morsel that goes into their child's mouth and when it becomes appropriate for a child to have some say in these decisions. The prevailing opinion is that children are apt to make the right choice when parents do three things: set a good example, let children know why the family is vegetarian, and let the child have some say in what is consumed outside the home. Happily, some parents have noted that even though children might complain about not eating meat, they don't choose it when given the chance.

There are other problems that vegetarian parents face. Your own parents may be unhappy that their grandchildren are not eating meat; they're likely to be positively aghast if they aren't receiving milk and eggs. After all, meat and dairy represent an entire half of the basic food groups that they raised you on. Grandparents and other family members may hinder your efforts to raise your family as vegetarians by feeding animal foods to your children when they are in their care. In many cases it is simply because they are worried about your child's health. In other cases, grandparents may react poorly to your decision to raise your children as vegetarians because it is perceived as a rejection of their values.

It helps if you can assure family members that a vegetarian diet is a healthy choice for children. Perhaps this chapter can help. You might also order a copy of the American Dietetic Association pamphlet *Eating Well the Vegetarian Way* (free by calling 800-366-1655), which includes a statement about the healthfulness of vegetarian diets for children.

Reassure your parents that this isn't a rejection of the way they raised you. Your decision is based on newer and better scientific information than what was available thirty years ago. You might also involve your parents by enlisting their assistance and taking advantage of their experience and wisdom. How did *they* get *you* to eat vegetables? Did they suffer over two-year-old picky eating habits and food jags?

SCHOOL LUNCH

Will your child ever get hummus, tofu tacos, and other vegetarian meals through the school-lunch program? Probably not. A little history of the school-lunch program helps to show why school lunches continue to stay off the menu for vegetarian and other health-conscious families.

The National School Lunch Program (NSLP) was started in the 1940s as an outgrowth of the food programs of the Depression of the 1930s. Its aim was to provide low-cost, nutritious meals to hungry children. Today, at a cost of $4.7 billion, the NSLP serves 25 million students per day and is critically important to low-income children. Schools that participate in this program are bound by law to serve meals that provide a third of the RDA for protein and for several other nutrients. The NSLP is successful in providing nutrients; however, excessive fat, saturated fat, cholesterol, and a lack of fiber are persistent problems with school lunch. And, of importance to readers of this book, vegetarian meals are few and far between in the school-lunch program. Vegan meals are virtually nonexistent.

The NSLP is administered by the United States Department of Agriculture. According to USDA surveys, school lunches are on average 37 percent fat and 15 percent saturated fat. Children who eat school lunches have higher-fat diets than children who don't.[24]

High-fat diets are a critical childhood problem. An estimated 36 percent of American children have cholesterol levels that are too high, and 15 percent of adolescents are overweight.[25] The American Heart Association notes that one in five adolescents and one in twelve children have blood pressure levels that are too high.[26]

A number of factors work against healthy school lunches. School food-service directors must maintain an incredible balancing act in planning these meals. They need to administer cafeteria budgets that keep them in the black, develop menus that provide adequate levels of certain nutrients as mandated by the USDA, and, finally, they must provide meals that children will eat. Since childhood tastes in this country run toward burgers and tacos, those are the kinds of meals often seen along the cafeteria line.

But one of the biggest problems of school lunches is that they depend on $3 to $4 billion worth of surplus foods donated each year by the USDA. Meals are planned around these foods, which constitute 20 to 30 percent of the food served in school lunches and which are most likely to include eggs, high-fat cheese, butter, ground pork and beef, and whole milk. In fact, legislation passed in 1986 requires schools to offer whole milk, because farmers make more money from the sale of whole milk than from the sale of low-fat milk.

While the school-lunch program provides much-needed nutrition to some children, it

BROWN-BAG LUNCHES FOR CHILDREN

SANDWICH IDEAS

Pita stuffed with hummus spread, chopped tomatoes, and lettuce*

Shredded carrots with almond butter or peanut butter

Fluffy peanut-butter spreads (try peanut butter blended with tofu, ricotta cheese, or pureed dried fruits)

Missing-egg salad*

Avocado blended with chopped or shredded raw veggies, topped with alfalfa sprouts

Peanut butter mixed with crushed pineapple and raisins

Notuna salad*

Submarine sandwich with cheese, lettuce, tomatoes, and other sliced vegetables

Cheese with sliced apples

ON THE SIDE

Fresh fruit

Raw carrots, celery, and zucchini strips

Trail mix

Rice cakes

Carrot-and-raisin salad

BEVERAGES

Individual containers of soymilk, almond milk, or rice milk

Juice

TREATS

Cookies cut in animal shapes or decorated for a holiday

Cupcakes baked in ice-cream cones instead of muffin cups

Oatmeal cookies

Homemade mini–fruit pies

KEEP IT COLD

If a portable lunch includes perishable ingredients (such as tofu, bean spread, or soft cheeses) include a small ice pack. You can also freeze a small container of juice. It should keep the meal cold but defrost in time for lunch.

Recipe included in recipe section of this book.

does so through extremely unhealthy meals. And it does so largely because of USDA support of animal agriculture. While child health may be a motivator for those who administer the school-lunch program, it clearly is not a factor in USDA decisions about which foods to donate to the program.

In addition, the way that meals have been evaluated for nutritional adequacy has been problematic. For example, the USDA persists in not allowing tofu to be served as a protein food, despite recommendations by the American Dietetic Association as long ago as 1986 that this food be allowed and despite the consensus of opinion of protein experts that soy protein is equal in quality to meat and dairy protein.[27] Some school districts with a high percentage of Asian students would find tofu to be a popular school-lunch item. Also, the USDA evaluates meals based on servings from specific food groups. For example, school lunches must include milk. A better way to evaluate a meal would be to specify that it include a particular amount of calcium, since many foods other than milk provide calcium.

In late 1993, the USDA held nationwide hearings on the school-lunch program. People from nutrition programs, child-advocacy programs, and the food industry, as well as concerned parents, testified. Some recommendations made to the USDA included:

• Place upper limits on the amounts of fat, saturated fat, and cholesterol in school lunches.

• Require that more whole grains be served.

• Change the agricultural commodity programs so that healthier foods are donated to school-lunch programs.

• Repeal requirements that whole milk be offered in cafeterias.

• Allow soyfoods such as tofu to be used in some meals in place of meat.

• Evaluate school meals based on nutrient content—not on a set number of servings from specific food groups.

• Make more fresh fruits and vegetables available to school-lunch programs.

• Eliminate fruits and vegetables that have added fat.

It is reasonable to expect that some changes will occur in the school-lunch program over the next several years. In fact, some changes are already being set in motion. Several schools are part of a USDA program that will allow meals to be evaluated on the basis of their nutrient composition—not whether they include foods from certain food groups. This will make it easier to fit nonmeat items into menus. But we are a long way from changes that will be extensive enough to satisfy health-conscious parents and certainly not vegetarian parents. Right now, while there are occasional vegetarian offerings on the school-lunch menu, they are usually the fatty, cheesy kind.

Parents of vegetarian children have a few options. The easiest, of course, is to brown-bag it. See the sidebar "Brown-Bag Lunches for Children" for ideas.

You can also send your child to a school where fewer restrictions exist for school meals. Private schools are a good option for parents who worry about their child being the only vegetarian in the class. The Montessori and Waldorf schools are more supportive of healthy eating and are more likely to offer vegetarian meals in cafeterias than are the public schools. Seventh-day Adventist schools that do have cafeterias offer only vegetarian foods. And as many as 50 percent of the students in these schools are likely to be vegetarian.

HEALTHY VEGETARIAN CHILDREN

Feeding children takes extra care and consideration—whether they are vegetarian or not. Parents of vegetarian children may need to pay extra attention to food sources of some nutrients, such as calcium, zinc, and vitamins D and B$_{12}$. At the same time, your child's diet is likely to be lower in fat and cholesterol and especially rich in vitamin C, beta-carotene, and other nutrients. There is a special reward in knowing that your child has a better chance of avoiding chronic disease later in life because of the vegetarian food you serve in your home today.

TABLE 13.3 SAMPLE MEAL PLANS FOR VEGETARIAN CHILDREN

Vegan Plan for Toddlers and Preschoolers, Ages 1 to 4 years

BREAKFAST
½ cup Cheerios
½ cup fortified soymilk
½ banana

SNACK
Frozen juice bar

LUNCH
2 to 4 tablespoons tofu spread (tofu mashed with eggless mayonnaise)
4 whole-grain crackers
1 cup fortified soymilk
¼ to ½ cup strawberries
Carrot sticks

SNACK
½ English muffin, with ½ to 1 tablespoon almond butter
1 cup fortified soymilk

DINNER
½ cup soup, with ¼ cup beans and ¼ cup macaroni
2 to 4 tablespoons steamed kale, braised in 1 teaspoon oil
¼ to ½ cup watermelon cubes
¼ cup peas

SNACK
½ slice oatmeal bread, with ½ to 1 tablespoon tahini
½ cup fortified soymilk

Lacto-Ovo-Vegetarian Plan for Toddlers and Preschoolers, Ages 1 to 4 Years

BREAKFAST
Pancake, with 1 teaspoon margarine
2 to 4 tablespoons applesauce
1 cup 2% or whole milk

SNACK
¼ to ½ cup cantaloupe chunks

LUNCH
½ cup cheese ravioli with tomato sauce
2 to 4 tablespoons spinach, braised in 1 teaspoon oil
½ slice bread, with 1 teaspoon margarine
¼ to ½ cup orange juice

SNACK
Soymilk shake (1 cup soymilk, ¼ cup strawberries)

DINNER
½ tofu hot dog, with ½ hot-dog roll
¼ cup raw zucchini chunks
1 cup 2% or whole milk

SNACK
2 saltine crackers, with 1 or 2 tablespoons peanut butter

TABLE 13.3 SAMPLE MEAL PLANS FOR VEGETARIAN CHILDREN (cont.)

Vegan Plan for 5- and 6-year-olds

BREAKFAST

Slice vegan French toast, cooked in 1 teaspoon oil

½ cup applesauce

1 cup fortified soymilk

SNACK

Carrot sticks

Apple slices

LUNCH

Pureed-peanut-butter-and-tofu sandwich (1 tablespoon peanut butter, 2 ounces tofu, banana slices, 2 slices whole wheat bread)

Peach

1 cup fortified soymilk

SNACK

Zucchini muffin, with 1 tablespoon almond butter

1 cup fortified soymilk

DINNER

½ cup baked beans

¼ cup steamed kale, with 1 teaspoon margarine

½ cup white rice

Frozen juice bar

SNACK

½ bagel, with 2 tablespoons apricot spread

Lacto-Ovo-Vegetarian Plan for 5- and 6-year-olds

BREAKFAST

½ cup bran flakes, with 1 cup skim milk

½ cup orange juice

SNACK

2 tablespoons raisins

2 tablespoons peanuts

LUNCH

½ pita stuffed with ¼ cup hummus and sliced tomato

Kiwifruit

Oatmeal cookie

½ cup skim or 2% milk

SNACK

1 cup Vegelicious

4 graham crackers

DINNER

½ bean burrito

¼ cup spinach

Apple slices

¼ cup green beans, braised in 1 teaspoon margarine

SNACK

½ bagel

½ cup 2% milk

TABLE 13.3 SAMPLE MEAL PLANS FOR VEGETARIAN CHILDREN (cont.)

Vegan Plan for 7- to 10-year-olds

BREAKFAST

¾ cup oatmeal, with ¼ cup raisins, 1 cup fortified soymilk

Slice toast, with 1 teaspoon margarine

SNACK

Frozen bananas

LUNCH

Pita bread stuffed with missing-egg salad (4 ounces tofu, 2 teaspoons eggless mayonnaise, and tomato slices)

3 apricots

2 graham crackers

4 ounces apple juice

SNACK

2 oatmeal cookies

1 cup fortified soymilk

DINNER

1½ cups quinoa, black beans, and corn, sautéed in 1 teaspoon oil

½ cup broccoli

Slice whole wheat bread, with 1 teaspoon margarine

Tossed salad, with 2 tablespoons tahini dressing

1 cup fortified soymilk

SNACK

2 cups popcorn, cooked in 1 teaspoon oil

Lacto-Ovo-Vegetarian Plan for 7- to 10-year-olds

BREAKFAST

¾ cup 7-grain cereal, with 1 cup soymilk

½ cup sliced peaches

½ bagel, with 1 teaspoon margarine

SNACK

5 vanilla wafers

½ cup watermelon chunks

LUNCH

Cheese sandwich (1 ounce American cheese, lettuce, tomato, 2 slices whole wheat bread)

Carrot salad (½ cup shredded carrots, 2 tablespoons peanuts, 2 tablespoons raisins, 2 teaspoons mayonnaise)

1 cup 2% milk

SNACK

4 saltine crackers, with 2 tablespoons peanut butter

1 cup skim milk

DINNER

Vegetable stir-fry (¼ cup tofu, ¼ cup broccoli, ¼ cup carrots, ½ cup brown rice)

Salad (leaf lettuce, tomatoes, chopped carrots), with 2 tablespoons French dressing

½ cup grapes

SNACK

¼ cup soy nuts

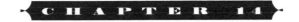

VEGETARIAN NUTRITION
FOR TEENAGERS

◆◆◆

*A plain, rigid, yet bountiful diet is
of itself a means of education that may
fortify the young person against the great
tempter who in later life usually
approaches him through the stomach.*

— *The Ann Arbor Cookbook, 1904*

◆

Vegetarianism is especially popular among teenagers. Parents are sometimes concerned about their vegetarian teens, since nutrient needs are high at this time, and teenagers are making many of their own food choices. But vegetarianism can be a very positive and healthy choice for teenagers.

The teenage years are a time of very rapid growth—faster than at any other time except for infancy. All nutrient needs are greater than they were during childhood. Needs go up dramatically for calories, protein, calcium, and, for girls, iron. Although most teens easily meet calorie and protein needs, many, vegetarian or not, may fall short for calcium and iron.

Unfortunately, we don't have much information about the eating habits of vegetarian teens. We do know that among average American teenagers, diets are generally too high in fat from favorite foods like hamburgers, pizza, snack chips, and sweets. The average teenager eats a diet high in fat and sugar and low in fiber and complex carbohydrates.[1] Obesity is a significant problem among American teenagers. Approximately 15 percent of American teens are overweight.[2] Teen diets are also low in a number of important nutrients, including folic acid, calcium, iron, vitamin B6, and magnesium.[3]

Vegetarian teens may have the nutritional edge. Those who were raised in vegetarian families are likely to be familiar with a wide array of whole foods that are rich in nutrients and lower in fat than meat and dairy products. Teens who are avoiding burgers and fried chicken at fast-food outlets are setting the stage for a lifetime of eating habits that will lower their risk for cancer and heart disease. Because these diets help to establish optimal eating habits, we believe that vegetarianism is an excellent choice for adolescents.

Teens who are new to vegetarianism, especially those who do not live in vegetarian families, are at some disadvantage. They may be largely unfamiliar with whole grains, leafy green vegetables, and beans. And if parents are unwilling to take an interest in their vegetarian diet, they are on their own for meal planning. But for teenagers who are willing to follow some very flexible guidelines and to explore new foods, meeting nutrient needs is really quite simple.

◆◆◆

GROWTH OF VEGETARIAN TEENS

Growth during adolescence is nothing short of phenomenal. During the two- to three-year growth spurt of the average adolescent male, a boy can add ten inches to his height. Nearly half of the total adult skeleton is created during adolescence, although bones continue to grow throughout the twenties. The average teenager also experiences a 50 percent increase in weight. However, because growth is erratic, it is very difficult to pin down nutrient needs at any one time. During the actual growth spurt, nutrient needs can be twice as high for protein, calcium, and iron.[4]

Boys grow faster and for a longer time than do girls. They also gain considerably more muscle mass than girls, who tend to gain more fat. For this reason, teenage boys need more iron, zinc, and protein than girls. They may need more calcium at certain times also, although that need isn't reflected in the RDAs.[5]

Fortunately, teens' appetites increase considerably when they are growing fastest. This almost guarantees adequate calories and protein in healthy teens. Calorie needs are actually quite high compared with nutrient needs, which makes it somewhat easier to get adequate nutrition.

The few studies that have been done on the growth of vegetarian teenagers show that there is little difference in growth between vegetarians and nonvegetarians. In a study of 1,800 children between the ages of seven and eighteen, lacto-ovo-vegetarian children and adolescents were slightly taller than nonvegetarian children.[6] This finding was especially interesting because the nonvegetarians in the study were from southern California, where children are somewhat taller than average.

One exception was that eleven- and twelve-year-old vegetarian girls were a little bit shorter than their nonvegetarian peers. This isn't at all surprising, since vegetarian girls tend to mature later and therefore have a later growth spurt. One study of Seventh-day Adventists shows that vegetarian girls have a later menarche—or onset of menstruation—than nonvegetarian girls.[7] This later development for girls is probably a health advantage, as a later age of menarche is associated with a lower risk of breast cancer later in life.[8]

NUTRIENTS FOR SPECIAL CONSIDERATION IN TEENAGE DIETS

Although the needs for all nutrients increase during adolescence, teens do have one particular advantage: they tend to be hungry and therefore they eat more. This is especially true of teenage boys, since girls may sometimes restrict calories to control their weight. Unfortunately, teenagers are notorious for making poor food choices. But when healthy foods are included in the diet, it is relatively easy for all adolescents to meet nutrient needs. A few areas require special consideration in the diets of all teenagers: calories, calcium, iron, vitamin B_{12}, and zinc.

Calories
On a body-weight basis, teens actually need about 50 percent more calories than adults. Teens who skip meals—a common practice

in adolescence—or who diet for weight loss can have trouble meeting calorie needs. Of course, much of what we know about adolescent health belies this concern. American teens tend to ingest too many calories or to be too inactive, and obesity is a common problem of adolescence.

Vegetarian teenagers who have trouble meeting energy needs can include some high-calorie foods in their diet, such as milk shakes, nuts, nut butters spread on toast or bagels, and trail mix made with dried fruit and nuts. As is true for adults, however, adolescents should not emphasize fatty foods. Our meal-planning guidelines (table 14.1) describe a diet that is about 20 percent fat, with most or all of the fat from plant sources, so that cholesterol and saturated fat are kept low. Several studies indicate that teenagers in developed countries, including the United States, exhibit the earliest stages of artery disease; that is, they already are forming plaques in their arteries, which can eventually lead to heart disease.[9] Lacto-ovo vegetarians in particular who depend on cheese and other high-fat dairy products for many of their meals can end up consuming diets that are too high in saturated fat and cholesterol. A healthy teenage diet should be low in fat. As long as teens are eating enough calories to maintain appropriate growth and development, low-fat diets are fine for teenagers.

To meet calorie needs, teenagers probably need to eat more frequently. Three meals a day plus several snacks is a good pattern for most teens.

Calcium

For teenagers, the RDA for calcium is 1,200 milligrams per day. Some health experts believe the need is even higher—as high as 1,600 milligrams per day. But in other parts of the world, recommendations for calcium are as low as 650 to 700 milligrams per day. As we noted in chapter 7, calcium needs vary, depending on many factors.

Including cow's milk in the diet doesn't automatically ensure adequate calcium intake. Some surveys indicate that omnivore American teens generally don't meet requirements for this nutrient.[10] In addition, omnivore teens are likely to have high intakes of animal protein and sodium, which can raise calcium needs. But we don't have studies on the effects of protein on calcium during the growth years. Studies exist only for adults who are not growing. Until we have a clear indication that vegetarian teens need less calcium, we recommend that American vegetarian teenagers strive to consume 1,200 milligrams of calcium per day.

Fortunately, a high calcium intake is very easily achieved on a plant-based diet. We recommend continued use of three cups of fortified soymilk or fortified vegetable milks throughout the teenage years as excellent sources of many nutrients for adolescents. Teens should include other calcium-rich plant foods in addition to soymilk in their diet. Vegan teenagers who don't drink three cups of soymilk a day need to place even greater emphasis on other calcium-rich plant foods in their diet, such as tahini, almond butter, greens, figs, and tofu. Calcium-fortified orange juice is another good choice, and it is well liked by most teenagers.

Lacto-ovo-vegetarian teens need to be careful of overdependence on dairy products to meet calcium needs. Dairy foods are lacking in iron, a problem nutrient for teenage girls in particular. And when whole or 2 percent milk, cheese, and other high-fat dairy products are used, a teenager's diet can become too high in saturated fat and cholesterol. Therefore, even lacto-ovo-vegetarian teens should consider including some fortified soymilk or other plant sources of calcium in their diet.

Iron

Iron deficiency is a common nutritional problem among teens, especially among teenage girls. Girls have higher iron needs than boys, since they begin to lose significant amounts of iron through menstruation. And because teenage girls consume less food than teenage boys (they eat between three hundred and eight hundred fewer calories), they need a diet that is rather iron dense. But teenage boys need to pay attention to iron also, as their needs are higher than an adult's. There is no evidence that vegetarian teens are any more or less likely to be iron deficient than teens who eat meat. Again, lacto-ovo-vegetarian teens who have exceptionally high dairy intake may be at some disadvantage because these foods are so low in iron.

Teenage boys need twelve milligrams of iron a day, and girls need fifteen. These needs can be met with very little effort, as long as a few good sources of iron are included in the diet every day. For example, a cup of bran flakes provides twelve milligrams of iron, three-fourths cup of instant oatmeal provides six to eight milligrams (although whole oats provide much less), and a slice of bread provides about one milligram. As is true at other stages of the life cycle, vegetarian teens can make the best use of the iron in their foods by consuming a source of vitamin C along with iron-rich foods.

Vitamin B12

A teenager's need for vitamin B_{12} is 50 percent higher than that for young children. Lacto-ovo vegetarians who consume at least two servings of dairy foods a day will easily meet those needs. Vegan teens must make a special effort to include B_{12}-rich foods in their diets. Many brands of soymilk are fortified with this nutrient. Other foods that are especially appealing to teens are fortified breakfast cereals and some meat analogues. If a teenager doesn't use these foods on a daily basis, a vitamin B_{12} supplement is imperative.

Zinc

Zinc is of special importance in adolescence, since it is crucial in both growth and sexual maturation. High levels of protein and phosphorus, both common in the diets of omnivores, may raise zinc needs.[11] Since vegetarian diets are lower in these nutrients, vegetarian teens may have lower zinc requirements. But absorption of zinc from plant foods is also lower, so all teens need to include good sources of this nutrient in their meals. Three cups of soymilk per day provide 24 percent of a teenage boy's zinc requirement and more than 30 percent of a teenage girl's. But the zinc in soymilk seems to be absorbed poorly, so the actual contribution to zinc intake might not be that significant. The zinc in other types of vegetable milks might be absorbed better. The zinc in cow's milk is absorbed better, but the quantity is much lower. Other good sources of zinc include legumes (particularly adzuki beans, vegetarian baked beans, refried beans, and black-eyed peas), oatmeal, bran flakes, nuts, and leafy green vegetables. If teens aren't consuming several servings a day of foods that are very rich in zinc, then a zinc supplement might be a good idea. Because high doses of one mineral can affect the absorption of others, we don't recommend taking supplements that contain more than the RDA for zinc.

Teenagers can follow the same general guidelines for meal planning that we've outlined for adults. They will need more servings from each of the food groups, but serving sizes are the same as those in chapter 10. There is a great deal of flexibility here. The amount of

TABLE 14.1 MEAL-PLANNING GUIDELINES FOR TEENAGERS

Food Group	Number of Servings per Day
Grains, breads, cereals	10–12
Leafy green vegetables	1 or 2
Other vegetables	3–4
Fruits	4–6
Legumes	2 or 3
Nuts and seeds	1
Fortified soymilk, Vegelicious, Take Care, or cow's milk	3
Fats	4–6

food that teens eat will vary, depending on where they are in their growth spurt, the amount of physical activity engaged in, and the teen's body size. Teenage girls can aim for the lower number of servings in food groups where we give a range, and boys can aim for the higher number.

MEALS ON THE GO FOR TEENAGERS

With school, extracurricular events, and social activities, teens can be busy people. Skipping meals, snacking, and eating at restaurants are all typical teenage eating habits. We've noted that teens should eat frequently—at least three meals a day, plus snacks. Obviously some of these meals are going to be consumed away from home or eaten on the go. Parents can help by making sure that the kitchen is stocked with healthy foods that teenagers can grab and eat as they are headed out the door.

Breakfasts that are fast and portable are

especially important, as many teens skip breakfast because they don't have time in the morning. Fast breakfasts or snacks include muffins, individual containers of yogurt, frozen or leftover pizza that can be heated in the microwave or toaster oven, fruit-flavored milk shakes with soymilk or cow's milk, hummus in pita bread, bagels with peanut butter, and peanut-butter-and-banana sandwiches.

VEGETARIAN TEENS ON THEIR OWN

Children raised in vegetarian families might be tempted to stray from that vegetarian pattern once they arrive at their teenage years. Adolescence is a time to express independence from parents and family, and food is an attractive way to do this. Because fitting in with peers is important to teenagers, and food plays a big role in teenage social activities, some adolescents might be tempted to shed vegetarian habits in order to be an active part of their social group. Teens might also simply be curious about foods that their friends eat and that they have never tasted.

We have no studies to show us what happens to vegetarian children as they enter the teenage years—though we do have individual reports from vegetarian families. It's a safe guess that some teens may completely reject their family's vegetarianism. But this is likely to be less and less true as vegetarianism becomes more popular among teens. Also, children who are raised in families in which vegetarianism is a strong part of the family's values (regardless of the reasons) may be more likely to adhere to a meatless diet. Even if they choose to experiment a bit during their adolescent years, there is proba-

bly a good chance that they will remain vegetarian over the long run.

At the very least, children raised in vegetarian households are likely to be more familiar with a wide variety of healthy plant foods and to have more extensive food likes among these health-promoting foods. This should serve them well as they head out the door to make their own food decisions.

TEENS IN A NONVEGETARIAN HOUSEHOLD

During the teenage years, we see an interesting—and we think exciting—phenomenon. Many teens are choosing vegetarianism even though their families eat meat. Of course, many parents do not find it particularly exciting when their teenage son or daughter announces that he or she has gone meatless. Suddenly, you are faced with feeding your child a diet that is completely unfamiliar to you—while keeping the rest of the family members happy with the foods that they enjoy. What will you feed this rapidly growing, ravenous almost-adult when she turns her nose up at what used to be her favorite—spaghetti with meat sauce?

Some parents agree not to make a big fuss about their child's new eating habits. They are willing to be open-minded about a vegetarian diet—as long as the teen is responsible for his or her own food. We'd like to make a plea for a slightly more generous attitude than that. First of all, if you suddenly stop shopping and cooking for your child, your attitude can be perceived as rather negative toward his or her new eating habits. Second, teens have a lot of things on their minds. Generally, planning well-balanced meals isn't one of them. If you want your vegetarian teen to be healthy, you may need to pitch in by buying some special foods and, at least several times a week, prepare meals that the whole family can enjoy or that can be made vegetarian with slight modification (see "Meals for Mixed Households," page 275). Of course, in most families, older children might help with meal preparation anyway, especially if both parents work outside the home. This is a good time for parents and vegetarian teens to explore some new cuisines together.

While this change in family menus may seem like a problem, there are some very positive points to consider. First, your teen has chosen a diet that can reduce his or her risk of getting cancer, heart disease, and many other chronic problems later in life. What parents wouldn't want that for their child? Second, while some teens might choose a vegetarian diet because it's "cool," many are sincerely concerned about the environment or about animal welfare. Parents can feel especially proud of a child who is socially responsible and compassionate. Finally, you may find yourself swept up in this vegetarian adventure. Many families who become vegetarian or at least adopt healthier meals do so because a child gave up eating meat. You could end up eating meals that help you lose weight and lower your blood cholesterol, thanks to your child.

However, it is certainly fair to ask for some ground rules. For your part, you can stock the kitchen with the vegetarian foods that your child likes. Other family members need to be respectful toward the vegetarian teen's beliefs and diet. In exchange, you can ask that your teen not badger and harass other family members about what *they* eat.

EATING DISORDERS

Eating disorders are a serious problem seen mostly in adolescent girls and young women. The two common eating disorders are anorexia nervosa, which is self-starvation, and bulimia, which is a syndrome of overeating and then purging either by self-induced vomiting or excessive laxative use. It is estimated that 4 percent of girls between the ages of thirteen and eighteen are anorexic, and 8 percent of young women between the ages of thirteen and twenty-four are bulimic.[12] The consequences of eating disorders can include osteoporosis, gastrointestinal problems, and even heart failure. Untreated anorexia nervosa is especially serious. Approximately 5 percent of patients with anorexia die. Signs of an eating disorder include dramatic weight loss, a distorted body image, preoccupation with food, and evidence of purging.

Teens with eating disorders may show an obsessive preoccupation with food. In efforts to control the amounts and types of food that they eat, teens with eating disorders adopt a variety of eating patterns. Vegetarianism is somewhat common among anorexics in particular.[13] However, eating-disorder experts suggest that the avoidance of meat may actually be one result of advanced anorexia. Patients who suffer symptoms of wasting disease and starvation often lose their "taste for meat."[14]

There is *no* relationship between a vegetarian diet and the risk of developing an eating disorder. In fact, the causes of eating

TABLE 14.2 SAMPLE MENU PLANS FOR TEENAGERS

Vegan Menu for Teenage Girl

BREAKFAST
Strawberry soymilk shake (8 ounces fortified soymilk, ½ cup frozen strawberries)
Bran muffin

LUNCH
2 small pitas, each stuffed with ¼ cup hummus and chopped tomatoes and lettuce
Carrot sticks
Banana
2 oatmeal cookies
6 ounces orange juice

AFTERNOON SNACK
Bagel, with 1 tablespoon peanut butter
8 ounces fortified soymilk

DINNER WITH FRIENDS
3 slices cheeseless pizza, topped with mushrooms
Salad (1 cup mixed lettuce and spinach, ½ cup raw broccoli, ½ cup soy nuts, tomatoes, 2 tablespoons oil-and-vinegar dressing)
Coke

EVENING SNACK
Bran flakes, with 1 cup soymilk and ½ banana, sliced

Lacto-Ovo-Vegetarian Menu for Teenage Girl

BREAKFAST
3 pancakes, topped with applesauce
6 ounces orange juice

LUNCH AT THE MALL
Baked potato, topped with ½ cup steamed broccoli and 2 tablespoons cheese sauce
Salad (1 cup lettuce, ¼ cup chopped tomatoes, diet Thousand Island dressing)

SNACK AT HOME
English muffin, with 2 tablespoons peanut butter
1 cup skim milk

DINNER WITH FAMILY
4 ounces grilled tofu, with barbecue sauce
1 cup brown rice
½ cup steamed kale
½ cup baked beans
Apple crisp (½ apple, ¼ cup oats, ¼ cup brown sugar, 1 teaspoon oil)
1 cup skim milk

SNACK
1 cup fortified soymilk
Bran muffin

---

disorders are complex and multifaceted. Although a preoccupation with weight is a fundamental characteristic of eating disorders, the true causes of this problem are much more deeply rooted than that.

In the past, some eating-disorder-treatment programs have not allowed patients to follow vegetarian diets for a variety of reasons. Current recommendations are to adjust diets for recovering eating-disorder patients to allow them to follow a vegetarian diet if they wish.[15]

TABLE 14.2 SAMPLE MENU PLANS FOR TEENAGERS (cont.)

Vegan Menu for Teenage Boy

BREAKFAST

4 ounces tofu, scrambled in 1 teaspoon oil

2 slices whole wheat bread, with 2 teaspoons margarine

Soymilk shake (8 ounces fortified soymilk, 1 banana, 4 ounces pineapple juice)

LUNCH

4-ounce tempeh burger, with 1 slice tomato, 1 leaf lettuce, 1 hamburger roll

Carrot sticks (1 carrot)

2 peaches

8 ounces calcium-fortified orange juice

SNACK

English muffin, with 2 tablespoons almond butter

1 cup fortified soymilk

DINNER

2 cups vegetarian chili, with textured vegetable protein and tomato sauce

2 cups brown rice

1 cup steamed broccoli

Salad (1 cup lettuce, ¼ cup sliced mushrooms, 1 teaspoon sunflower seeds)

2 slices whole wheat bread, with 2 teaspoons margarine

Baked pear

SNACK

1 cup bran flakes, with 1 cup fortified soymilk

Lacto-Ovo-Vegetarian Menu for Teenage Boy

BREAKFAST

2 cups corn flakes, with 1 cup skim milk

2 slices whole wheat toast, with 2 teaspoons margarine

6 ounces orange juice

LUNCH

1½ cups macaroni and cheese

Slice whole wheat bread

½ cup green beans

Tossed salad, with oil-and-vinegar dressing

1 cup 2% milk

Apple

SNACK

Soymilk shake (1 cup soymilk, ½ banana, 4 ounces orange juice)

DINNER

2 cups lentil soup

3 slices bread, with 3 teaspoons margarine

½ cup kale

½ cup steamed carrots

2 date-oat bars

SNACK

¼ cup trail mix

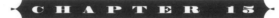

THE OLDER VEGETARIAN

I have better health today, notwithstanding I am seventy-six years old, than I had in my younger days. I thank God for the principles of health reform.

—ELLEN WHITE, *Counsels on Diet and Foods,* 1904

◆

Because vegetarian diets still have a bit of an alternative aura about them, they are likely to be associated with younger people. Surprisingly, though, the vegetarian population is slightly skewed toward the over-forty crowd. According to a poll conducted for *Vegetarian Times* magazine, 55 percent of the vegetarian population is over forty.[1]

We don't have any specific information about the number of vegetarians who are age sixty-five and older. But a number of factors lead us to believe that vegetarianism will be increasingly important for older people. For one thing, the number of senior citizens is growing. Census takers expect that by the twenty-first century 20 percent of our population, or about sixty million people, will be sixty-five and older.[2] Americans over the age of eighty-five represent the fastest-growing age group in the United States and in other industrialized countries.[3]

We already discussed that the number of vegetarians in this country is growing.

Those who choose a vegetarian diet are also likely to maintain it—about one-quarter of all vegetarians have consumed a meatless diet for more than twenty years.[4] And though many would argue that a vegetarian diet challenges the aging process, the inescapable fact is that vegetarians do grow older, just like everyone else. So we can certainly expect to see the number of older vegetarians rise as this population group expands.

Nutrient needs and diet adequacy are real issues for all older Americans. Dietary surveys show that older people have a relatively high incidence of poor nutrition compared with other age groups. Generally speaking, various studies suggest that older vegetarians surpass or equal their meat-eating peers in meeting nutrient needs. For example:

• Dutch vegetarians age sixty-five to ninety-nine had intakes of fiber, carbohydrates, fat, and protein that were closer to recommended guidelines than those of older omnivores, although their intake of zinc was somewhat low.[5]

• Seventh-day Adventist vegetarian women in their early seventies consumed less saturated fat and cholesterol than omnivores and more carbohydrates, fiber, vitamin A, vitamin E, copper, folacin, and magnesium. According to this study, meat eaters were more likely to be deficient in vitamins B6 and E.[6]

• Sixty-five-year-old Seventh-day Adventist vegetarian women had better nutrient intakes overall than nonvegetarian women of the same age, although, again, zinc intake was low.[7]

There are some real problems in evaluating these needs for both omnivores and vegetarians. One is that the most recently published RDAs, in 1989, lump all older people into one age group—fifty-one and older. But nutrient needs are likely quite different for people in their eighties than for people in their fifties. Earlier editions of the RDAs did include separate recommendations for people over the age of seventy-five, providing much more useful information.

Also, the most recent RDAs were determined when there was relatively little information available about the nutrient needs of older people. Since then, there has been much more research on these needs, so future editions of the RDAs should be more helpful in this regard.

Although we have some understanding of the kind of physiological changes that take place in aging, we have much less knowledge of how these changes affect nutrient needs. We have even less insight into the nutrient needs of older vegetarians, which may differ from those of omnivores.

NUTRIENT NEEDS OF OLDER PEOPLE

Calories

Body composition shifts with aging—the amount of muscle tissue decreases, and the amount of fat increases, although actual body weight might stay the same.

The changes in body composition can be fairly dramatic. The average man in his late sixties has twenty-six pounds less muscle tissue than he did at age twenty-five. Women have about eleven pounds less, since they start out with much less muscle tissue than men do.[8] The less muscle on the body, the fewer calories you burn, so, not surprisingly, this results in a significant drop in calorie needs. Many older people also need fewer calories because they are less physically active.

Needs for vitamins and minerals stay about the same as people age, which presents somewhat of a problem. If calorie needs drop but nutrient needs stay the same, then older people must squeeze more nutrition into less food. Wise food choices are crucial at this time of life. In addition, there is some indication that despite a drop in calorie needs, many older people still don't meet those needs.[9] This is a potential problem. Although the RDAs for most nutrients include a considerable margin of safety, this isn't true for calories. Calorie levels are set at averages. This means that many people will actually need quite a bit more than the levels specified by the RDAs, and some elderly people who don't meet the RDAs may be undereating by a lot.

Many older people have calorie intakes that are so low that meeting nutrient needs without supplements could be extremely difficult.[10] Boosting calorie intake could be even more of a challenge for older vegetarians, since vegetarian diets are higher in fiber and are therefore often filling and lower in calories.

Protein

People may actually use protein less efficiently as they age. Although their reduced muscle mass somewhat compensates for this, research indicates that people need more protein as they age. Younger adults need 0.8 grams of protein for each kilogram of body weight. Older people may need as much as 1 to 1.25 grams of protein per kilogram of weight.[11] Also, low calorie intake can boost protein requirements quite a bit. So older people who don't get enough calories may have even higher protein needs.

Studies show that many older nonvegetarians may not eat enough protein.[12] Since vegetarians typically eat less protein than nonvegetarians, we can assume that older vegetarians may also not be getting enough protein. Clearly, it is important for older vegetarians to eat more protein-dense foods.

Soy products are an especially good choice for older people because they are so rich in high-quality protein. At the same time, they don't stress the kidneys or produce bone loss, compared with animal proteins. Products like tofu are easily digested and are easy to eat, and some brands of tofu will also give your diet a calcium boost. Textured vegetable protein is a good choice for people who may be weaning themselves from a lifetime of meat-based dinners but want to try more meatless meals in an effort to lower cholesterol levels, improve diabetic control, or cut down on food costs. The meaty texture of this low-fat, protein-rich food makes it a good choice in spaghetti sauce or stews.

Of course, older vegetarians who get all or most of their protein from plant foods may have an advantage. We discussed the problems associated with excessive protein intake in chapter 6. Some of these could be much more pronounced in older people. Kidney function tends to decline with aging, and you may remember that excessive animal protein taxes the kidneys. Depending more on protein from plants may preserve kidney function in older people.

Calcium

Protecting the health of your bones in later years is important to your overall health. It's true that the amount of bone you start out with is one of the most important influences on later bone health—and there is little we can do to increase this bone mass once we hit our thirties. But holding on to the bone you've got, by reducing loss of calcium, is just as crucial.

Bone loss begins around the age of forty, but it steps up with advancing age. As the bones lose calcium and other components, they become porous and weak. Older women are at particular risk for osteoporosis, since they have less bone matter than men *and* they lose more as they age. In their twenties women have about 76 percent as much bone as men do; by their seventies that has dropped to about 60 percent.[13]

Can you protect your bones in later years by boosting your calcium intake? There is much debate over this question, and the answer is even more elusive for vegetarians. First, people do absorb calcium less efficiently as they get older, so it would seem to make sense that older people—women in particular—need more calcium in their diet. Several studies show that boosting calcium intake well above the RDA can delay loss of bone in women past the age of menopause.[14]

But in these studies calcium intakes were as high as 1,500 milligrams a day. It is unlikely that most women, vegetarian or not, can get this much calcium into their diets without using supplements. If this is truly the amount of calcium that older women need, then it really isn't a dietary issue. Anyone, regardless of the type of diet they eat, can take a calcium pill every day.

In chapter 7 we saw that osteoporosis is a complex disease. There is more to healthy bones than getting adequate calcium. Exercising regularly and avoiding excessive intake of animal protein and sodium could be just as important as dosing yourself up with calcium. However, there may be some merit to using calcium supplements, especially for older women who are at particularly high risk for osteoporosis. For vegetarians, a smaller dose—perhaps six hundred to eight hundred milligrams—in addition to including calcium-rich foods in the diet, may be enough. Many people use antacids as calcium supplements. Be sure to read the label, since there are many kinds of antacids. Not all are high in calcium; some may be high in less desirable ingredients, such as aluminum.

Be sure to include calcium-rich foods in your diet as well. Cooked dried beans, tofu, fortified soymilk, fortified orange juice, dark leafy greens, and skim milk are some good choices.

Vitamin D

Getting adequate vitamin D is important throughout life, but it may be more so for older people because vitamin D promotes bone health. Remember that we don't necessarily need vitamin D in the diet; we can make it when the skin is exposed to the sun's ultraviolet rays. But older people seem to make less. In one study of older people, although the average intake of vitamin D was two times the RDA, 30 percent had low blood levels of vitamin D.[15] Since the kidneys are involved in making vitamin D in the body, it is possible that decreased kidney function in later years affects the amount of vitamin D synthesized.

For some people decreased exposure to sunlight is also a problem. If you while away your retirement years in sunny Florida or Arizona, then getting adequate vitamin D will be less of a problem. But older people living in cold climates, especially in urban areas, may not get adequate exposure to the sun. This is a special problem for older people who have become housebound. Also, some drugs like Dilantin can increase the need for vitamin D.

Some researchers believe that older people could need as much as ten milligrams of vitamin D a day, which is twice the RDA. Since there is little vitamin D in foods, the only way to get enough of this nutrient in the diet is from fortified foods, supplements, or sun exposure.

Few foods are good sources of vitamin D, although milk is typically fortified with it. However, people are less likely to drink milk as they grow older. Lactose intolerance—the inability to digest milk sugar—can be one reason, especially in people of Asian, Native American, African, or Hispanic background. Soymilks that are fortified with calcium and vitamin D are very good choices for boosting intake of both these nutrients. Some breakfast cereals are also vitamin D fortified. If you don't use fortified foods and you don't get much sun exposure, a supplement is a good idea.

Vitamin B12

Although the RDA for vitamin B12 doesn't change as people age, some older people may need more because of changes in the digestive system. About 30 percent of people over the age of sixty have reduced acid secretion in their stomachs.[16] Acid is needed to free vitamin B12 from the protein to which it is bound in foods. If B12 isn't detached from the protein, it can't be absorbed and is virtually useless to the body. Also, bacteria are likely to flourish in the intestines when acid secretion is low, and these bacteria can use up some of the B12 you ingest, which will increase the need for this vitamin.

Since reduced acid affects B12 absorption, some researchers think that consuming more B12 doesn't help at all.[17] Others feel that if you consume large amounts of B12, then eventually enough will be absorbed to meet needs.[18] Of course, if no vitamin B12 is being absorbed at all, then all the dietary B12 in the world won't help you to meet needs. In this case, injections of the vitamin are necessary. Your health care provider can determine this.

We don't know how common B12 deficiency is in the elderly. Remember that in addition to anemia, B12 deficiency affects the neurological system. In fact, some nutritionists believe that symptoms we might write off as being related to old age could actually be symptoms of B12 deficiency. They include confusion, disorientation, depression, mood swings, impotence, crankiness, memory loss, concentration difficulties, dementia, chronic fatigue, apathy, insomnia, and perhaps even phobic disorders, hallucinatory episodes, and epileptic attacks.[19]

Of course, this doesn't mean that every person who suffers one or more of these symptoms is B12 deficient. After all, who doesn't experience some crankiness now and then, regardless of age? However, it does mean that physicians should not be too quick to write off symptoms as age related. Problems with vitamin B12 absorption are common in older people and should always be considered as a possible cause of symptoms.

Since vitamin B12 is found only in animal foods, older vegetarians are obviously at a somewhat-higher risk for inadequate intake. The older vegetarian has the potential dual problem of low intake and poor absorption. So attention to vitamin B12 is especially important in this age group. Ready-to-eat cereals are often fortified with this vitamin and are a good choice. Most cooked cereals are not fortified. Long-time vegetarians will probably be familiar with nutritional yeast (remember that Red Star brand T-6635+ is the only one that is a reliable source of B12). Older Seventh-day Adventist vegetarians are likely to use some meat analogues in their diet, which are often fortified. Lacto-ovo vegetarians can get considerable amounts of vitamin B12 from dairy foods and from eggs. However, for vegans who don't use fortified products, a vitamin B12 supplement several times a week is really a good idea.

Zinc

Older people sometimes have a lower zinc intake. In this age group, inadequate zinc intake impairs the immune system.[20] There isn't much information available on the zinc intake of older vegetarians, but the little bit there is suggests that zinc intake is low in this group.[21] It seems that all older people need to pay special attention to eating foods that are rich in zinc.

Riboflavin

According to the RDAs, riboflavin needs decrease with aging, mostly because your need for riboflavin is closely tied to the number of calories you consume. However, there is some evidence that older people need just as much riboflavin as younger people.[22] Also, older people who exercise may need more riboflavin.[23] On the other hand, a vegetarian diet may actually reduce your riboflavin needs. It seems that a high-carbohydrate intake changes the nature of the bacterial colony that lives inside all healthy people so that some riboflavin is manufactured in your intestines.[24] Since vegetarians typically eat a high-carbohydrate diet, they may need less of this B vitamin. Vegetarians can easily meet riboflavin needs, since whole grains, enriched refined grains, and leafy green vegetables are rich in this nutrient.

Vitamin B6

Older people have lower blood levels of vitamin B6 than younger people. Until recently, it was thought that absorption of this nutrient was poorer as people aged. But recent evidence is that absorption rates of B6 are no different for older people than for younger ones.[25] There is some evidence that people need less B6 as they age, even with higher protein intake.[26] And studies of vitamin B6 intake in older vegetarians show that they get enough of this vitamin.[27]

EXERCISE

Everyone knows that exercise is an important component of a healthy lifestyle, but we often think that as people age, exercise is no longer a viable option for them. But most older people can and should do some exercise. Walking, swimming, treadmills, and exercise bikes are all good choices for older people. Just be sure to set a reasonable pace with whatever exercise program you choose. Light weight training can also be helpful. Even people in their nineties can increase their muscle mass with this type of exercise.[28] Exercise raises your calorie needs and can improve appetite, making it easier to meet nutrient needs. In addition, exercise is crucial for older people, since it slows the loss of calcium from bones and helps to protect bone health. The list of benefits of exercise is extensive. It's good for your heart and circulation, can help to lower blood pressure, helps to regulate blood sugar levels, and promotes a general sense of well-being. Exercise is good for people of all ages. Many communities have exercise programs geared specifically to the needs of older people.

HEALTHY VEGETARIAN DIETS FOR OLDER PEOPLE

There are challenges to planning healthy diets at any stage of the life cycle, and the golden years are no different. The food guide in chapter 10 is a good place to start—its guidelines will help you plan a diet that provides minimal nutrient needs. Older vegetarians need to make sure that they choose foods that are nutrient dense. This means avoiding empty calories—foods that provide plenty of calories but not much nutrition. If your appetite is poor and you have problems getting enough calories into your diet, you probably need more than three meals a day. Some ideas for snacks that are nutrient rich but easy to prepare include:

Potatoes baked in the microwave

Fruit juice blended with a banana in the blender to make a smoothie

Instant cups of soup (the kind to which you just add hot water)

Toasted bagel with fruit spread

Cereal with milk

Instant oatmeal

If you find that you undereat, exercise can help. We usually think of exercise as a way to lose weight, but it can also perk up a sluggish appetite and increase your interest in food.

Some people have just the opposite problem, of course. If you are overweight and need to cut back on food intake, be sure that you aren't skimping on nutritious foods. Grains, beans, fruits, and vegetables won't make you fat, but added fats, sweets, and fatty snacks will. Cutting these foods from your diet can help you lose weight without sacrificing nutrient intake.

Some older people experience difficulties with cooking for a variety of reasons, including tremors, arthritis, poor vision, or just general decreased mobility. Of course, this tends to be a problem in very advanced age and affects only a small percentage of people in their sixties and seventies. But as many as 17 percent of people over the age of eighty-five cannot prepare their own meals because of a health problem or physical disability.[29] If food preparation is tiring or a burden, you'll need to find ways to simplify your cooking as much as possible. Remember first of all that meals don't need to be elaborate to be healthy. These meals are simple to prepare and nutritious:

Spaghetti with sauce from a jar

Canned vegetable soup with toast

Textured vegetable protein with canned sloppy joe sauce, heated and poured over rolls

Veggie burgers from the frozen-food section (you'll find many of these in a natural-foods store, but most supermarkets carry a few also)

Instant brown rice or white rice with canned vegetarian baked beans

Baked potato with steamed frozen vegetables and a sprinkle of nutritional yeast or Parmesan cheese

Peanut-butter-and-sliced-banana sandwich

Keep plenty of frozen vegetables on hand that don't require any chopping or slicing. You can also buy packages of fresh vegetables in the produce section that are already pared, cut up, and ready to use. Check the salad bar for vegetables that are already prepared, too.

Seasoning foods so that they are acceptable is another problem because taste acuity diminishes with aging. This is a very real physiological phenomenon. At age seventy, people have only 30 percent of the number of taste buds that they had as young adults.[30] Loss of smell begins in middle age and progresses as people get older also. As a result of diminishing sense of smell and loss of taste buds, many people have trouble distinguishing weak tastes by age sixty.[31] When food is bland, it is unappetizing, and that makes it harder to eat enough to satisfy your nutrient needs. You may also find that you gravitate toward sweets. The more intense flavor of very sweet foods may be especially attractive when other foods taste bland. Too many sweets in the diet can take the place of more nutritious foods and compromise nutritional status.

If food tastes generally bland to you, you need to perk it up with some more intense flavors. Add dried fruits like raisins, apricots, dates, or chopped prunes to lentil or rice dishes for a flavor that is both healthy and sweet. Use fresh lemon juice on vegetables and other dishes. Try spicy foods like chili and curry if you enjoy them. If you like to cook, use fresh herbs whenever possible. They tend to have a more intense flavor than dried ones, which quickly lose their flavor.

You might be tempted to add more salt to dishes to perk up your taste buds a little. While some salt is fine, be careful not to overdo it. Low-sodium soy sauce gives a pleasant taste to foods. You might try one of the herb mixes, like Mrs. Dash. These are designed to reduce the need for salt. A few drops of herb-flavored vinegar or fresh lemon juice can be used on vegetables instead of salt. You can also give vegetables more flavor by simmering them with leeks, herbs, and pepper to blend flavors and create a savory, low-sodium dish.

You may also find that certain foods that used to appeal to you are no longer easy to eat. Problems with chewing can keep you from eating some items and can greatly eliminate the variety in your diet and the enjoyment of eating. If you lean more toward refined foods, which are softer and easier to chew, your diet may lack fiber, and you might find constipation is a problem. Vegetarians have some real advantages here, since meat is one of the toughest foods for people who don't chew easily. Plant foods can also be difficult to eat, but choosing the right foods and cooking them well can make it easier. Many fiber-rich foods are easy to eat. Even without the skins, boiled or baked potatoes are fiber rich. Sweet potatoes are especially so. Many cooked cereals, such as oatmeal, multigrain cereals, or Wheatena, are easy to eat and nutritious and rich in fiber. Cook vegetables just to the point at which they are easy to eat. It's true that prolonged cooking of vegetables reduces the nutrient content, but it isn't true that it completely destroys it. Even well-cooked fruits and vegetables can offer you good nutrition.

Cooked fruits are also a good way to go for people who have problems chewing. Try baked apples or pears, or simply stew any of your favorite fruits. Also cook beans more thoroughly and serve them in soups to make them easy to chew. Canned beans tend to be quite soft. Blended tofu is a wonderful way to boost the nutrient intake of people who can't chew well. (See page 311 for some hints on ways to use this food.) Other foods that are easy to eat and nutritious include pasta, nut butters, textured vegetable protein, and cream of vegetable soups.

Many people find that digestive problems accompany aging, so foods that produce gas—beans and some vegetables—make them uncomfortable. A product called Beano, which is available in drugstores, can help. Just add a few drops to your first forkful of beans or vegetables, and it will aid with digestion. If you make your own beans from scratch, check our instructions on page 309 for cooking beans to reduce gas. You might also concentrate on beans and bean products that are less likely to produce gas, like lentils and split peas.

Attitude, outlook on life, and general well-being can have a profound effect on diet. Older people are likely to have suffered some losses in life—of friends or a spouse—which can lead to depression. People who are housebound or less mobile because of physical constraints might feel isolated and depressed. Under those circumstances, developing enthusiasm for cooking and eating can be difficult. Those who find themselves living alone for the first time may find it hard to cook for just themselves.

Most communities offer hot lunches for senior citizens either at a senior center or church. Many provide transportation to these meals. Rarely will these meals be vegetarian, and cost constraints make "special meals" for individuals somewhat difficult. But if you are a regular attendee, you might be able to arrange to get an extra portion of rice and vegetables on your plate and skip the meat. You might also call a local Seventh-day Adventist church to see if any vegetarian meals are offered for seniors in your area.

Most communities provide meals-on-wheels—a hot lunch delivered to your home if you can't get out. Again, these are rarely, if ever, vegetarian, but there might be portions of the meals that you can eat.

If you spend a lot of time alone, sharing occasional meals can do a lot to make mealtime more pleasant and to improve your appetite. If other people in your neighborhood live alone, see if they want to get together for lunch several times a week. You can keep it simple by brown-bagging and meeting at a different person's house each time, or take turns cooking up a big pot of soup for everyone. Your lunch mates may not be vegetarians, but will probably be happy to accommodate you by sticking to vegetable soups and salads.

Finally, although the retirement years are carefree ones for many people, they can be a time of great financial stress for others, especially for older women who live alone. Food is one area in which people cut down on expenses. This doesn't have to compromise nutrition, but it can.

If food dollars are limited, choose foods that give you the most nutritional bang for your buck. Some fantastic nutritional buys include potatoes, beans, fresh greens,

TABLE 15.1 SAMPLE MENU PLANS FOR OLDER PEOPLE

Day 1

BREAKFAST

1 package instant oatmeal, with ½ cup fortified soymilk and ½ banana, sliced

1 cup calcium-fortified orange juice

SNACK

½ cup canned pears

Bran muffin

LUNCH

Sloppy joe (½ cup textured vegetable protein, ½ cup Manwich sauce, with 1 whole wheat hamburger bun)

½ cup canned carrots

SNACK

Slice toast, with 2 tablespoons almond butter

DINNER

Small baked sweet potato

½ cup vegetarian baked beans

1 cup steamed frozen or fresh broccoli

Day 2

BREAKFAST

1 cup corn flakes, with ½ cup fortified soymilk

Fruit smoothie (½ cup calcium-fortified orange juice, ½ banana, ¼ cup strawberries)

LUNCH

1 cup rotini, with 1 cup spaghetti sauce

1 cup steamed collards

SNACK

4 saltine crackers, with 2 tablespoons peanut butter

DINNER

1 cup canned or instant split-pea soup

4 crackers

1 cup steamed frozen or fresh asparagus

Sliced tomatoes

½ cup canned apricots

½ cup fortified soymilk

---

peanut butter, rice, and oatmeal. If you are really on a tight food budget, there are ways to economize without sacrificing your overall diet. For example, if you get plenty of fiber from cereals, fruits, vegetables, potatoes, and beans, then who says you *have* to use whole wheat bread? As long as you like it, white refined bread is much less expensive, and there is no reason why you can't have one or two refined foods in your diet, as long as the overall emphasis is on whole foods.

Consider growing some of your own produce. Gardening is wonderful physical activity and is a favorite pastime of many retirees. If you have limited space or don't feel you can take care of a big garden, try potted tomatoes, strawberries, peppers, or greens on a patio or deck.

Of course, many older people are healthy and active and consider their golden years the best time of their lives. And most constraints to healthy eating can be overcome by making some adjustments in the way you cook and eat and by asking for help when you need it.

Vegetarians will find that a meatless diet

offers many benefits at this time of life, just as it does for younger people. As is true in all stages of the life cycle, older vegetarians have lower blood cholesterol than omnivores.[32] The lower fat content of vegetarian diets can make it easier to control blood sugar in diabetes, and in fact vegetarians are less likely to get diabetes.[33] Vegetarians consume two or three times more fiber than nonvegetarians, which helps them avoid some of the digestive problems that are common in older people, such as constipation.

THE FOUNTAIN OF YOUTH

We can't stop the march of time. All the skin creams, face-lifts, good food, and positive thinking in the world won't change the fact that everyone ages. But it may be possible to slow down aging a little bit with healthful living.

Like everything that happens in our body, aging is a complex, imperfectly understood process. We know that free radicals have a lot to do with the aging process. They may raise the risk for heart disease and cancer and speed up aging.

Free radicals usually form in the cells as a part of normal cell activity. But exposing the skin to sunlight results in increased formation of these compounds. You can't completely stop free-radical production, but you can minimize the damage. One way is to avoid the sun as much as possible. Small amounts of sun exposure are healthy and are important for the creation of vitamin D. But too much sunlight—especially to the point where your skin begins to darken—is dangerous. If you are outside in the summer for an extended time, using a sun block is one of the most important things you can do to slow aging and protect your health.

Antioxidants also will neutralize the effects of free radicals. The three most common of these compounds are vitamins: vitamin C, vitamin E, and beta-carotene. Vegetarians consume more of all three of these antioxidants than do omnivores.

Other dietary components can *encourage* the formation of free radicals. The one that has most recently come under scrutiny is iron. Since iron is a nutrient, we obviously can't eliminate it from the diet, but we're now beginning to see that too much iron can be harmful.

While we can't promise that a vegetarian diet will keep you young forever, plant foods may have some influence in slowing the aging process. First, while they provide plenty of iron to meet needs, they are much lower in iron than meats, and the iron is not as well absorbed. So depending on plant foods that are rich in iron is one way to get plenty of this mineral without overdoing it. Also, plant foods are rich in antioxidants. Vitamin C is found almost exclusively in fruits and vegetables, and so is beta-carotene. Vitamin E is found in a wide variety of foods, but nuts, seeds, and whole grains are especially rich in it.

Whether or not a vegetarian diet offers any protection against the ravages of time, it probably can help you enjoy your golden years more. Because plant-based diets reduce the risk for heart disease, diabetes, hypertension, and other chronic conditions, those who eat this way are likely to stay healthier and active longer.

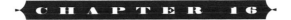
THE VEGETARIAN DIABETIC

*It is now known, that a meat diet
does not cure diabetes, but actually
aggravates the disease.*

—JOHN HARVEY KELLOGG,
The Natural Diet of Man, 1923

◆

*Further advantages to diabetics in the use
of the high carbohydrate–low fat diet are:
it is less expensive; it is more palatable and
permits greater variety; it is much more
likely to be nutritionally adequate.*

—DOROTHY DEMAREST, M.S.,
Journal of American Dietetic Association, 1929

◆

While vegetarianism was taboo for diabetics in the past, it is now clear that it comes closer to the perfect diabetic diet than any other way of eating. Old ideas about consuming a lot of protein and avoiding carbohydrates are forever gone. In fact, diabetics don't even need to stay away from sugar. Reaching this new understanding of diabetes has taken centuries, and, in the process, ideas about how to treat diabetes have swung from one extreme to another.

The incidence of diabetes varies quite a bit throughout the world. In some areas or cultural groups, nearly 50 percent of the population has it; in other groups the disease is practically nonexistent. Amazingly, between one-third and one-half of all diabetics in the world live in the United States. Somewhere between 5 and 10 percent of Americans are diabetic—though many people don't know they have this disease.[1]

Clearly, some groups of people are genetically susceptible to diabetes. But physicians have known for centuries that lifestyle and diet have a profound impact on whether or not you get this disease.

People with high cholesterol levels and high intakes of fat, animal fat, and animal protein are more likely to have diabetes; people with a high carbohydrate intake are less likely to have it.[2]

DIABETES DEFINED

Although the disease was known for thousands of years, Greek physicians were the first to give it a name. The Greek word *diabētēs* means "siphon," since the clearest sign of the disease is increased urination. An early and intriguing observation about the urine of diabetics was that ants were especially attracted to it. Around 1650, a rather heroic doctor decided to find out why. When he tasted the urine of a diabetic patient, he declared it "wondrous sweet," and the disease was renamed diabetes mellitus, which means "honey siphon."[3]

The fundamental problem of diabetes is that cells can't absorb glucose, their preferred fuel source. Glucose is absorbed into the bloodstream when dietary carbohydrates are digested. The glucose eventually enters individual cells and provides them with nourishment.

But cells need the hormone insulin in order to absorb glucose from the blood. Insulin, which is produced by the pancreas, hooks up to certain receptors on the surface of the cell and acts as a sort of calling card for glucose. When the cell recognizes insulin, glucose is ushered in. Without insulin, glucose levels in the blood rise because the glucose can't get into the cells. Some early signs of diabetes are frequent urination and thirst, as the kidneys work overtime to excrete excess glucose. In the meantime, surrounded by this sea of glucose, the cells starve for a lack of fuel.

Diabetes is actually two separate diseases. Type I diabetes (also called insulin-dependent diabetes, or IDDM) can occur at any time in life. However, it tends to be diagnosed in younger people and therefore used to be called juvenile-onset diabetes. There is a strong hereditary component to this type of diabetes, but environment has an effect, too. People who move from areas where Type I diabetes is uncommon to countries where it is more prevalent have a greater risk of developing this type of diabetes.[4]

People with Type I diabetes produce very little insulin or no insulin at all. They must have insulin injections to live. Before insulin was discovered, all people with this type of diabetes died fairly quickly from the disease. One cause of Type I diabetes is a viral infection that attacks the cells of the pancreas and causes them to stop producing insulin.[5] Also, as we noted in chapter 2, consuming cow's milk in infancy may destroy cells in the pancreas and eventually lead to diabetes in some individuals.[6]

Type I diabetes is the most common chronic disease of American children, with more than thirteen thousand new cases each year. More than three hundred thousand people have it in the United States.[7] There are some disturbing observations about Type I diabetes: its incidence has increased since the 1960s, and some evidence indicates that in the late 1980s there was an increase of almost epidemic proportions among young children. It's been especially pronounced in boys and nonwhite children.[8]

Despite the recent upswing in the occurrence of this disease, it is far outranked by Type II diabetes, also called noninsulin dependent diabetes (NIDDM). More than 90 percent of the diabetics in this country have this form of the disease.[9] It occurs most often in older people and used to be called adult-onset diabetes. About 10 percent of people over the age of sixty-five have Type II diabetes. About 6 million Americans have been diagnosed with this disease, and probably an additional 4 to 5 million have it but haven't been diagnosed.[10]

If the number of children with Type I diabetes is disturbing, the rise in Type II diabetes is nothing less than astounding. In the last fifty years, the number of people with this disease has increased between five- and tenfold. For the most part, this is probably because Americans have gotten fatter, and Type II diabetics tend to be overweight.[11] The location of accumulated fat on the body has a great impact on risk. Those who carry weight around their middle and in the belly—commonly referred to as "apples"—are much more likely to develop diabetes than are "pears," those people who carry extra fat in their hips and thighs.[12] In fact, the best way to control the disease, or even to cure it, is to lose weight.[13]

The surprising observation about Type II diabetes is that the pancreas pumps out plenty of insulin. In fact, sometimes these diabetics have high levels of insulin in their blood, but the problem is that insulin can't do its job. The receptors on the cell seem to have lost their memory. They don't recognize the insulin and won't allow glucose into the cell. In some cases, the number of receptors has decreased so that less insulin gets in.

Conditions and treatments vary widely in Type II diabetes. In some cases insulin injections help. But Type II diabetics don't need insulin shots to survive. Many control their disease through diet and exercise and sometimes through the use of pills called oral hypoglycemic agents.

Insulin does a lot more than escort glucose into the cell. It plays major roles in cell growth, fat metabolism, and the creation of new proteins. As a result, the effects of diabetes—regardless of the type—are far-reaching and insidious. Diabetics are at higher risk for elevated blood cholesterol and are much more likely to develop artery disease.[14] Uncontrolled diabetes can also cause nerve damage and can affect the reproductive organs, kidneys, eyes, and limbs.

DIET AND DIABETES

One early observation about diabetes was that restricting food intake seemed to improve it. During both world wars in Europe, when food was scarce and fat intake was low, deaths from diabetes-related symptoms decreased by half.[15] Many early physicians already knew about the positive effects of food restrictions. In some cases they took the curative powers of fasting to extremes. The German physician Bernard Naunyn ran a successful diabetic clinic in Strasbourg during the 1800s. He "encouraged" his patients to fast by locking them in their rooms.[16]

Ideas about the best diet for diabetes have changed throughout the centuries. Early Egyptian physicians recommended a very high carbohydrate diet consisting of "wheat, fresh grits, grapes, honey, berries, and sweet beer."[17] The Greeks agreed with that prescription and added milk and wine to it.[18]

But by the 1800s physicians were convinced that carbohydrates were deadly for diabetics and that high-protein meals were best. That belief persisted well into the twentieth century—until doctors began to make some surprising observations. That is, in cultures where diabetes is rare, people consume a diet that is largely plant based and therefore high in carbohydrates. In a study of inhabitants of several West African villages where the diet is more than 80 percent carbohydrates, not one of the 1,381 inhabitants had diabetes.[19]

As early as 1940, researchers had shown that a high-carbohydrate diet had a positive effect on glucose levels.[20] In 1979, the American Diabetes Association recommended that diabetics abandon the old high-protein regimen in favor of a diet that is rich in complex carbohydrates like starch and fiber and low in fat.[21] Avoidance of saturated fat and cholesterol has become especially important.

VEGETARIANS AND DIABETES

We saw in chapter 2 that vegetarians are less likely to develop diabetes than the general population. This isn't surprising; people who are lean and who eat low-fat diets are less likely to get diabetes. Vegetarian diets have, in fact, been used with success to treat diabetes.[22]

As we look at the basic components of a diabetic diet, we'll see that a vegetarian diet is a perfect choice for controlling this disease.

DIABETIC DIET

Fat

Ask average people what foods a diabetic should avoid, and most will tell you sugar. But, in fact, one of the most important issues for diabetics is fat. A low-fat diet is important for several reasons. First, because all diabetics are at very high risk for heart disease, meals that are low in saturated fat and cholesterol are essential for them. Second, we'll see in the next chapter that reducing fat intake is the most important

thing you can do to lose weight. In most cases, Type II diabetes is improved when people lose weight. Finally, fat can directly affect control of blood glucose.

One of the primary goals of dietary treatment for diabetes is to keep blood cholesterol levels low. Thus, a diet that is low in saturated fat and cholesterol, and therefore that greatly limits meat, is crucial for diabetics. The traditional approach to diabetes control is a diet that is 30 percent fat. As we noted in chapter 5, standard recommendations like this are often shaped by what authorities believe people will eat. Most nutritionists believe that many Americans won't eat a diet that is less than 30 percent fat.

But a 30-percent-fat diet is too high for diabetics. Reducing fat intake to 15 to 20 percent of calories can improve the way your body uses insulin and can help lower blood glucose.[23] It will certainly protect against some of the complications of diabetes. However, it also appears that monounsaturated fat—the kind found in olive and canola oils and in avocados and nuts—might help control diabetes. This doesn't mean you should go out of your way to add these fats to your diet. But when you do use added fats, olive oil and canola oil might be the best choices.[24]

Carbohydrates

It's easy to see why in the past carbohydrates were restricted in the diets of diabetics. A high blood level of glucose is the hallmark of diabetes. And glucose comes from carbohydrates. It makes intuitive sense that eating lots of carbohydrates would raise your blood glucose—but the reality is just the opposite. Many studies show that high-carbohydrate diets help to control blood glucose.[25]

It is probably the combination of high carbohydrate and low fat that does the trick. Therefore, in the diabetic diet, the bulk of calories should come from complex carbohydrates (starch and fiber).

Fiber

Fiber can help normalize blood glucose levels somewhat. It takes a lot of fiber to do this, however—about three times the amount the average American consumes. Some diabetes experts consider it unrealistic to expect people to consume enough fiber to help control diabetes. This certainly isn't true for vegetarians, who already consume two or three times as much fiber as the typical American.

Generally, eating a diet low in fat and high in fiber helps to reduce blood glucose levels. Low-fat diets that are not fiber rich have much less effect.[26] But not all studies show a benefit from fiber. One reason may be that only certain types of fiber seem to help in controlling diabetes. Soluble fiber, which is especially abundant in legumes, oats, and many fruits and vegetables, helps lower blood glucose levels.[27] It forms a gel in the intestines that slows the absorption of glucose from the intestines into the blood. In addition, it seems to help make cells more sensitive to insulin so that they take up glucose more easily.[28]

Another type of fiber, called insoluble fiber, doesn't have these beneficial effects in diabetes (although it has other health benefits). Insoluble fiber is the kind that is found in wheat bran and many other grains. Diabetics should include generous amounts of whole fruits and vegetables, legumes, oats, and barley in their diet to increase their intake of soluble fiber.

Protein

Diabetic diets in the past have stressed high protein intakes at each meal to control blood glucose. Actually there is no advantage to a high protein intake. In addition, when much of the protein comes from animal foods, there is the danger that the diet will be too high in fat. Current recommendations are for a protein intake that is between 10 and 20 percent of calories. Vegetarians fall into this range.

Excessive protein is never good for anyone, but it is especially harmful in kidney disease. Since diabetics are at a very high risk for kidney disease, the lower end of that protein range is best.

Sugar

Long taboo in the diets of diabetics, sugar is back on the menu for people with either type of diabetes. It was once thought to raise blood glucose levels more than other types of carbohydrate. But there is no evidence that this is true when sugar is included as part of a healthy diet. This doesn't mean that diabetics—or anyone for that matter—should have a free-for-all with sweets. For one thing, many sweetened foods are high in fat. And foods high in sugar are likely to take the place of other, more nutritious foods. However, for many diabetics it isn't realistic to expect that no sweetened foods will ever be consumed. According to the latest guidelines from the American Diabetes Association, there is no reason for completely avoiding sugar.[29]

MEAL PLANNING

In the past, diet prescriptions for diabetics were fairly standardized. The modern approach is to address the specific needs of each patient and to individualize the diet. There is really no longer any such thing as a diabetic diet. If you are a new diabetic or if you haven't been updated for a while on the best approach to managing your diabetes, you should definitely see a nutrition counselor who has expertise in diabetes. If your health care provider hands you a preprinted sheet outlining a diet, this isn't enough. We recommend that you see a registered dietitian who is a member of the American Dietetic Association's Vegetarian Nutrition Dietetic Practice Group. Before seeing a counselor, ask if he or she is knowledgeable about vegetarian diets. A good nutrition counselor will take into account your lifestyle needs and will have no trouble planning a lacto-ovo-vegetarian, vegan, or macrobiotic diet that meets your needs as a diabetic.

The goals of a diabetic diet are to provide good nutrition so that all of your nutrient needs are met, to help you lose weight if you are overweight, to lower blood cholesterol, and to normalize your blood glucose levels.

The best approach for most diabetics is to eat a low-fat, high-carbohydrate diet and to focus on complex carbohydrates. This means that a vegetarian diet is a perfect choice. Foods that are high in soluble fiber such as legumes, oats, fruits, and vegetables may offer some additional benefit, but as long as the overall focus is on fiber-rich foods, you really don't need to concern yourself too much with which type of fiber you are eating.

Some diabetics have high levels of a type of fat called triglycerides in their blood. In some cases, a diet too high in carbohydrates can aggravate this condition, and your health care practitioner might encourage you to avoid an excessively high carbohydrate diet. You can still follow a vegetarian diet, perhaps one that provides slightly more calories from foods with monounsaturated fats, because these fats don't raise blood cholesterol or triglyceride levels. Good sources of monounsaturated fats include avocados, nuts, and foods cooked in olive oil. Don't overdo it, though. The best approach to lowering triglycerides is to lose weight, which requires a low-fat diet. Exercise is also important. You might find that weight loss produces enough of a drop in your triglycerides that you don't need to worry about the amount of carbohydrate in your diet.

Physical exercise might be the most important factor in controlling diabetes. In addition to causing weight loss, it seems to act directly on the cells in some way to make them more sensitive to insulin. So in Type II diabetes, exercise may help your cells take up glucose from the blood, and just one session of exercise can produce these benefits.[30] In any event, exercise is a crucial part of the habits to control diabetes.

For Type II diabetics, keeping fat intake

down to 15 to 20 percent of calories and carbohydrates between 65 and 70 percent of calories is a good goal. In this type of diabetes, as we've already noted, eating a diet high in complex carbohydrates and shedding a few pounds may be all you need to do. Remember, though, that needs differ, and it is a good idea to discuss your diet on an individual basis with a nutritionist.

People who are using insulin injections, whether they have Type I or Type II diabetes, need dietary instruction from a professional. The total number of calories you eat is important in this case, and the timing of your meals is important, too. Most Type I diabetics will benefit from a diet that is low in fat and high in complex carbohydrates. If you have Type I diabetes, you will always need insulin injections. However, eating the right diet can help you manage your blood glucose and also can prevent serious complications.

Using the Exchange Lists for Meal Planning

In the old days, all people with diabetes were placed on what is called an exchange-list diet. The exchange lists are useful in helping people choose a varied diet that will control blood glucose. They also are often used to help people lose weight. Today, however, diabetics are not tied to the exchange lists. There are many ways to plan meals to help keep blood sugar under control. Your nutrition counselor can assist you in planning meals with or without the exchange lists.

Some people find the exchange lists rigid and cumbersome for long-term use. Initially, following them means measuring foods and keeping close track of everything you eat. On the other hand, they can provide needed structure for those who prefer it. And as structured as they are, they do permit great flexibility in food choices while allowing you to feel confident that your diet is well balanced and appropriate for your diabetic needs. For some diabetics, rigid calorie control is important, and the exchange lists are a reassuring guide.

Even if you prefer a more casual approach to menu planning, you might find that the exchange lists can set you on the right track. Using them for a few weeks can give you a good feeling for what your diet should look like. Once people have used them for a while, they usually find that they are familiar enough with the various foods and with serving sizes that they no longer need to measure foods or refer to the lists.

If you decide to use the exchange lists, you'll find that they are somewhat limited in their choices for vegetarians. While the protein group includes plant proteins like beans and tofu, it doesn't include tempeh or seitan. There are no vegan choices in the milk group. We've revised the exchange lists in table 16.1 to make them useful for both vegans and lacto-ovo vegetarians.

The exchange lists are a simple way to control the amounts of calories, fat, protein, and carbohydrate consumed and to assure that the diet is well balanced. Therefore, they are ideal for diabetics and for people who want to lose weight. Although they might look a little off-putting to someone who hasn't used them before, they are pretty simple once you get the hang of them. Diet planning is based on making food choices from six groups of food: starches, vegetables, fruits, protein foods, milk, and fats. Your diet prescription will tell you exactly how many servings you should eat from each group each day. Foods in one group are roughly similar to one another based on their calorie, carbohydrate, protein, and fat content. Therefore, you can "exchange" foods within a particular group. So if your diet calls for three servings of fruit a day, you can choose from any of the foods in the fruit list. But you *can't* exchange foods between different groups. That is, you can't substitute a food from the vegetable list for one of your fruit choices because fruits and vegetables are quite different in calorie and nutrient content.

Some foods span two groups. For example, a glass of skim milk is equal to one serving (or one exchange) from the milk group. But a glass of 2 percent milk counts as one milk exchange *plus* one fat exchange.

In using the exchange lists, vegans have two choices. You can use all six of the exchange lists and choose nondairy milks from the milk list. Or if you don't use any type of milk in your diet, you can omit the milk group completely and use the other five groups. Just be certain to choose calcium-rich foods in the other groups. (See chapters 7 and 10 for help in making those choices.) This approach is somewhat heretical in the world of diabetes. Conventional wisdom is that appropriate diets for diabetics include a variety of foods from all six of the exchange lists. But that idea is based on the old-fashioned notion that all people need milk in their diet to meet calcium needs. There is nothing about diabetes per se that makes milk an essential food. It isn't essential for anyone, diabetic or not. So if you've been following a diabetic exchange-list diet for a while and want to make some changes, don't be afraid to insist that your nutrition counselor help you to work out a diet that doesn't include milk. If you are following a vegan diet, don't forget to include some foods fortified with vitamin B_{12} or to use a supplement.

In addition to the revised exchange lists, we've provided some sample meal plans in table 16.2, based on using the exchanges at different calorie levels.

Table 16.1 Exchange Lists for Vegetarian Meal Planning

STARCHY FOODS

A starch exchange provides approximately 15 grams of carbohydrates, 3 grams of protein, a trace of fat, and 80 calories.

Breads
½ bagel
½ burger bun
½ English muffin
½ 6-inch pita
1 6-inch chapati (Indian bread)
1 6-inch poori (Indian bread)
1 dinner roll
1 slice whole-grain bread
1 6-inch corn or flour tortilla

Cereals, Grains
⅓ cup bran cereal
½ cup bran, corn, or other flakes
½ cup Shredded Wheat
1 Shredded Wheat biscuit
3 tablespoons Grape-Nuts
1½ cups puffed rice or wheat
½ cup cooked cereal (oatmeal, 7-grain, oat bran, Bear Mush, farina, Wheatena, etc.)
½ cup cooked grits
⅓ cup cooked white or brown rice
½ cup cooked bulgur
⅓ cup cooked couscous

⅓ cup cooked millet
⅓ cup cooked quinoa
½ cup cooked pasta
¾ cup mung-bean (cellophane) noodles
⅓ cup polenta
⅓ cup cooked wheat berries
3 cups air-popped popcorn
3 tablespoons wheat germ
5 tablespoons bran

Starchy Vegetables
½ cup corn
1 6-inch corn on the cob
½ cup lima beans
⅔ cup parsnips
½ cup green peas
½ cup plantain
1 3-ounce potato
½ cup mashed potatoes
1 cup winter squash
⅓ cup sweet potatoes or yams
¼ cup chestnuts

Dried Beans
½ cup vegetarian baked beans, cooked beans, peas, or lentils (count as 1 starch exchange plus 1 protein exchange)
3 tablespoons miso

Crackers and Cookies
4 RyKrisps
3 graham crackers
5 oblong melba toasts
2 rice cakes
¾ ounce matzo
8 animal crackers
2 thin bread sticks
2 Fig Newtons
3 gingersnaps
2 oatmeal cookies
6 vanilla wafers

Other Foods
Count each of the following as 1 exchange of a starchy food plus 1 exchange of fat.

¼ cup bread dressing
1 2½-inch biscuit
1 2-inch square corn bread
¼ cup granola
2 4-inch pancakes
2 4-inch crisp taco shells
½ cup chow-mein noodles

TABLE 16.1 EXCHANGE LISTS FOR VEGETARIAN MEAL PLANNING
(cont.)

VEGETABLES

An exchange provides approximately 5 grams of carbohydrates, 2 grams of protein, no fat, and 25 calories. One exchange is equal to ½ cup cooked or 1 cup raw vegetables selected from the following. Note that starchy vegetables like potatoes and corn are listed with "Starchy Foods."

Alfalfa sprouts
Artichoke
Asparagus
Bamboo shoots
Beans (green, wax, Italian)
Beets
Bok choy
Brussels sprouts
Cabbage
Carrots
Cauliflower

Eggplant
Greens (kale, collards, mustard greens, turnip greens, beet greens, Swiss chard)
Jicama
Kohlrabi
Leeks
Mushrooms
Okra
Onions
Pea pods

Pepper
Radicchio
Rutabagas
Sauerkraut
Sea vegetables
Spinach
Squash, summer, and zucchini
Tomatoes
Tomato or vegetable juice
Turnips
Water chestnuts

FRUITS

One exchange of fruit provides approximately 15 grams of carbohydrates, no protein or fat, and about 60 calories.

1 apple
½ cup unsweetened applesauce
4 fresh apricots
½ banana
¾ cup blackberries
¾ cup blueberries
1 cup cantaloupe chunks
12 cherries
½ grapefruit
15 grapes
⅛ honeydew melon, or 1 cup honeydew melon cubes
1 kiwifruit

½ mango
1 nectarine
1 orange
1 cup papaya chunks, or ½ papaya
1 peach
1 pear
¾ cup pineapple chunks
2 plums
1 cup raspberries
1¼ cups strawberries
2 tangerines
1¼ cups watermelon cubes

Dried Fruits
7 apricot halves
2½ dates
1½ figs
3 prunes
2 tablespoons raisins

Juices
½ cup apple juice or cider
⅓ cup cranberry juice cocktail
⅓ cup grape juice
½ cup grapefruit juice
½ cup orange juice
½ cup pineapple juice
⅓ cup prune juice

◆◆◆

TABLE 16.1 EXCHANGE LISTS FOR VEGETARIAN MEAL PLANNING (cont.)

PROTEIN FOODS

One protein exchange provides 7 grams of protein, 3 grams of fat, and 55 calories.

½ cup tofu

1 tofu hot dog

¼ cup tempeh

1 ounce seitan

¼ cup roasted soy nuts

¼ cup prepared textured vegetable protein

2 tablespoons Parmesan cheese

3 egg whites

1 whole egg

¼ cup egg substitute

½ cup cooked dried beans (count as 1 protein exchange *plus* 1 starch exchange)

1 ounce soy cheese (count as 1 protein *plus* 1 fat exchange)

1 ounce dairy cheese (count as 1 protein *plus* 1 fat exchange)

1 veggie burger (count as 1 protein *plus* 1 fat exchange)

2 tablespoons peanut butter, tahini, almond butter, or other nut or seed butters (count as 1 protein exchange *plus* 2 fat exchanges)

2 tablespoons nuts (count as 1 protein exchange *plus* 2 fat exchanges)

1 tablespoon seeds (count as 1 protein exchange *plus* 2 fat exchanges)

MILKS

One exchange provides approximately 12 grams of carbohydrates, 8 grams of protein, between zero and 2 grams of fat, and about 90 calories.

1 cup light soy milk

1 cup Vegelicious

1 cup Rice Dream

1 cup skim cow's milk

1 cup buttermilk

½ cup skim-milk cottage cheese

¾ cup plain nonfat yogurt

1 cup 2% cow's milk (count as 1 milk exchange *plus* 1 fat exchange)

1 cup whole cow's milk (count as 1 milk exchange *plus* 2 fat exchanges)

1 cup regular soymilk (count as 1 milk exchange *plus* 1 fat exchange)

¾ cup fruit-flavored nonfat yogurt (count as 1 milk exchange *plus* 1 fruit exchange)

FATS

One exchange provides approximately 5 grams fat and about 45 calories.

⅛ avocado

1 teaspoon mayonnaise

1 tablespoon reduced-calorie mayonnaise

1½ tablespoons tofu mayonnaise (Nayonaise)

1 teaspoon vegetable oil

10 small or 5 large olives

2 teaspoons mayonnaise-type salad dressing

2 tablespoons low-fat salad dressing

1 teaspoon margarine

1 teaspoon butter

1 tablespoon reduced-calorie margarine

1 tablespoon cream cheese

1 tablespoon tofu cream cheese

2 tablespoons sour cream

2 tablespoons shredded coconut

1 tablespoon coconut cream

1 tablespoon coconut milk

TABLE 16.2 SAMPLE MENU PLANS USING THE EXCHANGE LISTS

1,500-Calorie Vegan Plan

13 starch exchanges
4 vegetable exchanges
3 fruit exchanges
3 protein exchanges
3 fat exchanges

BREAKFAST
1 cup 7-grain cereal
½ cup grapefruit juice
Slice toast, with 1 teaspoon margarine

SNACK
English muffin, with 1 tablespoon almond
    butter

LUNCH
Small pita, stuffed with ½ cup hummus,
    sliced tomato, lettuce
Peach

SNACK
Carrot sticks
3 cups air-popped popcorn

DINNER
½ cup vegetarian baked beans
1 small potato
1 cup collards
Slice whole wheat bread

SNACK
2 plums
3 graham crackers

1,500-Calorie Vegan or Lacto-Ovo Plan

10 starch exchanges
4 vegetable exchanges
3 fruit exchanges
3 protein exchanges
2 milk exchanges
4 fat exchanges

BREAKFAST
1 cup corn flakes
1 cup soymilk or skim milk
Slice toast, with 1 teaspoon margarine
½ cup apricots

SNACK
½ bagel
1 ounce soy cheese or cow's-milk cheese

LUNCH
1 6-inch pita
½ cup tofu chunks, with herbs and 1½
    tablespoons tofu mayonnaise
Salad (1 cup lettuce, 1 cup raw
    vegetables), with 2 tablespoons low-fat
    dressing

SNACK
Peach

DINNER
⅔ cup couscous with ½ cup chickpeas,
    flavored with lemon juice and fresh
    mint
½ cup steamed carrots
½ cup steamed spinach

SNACK
1½ cups puffed wheat cereal
1 cup soymilk or skim cow's milk
½ cup apple juice

TABLE 16.2 SAMPLE MENU PLANS USING THE EXCHANGE LISTS (cont.)

2,000-Calorie Vegan Plan	2,000-Calorie Vegan or Lacto-Ovo Plan
17 starch exchanges	15 starch exchanges
4 vegetable exchanges	4 vegetable exchanges
3 fruit exchanges	4 fruit exchanges
5 protein exchanges	4 protein exchanges
4 fat exchanges	2 milk exchanges
	5 fat exchanges

2,000-Calorie Vegan Plan

BREAKFAST
1 cup oatmeal
English muffin, with 2 teaspoons reduced-fat margarine
½ banana
½ cup calcium-fortified orange juice

SNACK
2 oatmeal cookies
Herb tea

LUNCH
1 cup lentil soup
Garden salad (lettuce, tomato, carrots, broccoli), with 2 tablespoons nonfat dressing
2 small rolls

SNACK
Bran muffin
Apple

DINNER
1 cup rice
1 cup black beans, with ½ cup chopped tomatoes
1 cup steamed kale
2 dinner rolls

SNACK
Slice whole wheat bread, with 2 tablespoons almond butter

2,000-Calorie Vegan or Lacto-Ovo Plan

BREAKFAST
Milk shake (1 cup soy or cow's milk, ½ banana, ½ cup strawberries)
English muffin, with 2 teaspoons margarine

SNACK
Bagel, with 2 tablespoons almond butter

LUNCH
1 cup chili (½ cup textured vegetable protein, ½ cup tomatoes)
1 cup brown rice
½ cup steamed kale
Roll

SNACK
2 rice cakes

DINNER
Veggie burger, with 1 hamburger bun
1 cup steamed broccoli
1 cup corn
½ cup applesauce

SNACK
1½ cups bran flakes, with 1 cup milk, ½ cup strawberries

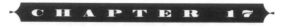

CHAPTER 17

WEIGHT CONTROL
VEGETARIAN-STYLE

◆◆◆

It's fun to count other people's
caloric intake.

—IRMA ROMBAUER, *The Joy of Cooking,* 1943

◆

In 1989, Americans spent more than $30 billion trying to get skinny.[1] Despite all that effort and money, we're fatter than ever. At least one out of every four Americans is significantly overweight.[2] At any given moment, 25 percent of all males and 50 percent of women are on a weight-loss diet.[3] And while we are very good at losing weight, keeping it off is another story. Most people regain between a third and two-thirds of the weight they lost within a year, and almost all of it is back within five years.[4] In fact, the very ineffectiveness of most of the diet programs out there is what keeps the dieting industry strong. Dieters hop from one program to another—from slimming shakes, pounds-off pills, to clinics where they can starve themselves to thinness under a physician's watchful eye—hoping to find the program that will finally work.

One thing that seems to help isn't a program at all. It's a vegetarian diet. Vegetarians are slimmer than meat eaters.[5]

Some people are surprised at the slenderness of vegetarians. Don't all those beans, potatoes, bread, and pasta make you fat? Everything we ever learned about dieting several decades ago told us to steer clear of starchy fare. Some of the most popular diet programs of the past involved counting grams of carbohydrates and avoiding them like the plague. But the vegetarian edge in weight control has become clear with a newer understanding of food and weight.

SUCCESSFUL WEIGHT CONTROL

The first step toward permanent weight control is to forget everything you've ever learned about dieting. Toss away those gruesome ideas of puny portions, endless calorie counting, and boring menus. Deprivation is out. So are counting calories and starvation plans. And you can hold on to your wallet. It doesn't cost money to lose weight because you don't need special foods or weigh-ins or a "diet counselor" to tell you how you are doing.

But those who fight the battle of the bulge do need to make some serious changes in the way they eat. If the way you eat now is making you fat, then it makes sense that you need to do something different to lose weight.

Also, patience is truly a virtue when it comes to weight control. On the road to permanent weight control, your best bet is to

◆◆◆

stay in the slow lane. You can take shortcuts and get the pounds off fast, but it is more difficult to keep them off. Seasoned dieters know that the faster the weight comes off, the faster it piles back on.

DON'T DIET!

To see why low-calorie diets are a bad idea, we need to understand the relationship of calories to weight gain. A calorie is actually a measure of energy in the same way that an inch is a measure of length and an ounce is a measure of weight. Your body takes in energy from food and uses it to fuel the various activities that keep you alive. Even when you think you aren't doing too much of anything—when you're staring out the window at work daydreaming, for example—your body is amazingly busy, working hard to keep your heart beating, your diaphragm moving so that you can breathe, and your brain cells functioning. The rate at which your body burns fuel (measured as calories) for all its activities when you are awake but not moving around or digesting food is called basal metabolism. Of course, you burn more calories throughout the day than what is needed to maintain basic functions. When you move your muscles, your fuel expenditure goes up. It increases when you digest food as well. But most of the calories you burn are due to your basal metabolism.

Some people have faster metabolisms than others—that is they burn more calories per minute and need more energy. Men tend to have higher metabolisms than women because they have more muscle tissue, and muscle burns calories. Fat doesn't burn calories very much so it doesn't add to your metabolic rate significantly. Even slender women usually have more fat tissue than the average man. Also, regular exercise tends to perk up metabolism a bit, so that active people burn somewhat more calories even when they aren't exercising.

The energy for your body's activities comes from foods. When you hear that a particular food is high in calories, it just means that this food contains a lot of energy that is available to the body as fuel. Fat, carbohydrates, protein, and alcohol all provide calories. If you take in the exact amount of energy you need, you're in good shape. If you take in too much energy from food, the body has no use for it, so it sends it off to its storage compartment—also known as fat tissue. When calorie intake gets too low, the body turns to its stores for fuel. It begins to break down body fat—and in some cases muscle tissue, too—and uses it for energy. The result is weight loss. You can force your body to break down that fat tissue by creating an energy deficit. This happens when you increase your caloric expenditure—by exercising—and/or when you reduce the amount of energy coming into the body by eating fewer calories.

But your body has a number of built-in defenses to preserve your life in threatening situations. When you drastically reduce your calorie intake, your body senses the threat of starvation. One reason that we can live for a long time without food is that the body is amazingly adept at dealing with a reduced intake of calories. It will break down fat, of course, and burn that for fuel. But it will also do two other things as it senses increasing danger of starvation. It will start to break down muscle tissue for fuel *and* it will slow the rate at which it burns calories. This produces a lowered metabolism, a common effect of chronic dieting. It explains why dieters shed five pounds a week and then suddenly hit that dreaded plateau, when they can't seem to ease another ounce off their hips despite an intake of eight hundred calories a day.

Exercise boosts your metabolism, although it probably does not increase metabolism much when calorie intake is too low. Exercise also maintains healthy muscle tissue while it eases off fat pounds. The best approach to keeping a normal metabolic rate is to reduce your calorie intake only moderately so that your body doesn't move into its starvation mode. You'll slim down slowly, especially if you don't have a great deal of weight to lose. This is frustrating to some people, but it is the only healthy and successful way to lose weight.

There is one more thing that you can do. Our explanation of calories and weight may be a little bit too simple. Recent research leads us to believe that the type of calories you eat may be as important as how many you eat. This might explain why vegetarians tend to be slimmer than meat eaters.

The Carbohydrate Connection

The old idea that people get fat simply because they eat too much food may not be the whole obesity story. In some cases, overweight people actually eat less.[6] But they eat too many fatty foods.

Fat is naturally fattening because it is

Table 17.1 Percentage of Calories from Fat in Foods	
Food	%
Baked potato	1
Black beans	3
Pasta	3
Brown rice	4
Banana	5
Broccoli	7
Whole wheat bread	16
Broiled skinless chicken breast	20
Broiled perch	30
2% milk	34
Whole milk	48
Sirloin steak	58
Egg	63
Cheddar cheese	73

higher in calories. A gram of carbohydrate or protein contains just four calories. An equal amount of fat has more than twice the calories, nine per gram. So the more fat in a food, the more calories it contains and the more fattening it is. Animal foods like meat, chicken, and dairy products tend to be higher in fat than plant foods. Look at the difference in the percentage of fat in plant and animal foods in table 17.1.

Because carbohydrate-rich foods are lower in fat, you can eat more food for fewer calories, which means that you are more apt to feel full. Look at the two meals in table 17.2. They both offer the same number of calories, but menu 2 is certainly more generous in food. You're likely to feel fuller and more satisfied after eating this meal.

TABLE 17.2 MENUS FOR WEIGHT CONTROL

Both of these menus provide the same number of calories—about 1,700. But menu 1 contains 75 grams of fat, whereas menu 2 has only 20 grams of fat. When you cut the fat, you can eat more.

Menu 1

BREAKFAST
4 ounces tofu, scrambled in 1 teaspoon margarine
Slice toast, with 1 teaspoon margarine
6 ounces orange juice

LUNCH
Pita, stuffed with ½ cup hummus
Tossed salad, (lettuce, tomato), with 2 tablespoons French dressing
Raw carrots
Banana

SNACK
Bran muffin

DINNER
Veggie burger, with 1 hamburger roll
½ cup French fries
½ cup steamed kale

SNACK
15 tortilla chips

Menu 2

BREAKFAST
4 ounces low-fat tofu, braised in vegetable broth
2 slices toast, with fruit spread
Strawberry shake (½ cup strawberries and 1 cup light soy milk)

SNACK
½ bagel, with fruit spread

LUNCH
Pita, stuffed with ½ cup chickpea salad, 1 tablespoon tofu mayonnaise
Tossed salad, with 2 tablespoons nonfat dressing
Raw carrots
6 vanilla wafers
Banana
6 ounces orange juice

SNACK
Soft pretzel, with mustard

DINNER
Veggie burger, with 1 hamburger roll
½ cup oven-fried potatoes
Dinner roll
½ cup steamed kale

SNACK
3 cups air-popped popcorn

Scientific studies support the idea that people who eat high-fat foods consume more calories.[7]

Theoretically it is possible to eat enough carbohydrate-rich foods that calories eventually add up to the point at which you gain weight. But that doesn't seem to happen when people eat low-fat diets.[8] For example, in a study of twenty-four women, subjects ate diets ranging in fat content from 15 to 50 percent of their calories. The ones who ate the lower-fat diets compensated somewhat by consuming slightly more food, but they never consumed as many calories as the women eating the higher-fat diets.[9] In a similar study at Cornell University, subjects who ate a low-fat diet (20 to 25 percent of their calories) also increased their food intake. But they never caught up to the subjects in the study whose diets were 35 to 40 percent fat.[10]

If the higher calorie content of fats were the whole story, it would be enough. But it turns out that those fat calories may actually be different. Traditionally, nutritionists have always believed that a calorie is a calorie. Eat too many of them, and you gain weight. But new studies are showing us that calorie for calorie, dietary fat turns into body fat more easily than carbohydrates do. The conversion of carbohydrates to body fat is just plain inefficient. For every hundred calories of carbohydrates that could potentially end up as fat, twenty-three get used up in the conversion process. However, dietary fat slips easily into body fat. We lose only three calories out of every hundred consumed in the process.[11]

These conversion factors may be irrelevant, though, in the face of one final virtue of carbohydrates. They seem to resist conversion to body fat. The reason is that carbohydrates are the preferred fuel source of the human body. Our body has evolved to burn carbohydrates for energy and seems to be very unlikely to turn it into fat. In one study, only 1 to 2 percent of the carbohydrates in subjects' diets were converted into fat.[12] Also, carbohydrates may give your metabolism a direct boost by activating a hormone that speeds up metabolism.[13] Perhaps for this reason, vegetarians have been shown to have a higher metabolic rate, so they burn up calories faster.[14]

Certainly, the total number of calories you consume is important, but it appears that the type of calories may be equally important. Consider the results of a Stanford University study. In 155 overweight men there was no relationship between the number of calories consumed and the amount of body fat. But the more fat the men ate, the more body fat they had.[15]

And, incidentally, you can't make up for a high-fat intake by boosting your exercise program. Subjects who consumed a high-fat diet burned fewer calories when they exercised.[16]

Protein is also inefficiently converted to fat. So theoretically a diet high in protein and low in fat will also help you to lose weight. But we can't recommend this as the best route to weight control. First, it is difficult to plan such a diet. The foods highest in protein—meat, dairy, and eggs—are often high in fat. A high-protein, low-fat diet would force you into a lifetime of eating broiled fish, skim milk, and egg whites. Second, we've seen throughout this book that diets high in animal protein are unhealthy and may raise your risk for heart

• Toss the word "diet" out of your vocabulary. When people think of diets, they generally think of a deviation from the way they usually eat in order to gain some benefit. The idea is that when you are done with your diet, you'll go back to your "real" way of eating. But permanent weight control means permanent changes in eating habits. It is about new, healthier habits, not a brief respite from old unhealthy ones.

• Choose high-fiber, whole foods whenever possible. Fiber has a well-earned reputation for helping people shed pounds.[17] Fiber provides few, if any, calories. It is also "bulky," so it seems to provide a feeling of fullness. These two factors make fiber a great aid to weight control. When subjects ate a low-fat, high-fiber diet, they reported that they felt full after eating only half as many calories as subjects who ate a low-fiber, high-fat meal.[18] Choose whole grains over refined and fruits over fruit juices to boost your fiber intake.

• Limit sugar. Sugar is a simple carbohydrate. Foods high in sugar tend to be very calorie dense. Even though carbohydrates are less likely to turn into fats, any calories will contribute to weight gain if you eat too many of them. Sugary foods are a surefire way to get the calorie content of your diet up. Also, sugar is often teamed up with fat in baked goods and candies. The foods we think of as sweets are more likely to be fats. For example, brownies are more than 40 percent fat, and cheesecake is more than 50 percent fat. These foods are likely to put the pounds on not because of the sugar they contain, but because they are so fatty. But even fat-free sweets like soft drinks, juices, and some of the new fat-free baked goods should be limited in the diet when you are watching your weight. It's also a good idea to avoid artificially sweetened foods, since they can perpetuate a craving for sweets. They also don't seem to help at all with weight control.[19]

• Avoid alcohol. It may actually suppress your body's ability to burn fat. Just three ounces of alcohol can reduce the body's ability to metabolize fat by as much as a third.[20] In addition, alcohol increases appetite, and its relaxing effects can weaken your resolve to stick to good eating habits.

• Get help if you need it. There is more to weight control than choosing the right foods. Many people suffer from problems associated with overeating, binge eating, food disorders, and body image. By all means, if you truly can't control your eating habits, for whatever reason, find some help. A trained counselor can help. So can Overeaters Anonymous, a twelve-step program for people with diet problems.

• Trade in your bathroom scale for a tape measure. Changes in weight aren't the best indicators of progress. Body fat is relatively light. This means that you can lose considerable amounts of fat and not have it register as anything significant on the scale. Muscle, on the other hand, is heavy and compact. As you change your eating behavior and begin to exercise, you will lose considerable amounts of light fat tissue and exchange it for small amounts of heavier, compact muscle tissue. The result will be a slimmer, firmer body—but the scale may not show much change in actual weight. Weigh-ins can be frustrating and depressing, and they really don't reflect the situation at all accurately. You'll know your body is changing, however, as you see changes in the way your clothing fits or when you take measurements with a tape measure.

• Believe that low-fat eating is wonderful. In the nutrition field there is a firmly held belief that low-fat diets are generally unacceptable to the public. However, several studies show low-fat eating plans to be very acceptable.[21] Not only that, but when people start eating low-fat foods, they begin to perceive fatty foods as unpleasant.[22] So if you despair of ever enjoying a baked potato without your usual topping of sour cream and chives, just give it a chance. Check some of the cookbooks in "Especially for Low-fat Cooks" in the resource section at the back of this book. After taking some time to experiment with low-fat cuisine, you'll probably find that you actually prefer eating this way.

disease, osteoporosis, kidney disease, and kidney stones. There are other ways to lose weight, but a high-carbohydrate diet is the only healthy, effective choice for permanent weight control.

EXERCISE

In addition to a low-fat eating plan, physical activity is crucial to keeping pounds off. It doesn't need to be a rigorous program, but it should pair up regular aerobic exercise, such as walking, jogging, or aerobic dancing with a moderate muscle-toning program. Aerobic exercise results in the breakdown of fat in your body. Also, while dieting can lead to loss of muscle tissue as well as fat, aerobic exercise helps to reduce muscle loss and results in more loss of fat. Toning exercise helps to firm muscles and increase muscle mass. Muscle burns calories, so the more muscle on your body, the more calories you burn at any given moment.

Look for activities that are a good fit to your lifestyle, and to both your physical and psychological comfort levels. If you don't feel comfortable in a gym, invest in a treadmill or exercise bike to use in the privacy of your home. The more simple your exercise program, the more likely you are to maintain it. Walking is probably the best choice. You can do it anywhere, and it doesn't require any more equipment than a good pair of shoes.

Your exercise program should be a good workout, but vigorous isn't necessarily better. Some studies show that moderate exercise burns more fat than vigorous exercise. You'll want to get your heart beating a little faster than usual, but walking is just as good as running for weight controls.[23]

WEIGHT CONTROL VEGETARIAN-STYLE

A good first step in a weight-control program is to adopt a vegetarian diet. For most people, this change alone will immediately produce an increase in carbohydrate intake and a drop in fat consumption. Animal foods tend to be higher in fat than plant foods, and complex carbohydrates are found *only* in plant foods. If you eat a diet that is 100 percent plant foods—a vegan diet—your meals are likely to be even lower in fat and higher in healthy carbohydrates.

But there are exceptions. Some plant foods are very fatty, including avocados, nuts, olives, and seeds, all of which are upward of 70 percent fat. Soybeans and tofu are about 50 percent fat. And, of course, you can be a vegan and still base your diet on the fattiest foods in town—French fries, potato chips, and sandwiches layered with slices of soy cheese. So while going vegetarian is a good first step toward permanent weight control, you need to use some wisdom in planning your vegetarian meals.

The best approach to planning low-fat meals for weight control is to follow the guide for meal planning that we outlined in chapter 10. You can lose weight without keeping track of serving sizes or total amounts of fat and calories as long as you follow the general guidelines in that chapter and always make smart choices within these food groups.

Grains. Choose whole grains whenever possible, since these high-fiber foods will fill you up. Watch out for hidden fat in breakfast cereals; cooked cereals tend to be more fiber rich and lower in fat than many cold cereals. Be cautious also with grain-based foods that may have a lot of added fat or are cooked in fat such as pancakes, waffles, tortillas, muffins, and biscuits.

Vegetables. Prepare them without added fats and serve with herbs, a squeeze of fresh lemon juice, or nonfat salad dressing. With the exception of avocados and olives, vegetables are almost fat free.

Fruits. Again, you can't go wrong with fruits, whether fresh, canned, or baked. Choose whole fruits over fruit juice whenever possible. Juices are much higher in calories than whole fruit. This makes sense when you consider that it takes three or four oranges to make one six-ounce glass of orange juice. And the juice also doesn't have the filling and healthful advantages of fiber.

Legumes. Nearly all beans are super-low-fat, high-carbohydrate foods. Except for textured vegetable protein, soyfoods tend to be quite a bit higher in fat than other foods in this group. Look for reduced-fat versions of tofu. Many commercial vegetarian products like tofu hot dogs, veggie burgers, and veggie breakfast patties are much lower in fat than the meats they replace, but they can still be fatty foods. There are a few nonfat and low-fat meat analogues on the market. Look for these or limit the amounts of analogues in your diet.

Nuts and seeds. Enjoy these foods in very small quantities, no more than a serving a day. They are the highest in fat of all natural, whole foods.

Milks. Lacto-ovo vegetarians who drink cow's milk should stick to skim or 1 percent milk. Soymilk contains about as much fat as 2 percent cow's milk, which makes it fairly high in fat for those who are trying to lose weight. Low-fat soymilk is becoming increasingly available, and you can also choose nonfat soymilk. You might also try rice milk on your morning breakfast cereal for a lower-fat beverage.

Fats. This is one case in which there is no

advantage to vegetable oil over its saturated-fat counterparts. All fats are fattening. You really don't need added fats in your diet. We include them in the food guide in chapter 10 to help vegetarians maintain an adequate calorie intake. You can eliminate them if you like or include just one or two teaspoons a day. Keep in mind that a teaspoon of added fat is a tiny amount but it contains forty-five calories and five grams of fat.

Other foods. These are foods to eliminate if you are watching your fat calories. Cheese, eggs, commercial baked goods, and snacks are all too high in fat for regular use, and you don't need any of them in your diet. For desserts, choose fruit ices or sorbets, baked whole fruit, or fresh fruit salad.

DEFATTING VEGETARIAN MEALS

How did carbohydrates get their fattening reputation? Well, it may have something to do with the way we eat them. We love to fatten up our healthy carbohydrates. We drench baked potatoes in butter, sour cream, and melted cheese. Bread gets slathered with butter, peanut butter, or piled high with cheese.

Since vegetarian diets are based on carbohydrate-rich plant foods, the most important step toward defatting them is to treat those foods with care in the way we prepare and serve them.

Bread Spreads
Reduce your use of fatty spreads like margarine, butter, peanut butter, and mayonnaise by trying the following:

- Mash soft, cooked beans with chopped onions and celery, herbs or spices, and your favorite condiments, such as lemon juice, salsa, mustard, or ketchup, to create your own tasty bean spreads for sandwiches or toast.

- Puree dried fruit for sweet toppings for toast.

- Blend low-fat tofu with herbs and lemon juice to create savory spreads.

Potato Toppers
A baked potato has just ninety-five calories and less than a gram of fat. But load it up with butter and melted cheese, and the calories skyrocket to more than three hundred, with as much as twenty-five grams of fat. When you give up the butter, sour cream, or cheese sauce on your potato, you'll find that there are still plenty of options. Try one of the following on your next baked potato:

Salsa

Steamed asparagus

Vegetarian chili

Vegetable stew

Vegetables and pineapple in a sweet-and-sour sauce

Sloppy joes made with textured vegetable protein

Baked beans

Vegetable curry

Stewed tomatoes

Baked Goods

You can reduce the fat in nearly any cake or cookie recipe by at least a quarter and sometimes much more. Keep cutting the fat down every time you make a favorite recipe until you reach the minimum amount that will produce a tasty product. Baking with whole wheat pastry flour or with unbleached white flour will keep low-fat baked goods more tender. You can also replace some of the fat with thick, pureed moist ingredients like mashed bananas, blended tofu, or pureed prunes. Since fat tends to intensify flavors, you may need to increase the amount of vanilla extract or spices in your lower-fat baked goods.

Dressings

There are a number of wonderful nonfat salad dressings on the market. Note that there is a difference between nonfat and low fat. Low-fat dressings still contain some fat, so you will need to watch the amounts you use. You can also make your own. Blend V-8 juice with vinegar, lime juice, and chunks of cucumbers or peppers to make a chunky, refreshing dressing for summer salads. Or blend nonfat yogurt or cottage cheese with lemon juice and herbs.

Cooking for Great Low-Fat Flavor

For dishes that call for onions or other ingredients to be sautéed in oil, try sautéing in sherry or dry wine instead. Vegetable broth, tomato juice, or even apple juice are other good choices. Perk up the flavors in your low-fat dishes by using fresh herbs, sun-dried tomatoes (not the kind packed in oil), fresh ginger, or freshly squeezed lemon or lime juice. Try a few drops of black-walnut extract in rice dishes.

Sauces and Gravies

Dishes that call for cream will never know the difference if you add blended tofu instead. It adds a rich, creamy texture and flavor to recipes. Thicken soups and stews with pureed vegetables or mashed potatoes. Pinto beans or chickpeas, pureed, diluted with water, and seasoned with a dash of salt, pepper, and herbs, make a perfect low-fat gravy. Low-fat tofu blended with cooked vegetables makes a rich sauce to serve over rice or pasta.

Lacto-Ovo Vegetarians, Watch Out!

Vegetarians who use generous amounts of milk, cheese, and eggs can get way too much fat in their diet. Use only skim or 1 percent milk and only small amounts of shredded cheese to flavor foods if you use it at all. One ounce of cheddar cheese contains more than nine grams of fat and gets nearly 75 percent of its calories from fat. Limit eggs to just one or two per week if you use them at all.

Smart Substitutions

In any food category, there will always be a best and a worst choice. When you want a snack, try fat-free pretzels, popcorn sprinkled with nutritional yeast or Parmesan cheese, or fat-free crackers. There are several fat-free potato chips and tortilla chips available now.

Stop and do some creative thinking when the first food that comes to mind is a fatty one. If you usually serve guacamole and chips at a party, try our spicy black-bean dip (see the recipe section at the back of the

HIGH-FAT VEGETARIAN FOODS

Not all plant foods are low fat. Beware of these fatty vegetarian food:

Many commercial veggie burgers

French fries

Falafel

Vegetable potpie

Tofu ice cream

Some meat analogues

Hummus

Soy cheese

Peanut butter

Almond butter

Regular soymilk

Tofu

Commercial vegan cookies and cakes

Tahini

Oils

Vegan mayonnaise

Avocados

Olives

Coconut

Potato chips

---

book) instead with home-baked pita chips. If you always have homemade French fries on Saturday night, opt for oven fries. Just cut potatoes in thick wedges, dust with chili pepper if you like, and bake on a cookie sheet spayed with nonstick spray at 450 degrees Fahrenheit until they are browned and puffed.

SNACKS FOR VEGETARIAN WEIGHT WATCHERS

It's easier to stick to low-fat eating when you include plenty of carbohydrate-rich snacks in your eating plan. These are super foods for people who are watching their weight. They're filling, satisfying, tasty, and simple. Stock your kitchen with them, and you'll always have something healthy and low fat on hand.

Potatoes, baked, broiled, grilled, or boiled

Steamed vegetables

Bean soups

Fresh salads with nonfat dressing

Fresh fruit salads

High-fiber ready-to-eat cereals for crunchy snacks

Whole-grain breads

Bagels

Pita bread

Nonfat crackers

Rice cakes

Air-popped popcorn

Soft pretzels with mustard

Baked fruit dusted with cinnamon

FIGURING OUT FAT

If you prefer to keep track of the amount of fat in your diet, there are two ways to do it. You can invest in a pocket-sized book that lists the amount of fat in foods and keep a daily tally of your fat intake. Try to keep your fat intake down to fewer than 35 grams per day.

Determining the percentage of calories in your diet that come from fat involves a bit more record keeping. You'll need to keep track of your total fat intake (in grams) and the number of calories you consume each day. Multiply the grams of fat by 9 (because there are 9 calories in a gram of fat), and divide by the total number of calories you consume. So if you eat 35 grams of fat a day and consume 1,800 calories, your diet is 17 percent fat:

$$\frac{35 \times 9}{1,800} = .17$$

A good goal for anyone who wants to lose weight is a diet that is between 10 and 15 percent fat. But don't get too wrapped up in numbers. If you find that your favorite reading material is food labels, then you may be placing too much emphasis on seeking out lower-fat versions of fatty processed foods. When you plan your meals around whole, unprocessed plant foods, and limit your intake of nuts, seeds, and oils, your diet will automatically be low in fat and rich in complex carbohydrates.

WERE YOU BORN TO BE FAT?

We know that to some extent weight is affected by genetics. This means that some of us will never be superslender models while others will seemingly stay slim no matter what they do. Despite how hard they try, some people simply remain heavier than others. It's good to have a realistic view of the situation—but it isn't an excuse for giving up. First, having heavy parents and siblings doesn't necessarily indicate a genetic tendency toward obesity. Weight problems run in families for a variety of reasons. Did your parents pass on fat genes to you, or did they pass along their favorite fatty recipes?

Second, don't blame your weight problems on your genes unless you are leading a healthy lifestyle. If you are eating a 10- to 15-percent-fat diet and exercising every day and your body still stays a stubborn twenty pounds away from your goal weight, then you might just as well accept that this is where you belong. Don't abandon your healthy eating habits and exercise program, though. They will keep you close to where you are meant to be weightwise—perhaps twenty pounds away from so-called ideal weight rather than sixty pounds away from it.

When it comes to weight control, there are no guarantees. Any program that promises that you can reach a particular weight is lying. We're all different, with different body types. Our advice is to eat a low-fat diet and to exercise. It may not get your weight where you wish it could be, but it will get it where it is right for you.

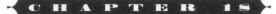
THE VEGETARIAN ATHLETE

Users of low-protein and the non-flesh dietaries have far greater endurance than those who are accustomed to the ordinary American diet.

—IRVING FISHER, PROFESSOR,
YALE UNIVERSITY, 1906

◆

For centuries, people believed that meat was important for athletes. It's easy to see why. If physical performance depends on strong muscles, doesn't it make sense to eat muscles? The nineteenth-century German chemist Liebig proposed that the energy for all muscular movement came from protein.

But by the 1850s, scientists knew that the important fuels for physical activity were actually carbohydrates and fat—not protein at all. Despite that, protein and meat continued to be favored by athletes well into the twentieth century; as recently as the 1970s the dinner of choice for any college football team was steak.

But long before meat-based diets fell out of favor for athletes, there were successful vegetarian athletes. Near the turn of the century Professor Irving Fisher of Yale University was intrigued with the physical endurance of "meat abstainer" athletes.[1] His studies were crude by today's standards but were interesting nonetheless. Dr. Fisher studied three groups of people: meat-eating athletes, vegetarian athletes, and a group of sedentary vegetarian nurses and physicians from the Battle Creek Sanitarium in Michigan. His results showed a remarkable superiority of vegetarians in three simple tests of endurance: (1) holding the arms horizontally as long as possible, (2) doing deep knee bends, and (3) raising the legs while lying on the back. Even the best members of the meat-eating group could hold his arms out horizontally only half as long as the vegetarians. Eighty percent of the vegetarians were able to do more than 325 knee bends, compared with just one-third of the omnivores. In some cases, even the sedentary vegetarian physicians and nurses outperformed the meat-eating athletes!

In a 1904 study, researchers tested endurance by measuring the number of times students could lift a weight by pulling on a handle. Nonvegetarians averaged thirty-eight times, whereas the vegetarians were able to lift the weight sixty-nine times.[2]

Early vegetarian athletes were excelling outside the laboratory as well:

• The London Vegetarian Society's athletic and cycling club, led by a member with the delightful name of James

VEGETARIAN ATHLETES

Think you need meat to compete? These superathletes—all vegetarians—are proof that vegetarian diets are a great choice for competition.

Surya Bonaly, French Olympic figure skater

Andreas Cahling, champion bodybuilder

Chris Campbell, Olympic medalist in wrestling

Desmond Howard, Heisman-trophy winner and professional football player

Billie Jean King, tennis champion

Bill Manetti, power-lifting champion

Martina Navratilova, tennis champion

Paavo Nurmi, long-distance runner with twenty world records

Bill Pearl, four-time Mr. Universe

Dave Scott, six-time triathlon winner

Parsley, won competitions over meat eaters in the 1890s. Parsley himself won the most prestigious hill-climbing race in England.[3]

• Around the same time, the West Ham Vegetarian Society formed a tug-of-war team that set records in that sport.

• Vegetarian American cyclist Will Brown thrashed all records for a 3,218-kilometer bicycle race in the 1890s.

• Vegetarian cyclist Margarita Gast established a women's record for a 1,606-kilometer race in the 1890s.

• In an 1893 walking race from Berlin to Vienna, the first two competitors to finish were vegetarians.

• A turn-of-the-century 100-kilometer race in Germany attracted attention because eleven of the fourteen competitors who finished the race were vegetarians.

• In 1912, a vegetarian was the first man to complete a marathon in less than two hours and thirty minutes.

According to historian James C. Whorton, meat eaters were reluctant to consider that vegetarianism might have some advantages. Instead, they credited the success of the vegetarians "not to their diets, but to their fanaticism."[4]

Today, some of the world's best athletes continue to defeat the idea that meat is essential for strength. Six-time triathlon winner Dave Scott, who reportedly trains eight hours a day, eats a diet that consists mainly of brown rice, tofu, low-fat dairy foods, and large amounts of fruits and vegetables, providing more than six thousand calories a day.[5]

As you can see in the sidebar "Vegetarian Athletes," the number of superathletes who eat a meatless diet is proof that vegetarianism can support athletic performance. But how do vegetarian athletes compare with nonvegetarian athletes today? Only two modern studies have tried to answer this question. In a 1986 Israeli study, researchers looked at criteria that can predict athletic performance, including strength, aerobic capacity, blood iron levels, and lung capacity. There was little difference between the vegetarian and nonvegetarian athletes.[6] A second study didn't use athletes but considered physiological factors that predict athletic performance in housewives and office workers. This study compared vegans with meat eaters and found essentially no difference in lung capacity, exercise performance on a stationary bicycle, and muscle development.[7]

These studies show that there is certainly no disadvantage to a vegetarian diet for athletes. But there may be some clear advantages to going meatless for competition, as we'll see later in this chapter.

MEETING THE NUTRIENT NEEDS OF ATHLETES ON A VEGETARIAN DIET

The specific nutrient needs of an athlete depend on how rigorously he or she trains. Generally speaking, a vegetarian diet comes closer to the recommendations for athletes than a standard Western diet. Both the American and Canadian Dietetic Associations recommend that the ideal diet for adult athletes include no more than 30 percent of calories from fat and between 60 and 70 percent of calories from carbohydrates.[8] For a diet to be high in carbohydrates it needs to make liberal use of plant foods, since carbohydrates are found only in these foods.

People who exercise are likely to have slightly increased nutrient needs. However, exercise also increases calorie needs, so athletes generally eat more. As long as food choices are made from the food groups we outlined in table 10.1, vegetarians should have no trouble meeting the increased nutrient needs of moderate exercise.

But while the casual jogger or Sunday tennis player can easily meet nutrient requirements, those needs are quite a bit higher for elite athletes who train rigorously. The following sections on nutrition are aimed at those athletes, including both endurance athletes, such as long-distance runners, and strength athletes, such as bodybuilders, who are in heavy training. This information is less relevant to you if you run three or four miles every day, attend aerobic dance classes, or do some moderate weight lifting for toning purposes. Under those circumstances, you won't have any problem meeting nutrient needs as long as you are eating the healthy, well-balanced vegetarian diet recommended in this book and meeting the increased calorie needs of exercise by choosing additional servings of whole grains, legumes, nuts, fruits, and vegetables.

Protein

Although muscle is mostly water, it does contain about 25 percent protein, so weight lifters and other athletes who want to bulk up often think first of this nutrient. Two recent surveys found that football players and triathletes consume more protein than the typical nonathlete—about two and half times the RDA for protein.[9] However, the amount of protein consumed varies widely among athletes.[10]

The National Research Council, which establishes the RDAs, notes that the recommendations for protein (and for all nutrients) include a margin of safety and that there is no reason to establish higher levels for athletes.[11] We think that research on protein needs of athletes suggests otherwise. As we discussed in chapter 6, individual protein needs are really based on body weight, and healthy adults need on average 0.8 grams of protein for every kilogram of body weight. However, athletes may actually need much more. According to the American and Canadian Dietetic Associations' position statement on nutrition for exercise, athletes should consume 1.5 grams of protein for every kilogram of body weight, or nearly two times the RDA.[12]

Most research on protein needs for exercise has been done on endurance athletes. In endurance sports, amino acids are catabolized—or used up—at a faster rate. In these athletes, protein needs are measured using nitrogen-balance studies. Since nitrogen is found almost exclusively in protein, these studies compare the amount of nitrogen in the diet with the amount lost in the urine and feces. When more nitrogen is lost than is consumed, protein needs are not met. This is called negative nitrogen balance (chapter 6 includes a more thorough discussion of nitrogen balance). Studies show that in some athletes who train very rigorously, protein needs can actually be quite a bit higher than expected. Endurance athletes

who consumed just 25 percent more than the RDA for protein were in negative nitrogen balance. They were just barely able to maintain nitrogen balance when they consumed two times the RDA for protein.[13] In a study of Polish weight lifters, five of the ten athletes studied were in negative nitrogen balance, even though they consumed two and a half times the RDA for protein.[14]

Of course these may be extreme cases. Clearly, protein needs vary considerably among athletes, depending on body size and intensity of exercise. Based on studies of nitrogen balance, it seems 1.5 grams of protein per kilogram of body weight would be adequate for most athletes. Although this is much higher than the RDA, it doesn't mean special protein drinks or supplements are needed. And it is perfectly reasonable to meet these needs on a vegetarian diet.

Let's consider the case of a 75-kilogram (165 pound) lacto-ovo-vegetarian male who consumes about 3,650 calories per day (that's 2,700 calories for normal activities plus 950 calories for training). About 13 percent of the calories in a typical lacto-ovo-vegetarian diet come from protein, so this athlete will consume about 119 grams of protein. (Thirteen percent of 3,650 means that 475 calories are coming from protein; divide that number by 4 because a gram of protein provides 4 calories.) The protein needs of this athlete—1.5 grams times 75 kilograms—are 113 grams of protein per day. You can see that this athlete would have no trouble meeting his protein needs.

Vegan athletes may not meet protein needs with quite as much ease. Typically, vegan diets are about 11 to 12 percent pro-

TABLE 18.1 FOOD GUIDE FOR
MALE AND FEMALE ATHLETES

2,500 CALORIES
13 percent protein
17 percent fat
70 percent carbohydrates

17 servings whole grains
3 servings legumes
1 serving nuts and seeds
3 servings milk (soymilk, Vegelicious,
  or cow's milk)
4 servings vegetables
4 servings fruit
6 servings fats

food to meet their requirements for protein than nonathletes. But strength athletes—weight lifters—are a different story. Although the need for increased protein is better supported in endurance athletes than in strength athletes, both need more protein than nonathletes. But it isn't the additional muscle that weight lifters are adding that raises protein needs. A very hardworking bodybuilder might be able to gain a half pound of muscle each week—though this rate of muscle gain would be a tremendous accomplishment. This is about 227 grams of *muscle* tissue. One quarter of that, or 57 grams, would be protein. So a weight lifter would require an additional 57 grams of protein per week and therefore would need only 8 additional grams of protein each day.

Clearly, it isn't the addition of muscle that raises protein needs for athletes. Rather, the extra demand for protein comes from the fact that exercise causes protein to be metabolized at a faster rate.

A one-and-a-half-hour weight-lifting session burns up fewer calories than running does. With the same type of calculations as used above, an 80-kilogram lacto-ovo-vegetarian weight lifter who required 3,750 calories per day (about 450 fewer than a runner) would consume 121 grams of protein. He requires about 120, so protein intake would be adequate. A vegan would consume about 102 grams of protein, or about 18 grams fewer than required. Again, this deficit can easily be made up by consuming additional sources of protein-rich plant foods. It's clear, however, that in the case of vegan strength athletes, meeting protein needs requires

tein. Therefore, our athlete above would consume only 100 grams of protein each day from his vegan diet. Although below recommendations, it is only 13 grams short—the amount of protein in about one cup of beans. With minor modifications, vegan athletes can also easily meet protein needs.

Of course, the above examples assume that athletes will meet their additional calorie needs by consuming more whole foods from the food groups in chapter 10. If athletes boost their calorie intake by consuming high-calorie, low-protein foods like pastries, candy bars, snack chips, soft drinks, and fruit juices, they may have trouble meeting protein needs. The guidelines in table 18.1 can help athletes choose diets that meet the protein needs of competition.

So far, we've been talking mainly about endurance athletes. They have high calorie needs, so it's easy for them to eat enough some thought. Our sample menu for a vegan weight lifter shows that it is certainly reasonable to meet those needs without the addition of protein supplements.

A few final thoughts on protein for athletes. We want to stress again that these recommendations are for elite, champion, or Olympic-level athletes. They are of much less concern to the average jogger or weight lifter whose protein needs will easily be met by consuming just the RDA for this nutrient. Also, while this discussion is based on sound research that supports a higher-protein requirement for athletes, it is certainly not the final word on the topic. There is widespread disagreement on protein needs of athletes. Some experts believe that protein needs are basically the same for athletes as for nonathletes. One of the world's experts on protein, Dr. Vernon Young of the Massachusetts Institute of Technology, suggests that athletes need between 1 and 1.5 grams of protein per kilogram of body weight.[15] However, some researchers suggest as much as 2 grams of protein per kilogram of weight.[16] This means that an 80-kilogram man would require 160 grams of protein each day.

Finally, the number of calories consumed affects protein needs. When calorie intake is too low, protein is not used efficiently, and protein needs are higher. And, of course, it is harder to meet those elevated protein needs on a low-calorie diet.

Even though vegetarian athletes may need to make an extra effort to include enough protein in their diet, they may have some real nutritional advantages. Remember that excess protein intake can be problematic. High animal-protein intakes are associated with loss of calcium (see chapter 7) and possibly increased risk of osteoporosis. But protein from legumes does not have the same calcium-wasting effect as animal protein. In particular, soy protein has been shown to reduce calcium loss compared with animal protein.[17] So athletes who boost their protein intake by eating more soy products may have some advantage.

An additional concern is the effect of high protein intake on the kidneys, since excess protein may be one factor in kidney disease.[18] Again, however, plant proteins such as soy don't have the same adverse effect as animal protein on kidneys.[19]

Given the higher protein needs of athletes and the adverse effects of animal proteins, vegetarian diets seem to make good sense for athletes. When the diet is plant based, meeting those high needs without danger of too much animal protein is possible.

Iron

Because iron is key to providing adequate oxygen for energy production, low levels of iron can hamper physical performance in athletes. This is especially true in aerobic exercise (walking, running, swimming, and so on) because these kinds of exercise depend on increased uptake of oxygen by the body.[20] Because exercise increases blood volume and muscle mass—both of which require iron—it makes sense that athletes might need more iron.[21] Iron is also lost from the body through sweat. In one study, subjects who sat in a sauna until their body temperatures were as high as those experienced by endurance athletes on a sunny day lost about 1.3 liters of sweat per hour for a loss of about a half milligram of iron.[22] Since only about 10 percent of the iron in the diet is absorbed, a loss of a half milligram theoretically raises dietary iron needs by 50 percent or more. It is likely that other factors increase iron needs for athletes as well.

The iron levels of both male and female athletes are below those of the general population.[23] Many athletes experience a phenomenon called sports anemia. This is a temporary iron deficiency that may be caused by hemodialysis—the destruction of red blood cells—which occurs with exercise.[24] Blood iron levels also decrease because of hemodilution; that is, blood volume increases so iron concentration decreases.[25]

Athletes' need for more iron is controversial. Poor iron status—even without true anemia—can impair performance.[26] But while iron levels drop during the initial weeks of training, they tend to climb back up to normal as training continues.[27] Also, because high levels of iron might increase the risk for heart disease and cancer (see chapter 9), it may not be wise to recommend routine supplements for iron.[28] However, there is no risk in increasing your iron intake by eating more plant-rich foods, since it appears to be iron from animal foods that primarily raises the risk for these diseases.

Female athletes are at a greater risk for low iron levels than are males. They tend to have smaller iron reserves, and they also lose iron through menstruation—although many elite female athletes stop menstruating. Clearly, if anemia is a problem, iron supplements will help. But the best advice is for athletes to have their iron levels monitored and to include iron-rich plant foods in their diet.

Carbohydrates

Carbohydrates are stored in the muscles and liver in the form of glycogen. Muscle glycogen is an important source of fuel for very intense exercise of short duration because it can be burned for energy without oxygen. In fact, during intense exercise, like sprinting, muscle glycogen is the only source of energy. Lower-intensity exercise, such as walking or jogging, is fueled by fatty acids and glucose in the blood via a process called aerobic metabolism.

High levels of muscle and liver glycogen offer an advantage to athletes. After a strenuous workout, glycogen stores are generally depleted, and a high-carbohydrate diet is necessary to build them up again. Athletes may need to consume as many as 2,000 to 3,200 calories in the form of carbohydrates in order to maintain glycogen stores and to achieve greater endurance.[29] For an athlete consuming 3,800 calories per day, this can mean that he or she may need to eat a diet that is, on average, 70 percent or even as much as 80 percent carbohydrate.

The carbohydrate intake of nonvegetarian athletes is around 45 to 50 percent of calories, which is much lower than is optimal for athletic performance.[30] Perhaps because of the age-old love affair with meat among athletes, some athletes who eat meat are still reluctant to increase their carbohydrate intake.[31] The higher carbohydrate intake of vegetarians and, in particular, vegans is a definite advantage of meatless eating for athletes.

Calories

Athletes have the enviable problem of needing to consume additional calories. Needs range considerably, depending on the type and intensity of training. An athlete can require anywhere from 2,000 to more than 6,000 calories per day to maintain appropriate weight and muscle mass.[32] Vegans in particular may need to make a special effort to consume adequate calories, since vegan diets are usually higher in fiber and lower in fat. Athletes can increase calorie intake by consuming frequent meals, high-calorie snacks, and some refined carbohydrates. The sample menu in table 18.4 shows what it might take to consume 5,500 calories on a vegan diet.

Other Nutrients

Athletes need greater amounts of other nutrients, including some of the B vitamins. Thiamin, riboflavin, niacin, vitamin B_6, and other B vitamins are used to metabolize protein, carbohydrates, and fat. Generally, the more calories you eat, the higher your need for these vitamins. Athletes have such high calorie needs that they are very likely to consume more of all the vitamins and minerals simply because they eat more food. Also, because the RDAs for these nutrients are quite a bit higher than what most people need, they will satisfy the nutrient needs of most athletes.

In some cases, however, it isn't clear that the RDAs are enough for athletes. Unfortunately, we have fairly limited information on the nutrient needs of elite athletes for many of the nutrients:

• The RDA for the B vitamin thiamin is 1.5 milligrams for men and 1.1 milligrams for women. While this is plenty of thiamin for most people, true thiamin needs are closely tied to calorie intake. People need about 0.5 milligrams for every 1,000 calories they consume. So an athlete who requires 4,000 calories a day actually needs 2 milligrams of thiamin, which is well above the RDA. But a vegetarian athlete who is including plenty of whole grains, enriched grains, legumes, nuts, seeds, fruits, and vegetables—all rich in thiamin—and who is meeting calorie needs, should have no trouble meeting those needs.

• The need for riboflavin is calculated at 0.6 milligrams per 1,000 calories. Again, athletes with high calorie needs might need more than the RDA of 1.7 milligrams for men and 1.3 milligrams for women. Several studies have shown that exercise generally increases riboflavin needs.[33] Vegetarian athletes can meet those increased needs by including plenty of leafy green vegetables and both whole and enriched grains in the diet.

• Although niacin is needed for fat and glucose metabolism—both of which are used as fuel during exercise—supplements of this vitamin don't seem to improve athletic performance.[34] The amino acid tryptophan in protein is actually converted into niacin. So athletes who meet their higher protein needs should also easily meet niacin needs.

• Vitamin B_6, pyridoxine, is needed for protein metabolism and also for the formation of hemoglobin and myoglobin. Vitamin B_6 needs are considerably higher when protein intake increases. However, the RDA for this vitamin has a very large margin of safety and should be enough to meet even the high protein intake of athletes.

• Vitamin B12 (cobalamin) and folic acid are both needed for red-blood-cell formation. Exercise speeds up the destruction of red blood cells so the need for both these nutrients is probably higher in athletes. Some athletes actually take B12 injections because they believe this speeds up the transport of oxygen to the muscles. But unless an athlete is actually deficient in B12, the use of supplements or injections doesn't seem to improve performance.[35] Because the RDA for B12 is actually about twice what most people need, athletes who meet that RDA should be in good shape. Of course, for vegans, this means using fortified foods or taking a supplement. Vegetarians generally have fairly high intakes of folic acid, which is abundant in whole grains, vegetables, and some fruits. Athletes may have higher needs, but they should easily meet them on a well-balanced vegetarian diet.

• Vitamin C needs are higher when people perform physical labor at high temperatures, so it makes sense that athletes may need more.[36] Again, we don't know how much vitamin C athletes actually need because requirements depend on the individual person and his or her exercise program. Most athletes can probably meet their nutrient needs by consuming a few additional sources of vitamin C–rich fruits or vegetables every day.

Vegetarians have higher intakes of vitamin C than nonvegetarians. Megadoses of vitamin C don't seem to help athletes perform any better.[37]

• Vitamin E helps to keep red blood cells healthy. When intake is too low, red blood cells are destroyed more rapidly. This may be especially important to athletes, since they generally experience faster red-blood-cell destruction. Exercise raises vitamin E needs, and exercise at high altitudes raises them even more.[38] But again, as long as athletes are choosing nutritious foods to meet their higher calorie needs, they should have no trouble getting adequate vitamin E, which is found in wheat germ, whole grains, vegetables, and vegetable oils.

• Both exercising strenuously and sweating raise the need for zinc.[39] Vegetarian athletes may need to make an effort to include several servings of zinc-rich foods in their diet every day, since this is one nutrient that is in short supply in carbohydrate-rich plant foods. The list of foods that are good sources of zinc in chapter 9 can be used as a guideline. Again, although zinc needs may be higher for athletes, supplementing the diet doesn't seem to help performance.[40]

The food guides in this chapter, designed to help athletes meet higher calorie, protein, and iron needs, automatically provide substantial amounts of all other nutrients. There doesn't seem to be any need for supplements when an athlete eats a well-balanced vegetarian diet.

MENSTRUAL PROBLEMS IN VEGETARIAN ATHLETES

A considerable number of women athletes who undergo intense training experience amenorrhea, which is loss of menstruation.[41] This is caused by changes that result in lower levels of estrogen in the blood. There is some risk involved here, since estrogen promotes bone health, and low levels of estrogen at any age can cause bone loss.[42] Of course, exercise itself protects bone health, so some experts have suggested that the benefits of exercise outweigh, or at least cancel, the risks of amenorrhea.[43] However, women athletes who stop menstruating do appear to lose bone matter in the vertebrae and other areas of the skeleton.[44] This might be especially harmful in teenage girls, whose bone development is just reaching its peak. Young women who miss 50 percent of their periods may end up with smaller bones by the age of twenty and could be at risk for osteoporosis later in life.[45]

Amenorrhea may be of special concern for vegetarian women. Compared with nonvegetarians, vegetarian women have lower levels of estrogen and of prolactin, another hormone that affects menstruation.[46] These differences in hormone levels may occur because vegetarians eat more fiber and less fat.[47]

Researchers at the Pennsylvania State University College of Medicine found that young vegetarians were about five times as likely as nonvegetarians to experience menstrual irregularities and to miss periods.[48] Since athletes are also more likely to stop menstruating, it isn't surprising that in vegetarian athletes the problem is compounded. In one study of amenorrheic athletes, 82 percent of the subjects were found to be vegetarians, while only 13 percent of the athletes who still menstruated were vegetarians.[49] In this study, both vegetarians and nonvegetarians had about the same amounts of body fat (low body fat is sometimes associated with menstrual irregularity), but the amenorrheic women did consume considerably less dietary fat than those who had their periods.

However, other research doesn't support a relationship of vegetarian diet to amenorrhea. In a study of participants in the 1982 Coors Classic bicycle race, twelve of thirty-six competitors were amenorrheic; all twelve were vegetarian or near vegetarian. But in this case twenty of the twenty-four competitors with regular menstrual cycles were also vegetarian.[50] In an Israeli study there was no difference in menstrual patterns between vegetarian and omnivore athletes.[51]

The relationship of diet and exercise to menstruation is somewhat of a mystery. Possibly, the menstrual cycle is directly affected by fiber, fat, and meat. It is also probable that many things affect menstruation in athletes, not just a vegetarian diet. Soyfoods in the diet provide components that are antiestrogens and that could theoretically affect menstruation.[52] However, in cultures where these foods are commonly consumed, there are no apparent problems with amenorrhea.

Whatever the cause, loss of menstruation is a concern. Female athletes who experience this problem may want to consider increasing their fat intake, cutting back on fiber, and perhaps reducing the intensity and duration of their exercise—although this may not always be a possibility for athletes who compete. Increasing calcium intake may help to maintain bone density.[53] Although some studies show that the addition of meat to the diet alleviates the problem, we're reluctant to recommend this except as a very last resort, since there are so many health benefits associated with a vegetarian diet.[54] Table 18.2 provides a food guide for young female athletes. It offers slightly more fat and high levels of calcium.

SUMMING UP:
THE BEST DIET FOR ATHLETES

There are particular issues that need to be addressed for vegetarian athletes. Amenorrhea in very young female athletes is probably the most serious. In addition, vegan athletes may need to make some effort to keep calorie intake high enough and to meet protein needs.

However, the advantages of a vegetarian eating pattern appear to outweigh most concerns. Athletes need diets that are very high in carbohydrates, which means their diets should be plant based. Meat eaters are much less likely to consume adequate amounts of carbohydrate for optimal performance. In addition, all elite endurance and strength athletes may have high protein needs. There are definite concerns about excessive intake of animal protein and the effect on bone and kidney health. Vegetarians have the advantage here, since plant proteins don't have the same harmful effects as animal proteins.

Professional and Olympic-level athletes have higher nutrient needs than sedentary people and those who perform only moderate exercise. In some cases the RDAs are already probably high enough to meet the needs of most athletes. In others, the RDAs may actually be too low, but the higher calorie intake of athletes almost ensures that needs will be met. For vegetarian athletes who follow the guidelines in chapter 10 and who choose additional servings from all those food groups to meet higher calorie needs or who use our guidelines in table 18.1, there is no reason for concern and no advantage to using supplements.

Finally, for those who are not professional athletes, but who enjoy regular moderate exercise, it is enough to meet the RDAs for all nutrients. We've already seen that vegetarians have no problem doing this.

TABLE 18.2 FOOD GUIDE FOR YOUNG FEMALE ATHLETES

2,000 CALORIES
13 percent protein
25 percent fat
62 percent carbohydrates
1,600 milligrams calcium

11 servings grains
2 servings leafy green vegetables
2 servings other vegetables
4 servings fruit
1 serving legumes
2 servings nuts and seeds
3 servings milk (calcium-fortified soymilk, Vegelicious, or 2% cow's milk)
4 servings fat

Table 18.3 Menu for Vegan Weight Lifter

3,450 CALORIES
14 percent protein
16 percent fat
70 percent carbohydrates

BREAKFAST
½ cup bran flakes, with 1 cup soymilk
Banana
3 slices toast, with 3 teaspoons
    margarine

LUNCH
2 tofu-salad sandwiches
Apple
Carrot sticks
Tossed salad, with 2 tablespoons dressing
2 oatmeal cookies
1 cup soymilk

DINNER
3 cups pasta, with 1 cup spaghetti sauce,
    with ½ cup textured vegetable protein
½ cup steamed broccoli
Roll, with 1 teaspoon margarine
1½ cups rice pudding, made with
    soymilk

SNACKS THROUGHOUT THE DAY
½ cup orange juice
Pear
5 gingersnap cookies
Bagel, with 2 tablespoons almond butter
½ cup soy nuts
Fat-free bran muffin

Table 18.4 5,500-Calorie Vegan Diet

13 percent protein
17 percent fat
70 percent carbohydrates

BREAKFAST
2 cups oatmeal, with 1 cup soymilk
4 slices toast, with 4 teaspoons
    margarine
Banana

LUNCH
2 hummus sandwiches
1½ cups potato salad
Tossed salad, with 2 tablespoons dressing
Carrot sticks
Apple
4 oatmeal cookies

DINNER
1 cup black beans
3 cups rice
2 rolls, with 2 teaspoons margarine
1 cup corn
1 cup broccoli
½ cup strawberries

SNACKS THROUGHOUT THE DAY
2 bagels, with fruit spread
½ cup bean soup
Pasta salad (2 cups pasta, with 1 cup
    steamed vegetables)
4 slices bread
Orange
Peach
Carrot sticks

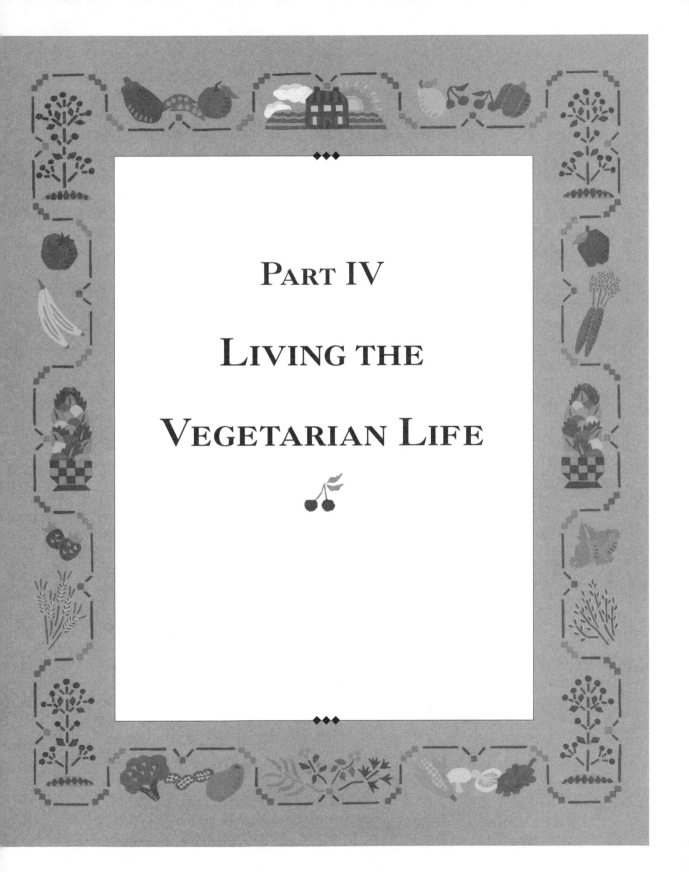

PART IV

LIVING THE

VEGETARIAN LIFE

CHAPTER 19

THE VEGETARIAN TRAVELER

Vegetable luncheon suggestions now appear on the main dining room menus of most of the Statler Hotels. . . . The salad plate combinations are very popular.

—J. L. HENNESSEY,
"PRACTICAL PROBLEMS IN FEEDING PEOPLE,"
Journal of the American Dietetic Association, 1929

◆

Tossing together tasty, healthy vegetarian meals in your own kitchen is one thing; tracking them down away from home and in restaurants is another. Happily, your healthy vegetarian habits don't have to hit the road when you do—it's becoming increasingly easy to find vegetarian fare in all types of restaurants, including fast-food establishments.

Your travel style will have a lot to do with where and what you end up eating. But you can travel vegetarian-style whether you prefer a week of dining at four-star restaurants or you pack the station wagon with kids, cooler, and camping gear.

BEST BETS FOR RESTAURANTS

Based upon the results of a 1991 Gallup poll, revealing that 20 percent of all people won't eat in restaurants that don't offer a vegetarian meal, the National Restaurant Association suggested to all its members that they add vegetarian entrées to their menus. Even if there is nothing vegetarian on the menu, the chef can almost always create something for you. The restaurants want your business and want you to be happy with your meal. Strict vegans do need to quiz the waiter a little, however, as eggs and cheese have a way of sneaking into even the most innocent-looking dishes. As long as you are pleasant about your request, there is every reason to feel perfectly comfortable about asking for something special.

Larger cities are more likely to have a selection of restaurants that cater specifically to vegetarians. If the local tourism office doesn't have any suggestions, find out if there is a natural-foods store or a food co-op in town. People who work at these stores are likely to have plenty of advice on where you can find a vegetarian meal. There are also some excellent restaurant guides available that will lead you to some of the best vegetarian restaurants around the country. See the resource section in the back of this book for some suggestions.

If you can't get a good restaurant recommendation, then the best bet for a vegetarian meal is a Chinese restaurant. Most larger towns have them, and they are among the few places where you can absolutely depend on finding wonderful vegetable stir-fries or other vegetable and rice dishes. Use a little caution when ordering from the "vegetable" section of the menu, though—sometimes these dishes feature vegetables but have tiny pieces of pork. Also, vegetable fried rice or vegetable lo mein can contain pieces of egg. Just make sure you specify to your waiter that you want no meat and, if you choose, no eggs in your dishes.

Indian restaurants have a variety of vegetarian dishes on their menus, although these restaurants are harder to find outside of cities. All Indian restaurants serve vegetable curries or curries made with chickpeas. Dal, a spicy lentil dish, is an Indian staple. Samosas are delightful appetizers that are usually vegetarian. A few of these pockets of pastry stuffed with potatoes, peas, and carrots can be a meal in themselves. Masala dosa is a delicious Indian "crepe" that is traditionally wrapped around potatoes and other vegetables.

Vegans should know that a fairly standard ingredient in Indian cooking is ghee, a type of clarified butter. You can ask for dishes to be prepared without it. Most restaurants are happy to accommodate that request.

Italian restaurants are also a good choice, since they generally have several vegetarian meals that will suit lacto-ovo vegetarians, as well as one or two dishes for vegans. Nearly every Italian restaurant offers a meatless marinara sauce over pasta or pasta primavera. Pasta fagioli is a standard Italian soup made with pasta and white beans. A bowl of soup with a salad and bread is a filling vegetarian meal. The soup is usually made with bean stock, but you may want to ask to be sure it doesn't use chicken broth.

Even the smallest towns generally have a pizzeria. Most will have a vegetarian pizza on the menu. A cheeseless pizza, topped with plenty of vegetables, is delicious; most restaurants will make one on request.

Diners or family-type restaurants normally have numerous offerings for lacto-ovo vegetarians, including grilled cheese, coleslaw, potato salad, macaroni and cheese, and waffles, eggs, or pancakes for breakfast. However, these are the trickiest places for vegans. Sometimes there is nothing on the menu except French fries. But if you are really stuck and really hungry, encourage the kitchen to take a creative approach. You might only have a baked potato and a side dish of corn or a plate of white rice topped with steamed vegetables, but it should be enough to hold you over until your next stop.

Slightly more upscale restaurants tend to offer a better selection for vegans. Some menus may offer several vegetable appetizers, fruit cups, pasta, and potato or rice side dishes. Even if there is no vegetarian entrée on the menu, you can make a meal of several appetizers or ask the chef to leave the meat out of one of the pasta dishes. Sometimes chefs will go all out. Some of the best vegetarian meals we've had have been at restaurants that don't normally offer any vegetarian entrées.

Oftentimes, the best restaurant in town turns out to be the local grocery store. Nose around the bakery, salad bar, and deli, and you are bound to find enough food to put together an impromptu, inexpensive picnic. Here are a couple of sample menus from the grocery store based on meals we've improvised on car trips:

Menu 1

Pasta salad with vegetables (from the deli)

Chickpea salad (chickpeas, chopped celery, chopped onion, black olives, nonfat dressing, from the salad bar)

Whole wheat pita bread

Peanut butter cookies (from the bakery)

Oranges

Menu 2

Hot mashed potatoes, with margarine (from the hot-food section of the deli)

Steamed mixed vegetables (from the hot-food section of the deli)

Biscuits

Tossed salad (from the salad bar)

Packaged oatmeal cookies

Apples

FAST FOOD

It may be just a matter of time before vegetarians can order a veggie burger at their favorite fast-food restaurant. McDonald's is currently test-marketing one overseas, while Burger King has already tested one in selected sites in the United States. It isn't all that surprising. In England, fast-food restaurants sell more than fifty thousand veggie burgers a year—which they purchase from the United States.

But until those burgers do become standard offerings at fast-food places, you can still find some vegetarian fare there. Bear in mind, though, that fast food is about convenience, not health. It represents the worst of American eating habits, and so the vegetarian meals that you find there may not be the healthiest options.

Fast-food Mexican restaurants are a good bet for finding something vegetarian, since most make their refried beans with vegetable fat. Taco Bell uses all-vegetable fat in cooking (as opposed to lard). At other Mexican restaurants it may be good to ask before you order. Most restaurants will be happy to omit the cheese from the burritos and tostadas. Usually, it can be replaced with guacamole (which may or may not contain mayonnaise; be sure to ask), chopped tomatoes, and lettuce. Vegans should also be warned that the flour tortillas in these restaurants often contain dairy products. Corn tortillas are generally free of animal ingredients.

Even burger joints have something for the vegetarian. Burger King offers a "vegetarian Whopper" at all of their restaurants. You won't see it on the menu, but the restaurant will make you one at any franchise if you ask. This is a Whopper without the burger—just all the fixings—and it is surprisingly good and filling. You can get it with or without cheese and mayonnaise.

Fast-food restaurants can provide some pleasant vegan surprises. For example, the French-toast sticks at Burger King include no eggs or milk in their ingredient list. McDonald's chocolate-chip cookies are vegan, and so are the refried beans available at some Wendy's salad bars. The French fries at most fast-food restaurants are vegetarian, since almost all are cooked in vegetable oil. Many of these restaurants also have salad bars or prepared salads. Look for fast-food restaurants that offer both baked potatoes and salad bars, so that you can create your own potato with toppings. It makes for a more hearty, stick-to-your-ribs fare than just a plain salad.

A number of fast-food restaurants offer hot- and cold-food buffets. They often include pasta and tomato sauce and ingredients to make your own tacos. But even if it looks like a vegetarian paradise, ask before you dive in. The tomato sauce might contain beef stock. Refried beans may be made with lard. Vegans might want to know whether the pasta is made with eggs.

PACKING A COOLER

This is a favorite way of traveling for many vacationers. With a cooler crammed full of vegetarian goodies you can snack your way across the country without having to worry about finding restaurants that will accommodate your needs. Meals eaten on the road can be fun as well as much healthier than what you'll find on restaurant menus.

A cooler packed with ice should keep perishables in good shape for one to two days—maybe longer if you are traveling where the nights are cool and you can leave the cooler in the car overnight.

Here are a few ideas for lunches that you can pack in a cooler and enjoy on the road:

• Instant hummus with pita bread and chopped tomatoes (Mixes for this wonderful Middle Eastern chickpea dip can be found in natural-foods stores and many grocery stores. Just add cold water and mix.)

• Instant cups of soup made with hot water from a thermos

• Canned vegetarian sandwich spreads (Look for these in natural-foods stores.)

• Sandwich spreads made at home and packed into a cooler (See the recipe section in the back of the book for some great ideas, including missing-egg salad, notuna salad, and hummus.)

• Peanut-butter sandwiches with sliced banana, sliced apple, or grated carrots

• Cheese or soy cheese with mustard, sliced tomatoes, and lettuce

• Bagels or muffins with almond butter

Many people travel with a cooler stocked with sandwiches and goodies for lunch and snacks and then rely on restaurants for breakfast and dinner. But if you are traveling where restaurants with vegetarian options are few and far between or if you are on a shoestring budget, it is easy enough to pack groceries for all your meals. With a hot pot to heat up soups and water you even have a safe, portable kitchen to take into motel rooms. Here are a few ideas for meals that can be whipped up in a hot pot in just a few minutes:

• For breakfast, instant oatmeal with diced apples and soymilk

- Instant soups

- Couscous

- Canned soups

- Canned vegetarian baked beans with instant brown rice or instant mashed potatoes

- Burritos (Heat up canned or instant vegetarian refried beans and serve them on flour tortillas with chopped tomatoes, lettuce, and shredded cheese.)

Snacks for the Road

Pack snacks that are high in nutrients. Make a special effort to include some calcium-rich snacks or meals such as dried figs, bagels, muffins with almond butter, or soy nuts to munch on. If you are a lacto-ovo vegetarian, some types of cheese, particularly processed ones like Velveeta, will travel well. Granola bars (try some of the fat-free brands), popcorn, and pretzels are all good snack choices, too.

Healthy cookies like oatmeal cookies and fig bars and lower-fat varieties like animal crackers and vanilla wafers make good sweet treats. Of course both fruit and raw vegetables are wonderful for long car trips when you can't fight the urge to constantly munch but don't want to load up on calories and fat.

CAMPING

Whether you are pitching a tent beside your car or backpacking into the wilderness, camping always makes food taste great. Campers are generally ravenous, and everything cooked over the campfire is delicious. Camping requires fast-cooking foods, and there are endless options for putting together great-tasting healthy meals over the cookstove or campfire.

Both natural-foods grocery stores and supermarkets boast a wonderful variety of foods that cook up fast and travel well. Instant soups cook in five minutes with the addition of boiling water. There are delicious vegetarian varieties of these soups, including black bean, curried pasta, pasta and bean, or minestrone. One advantage of the instant soups is that they are light and are a good option for backpackers. Since the packages themselves can be a little bulky, empty the contents into plastic bags for transport and then cook them in your own mug. For car campers there are many canned vegetarian soups. With a salad and rolls, these are a fast campfire meal.

Textured vegetable protein, a soy protein product, is a camper's dream. It's dried, so it is lightweight and nonperishable. Season it with canned sloppy joe sauce and serve over hamburger rolls or have it over instant brown rice with barbecue sauce. (See page 313 for more information on how to use TVP.)

For a fun evening of campfire cooking, try vegetarian hot dogs and hamburgers. Roast hot dogs over the fire on a stick. Children can enjoy a special treat of kosher marshmallows (they don't contain gelatin, which is derived from animal bones) to toast after dinner.

Soymilk is a great beverage for camping. Since it is usually packaged in aseptic cartons it doesn't require refrigeration and is

TABLE 19.1 CAMPING MENUS

Car Camping	Backpacking Menu
BREAKFAST Pancakes, with sliced bananas and syrup Juice	**BREAKFAST** Instant oatmeal, with raisins Hot chocolate, with soymilk
LUNCH Peanut butter sandwiches, with sliced banana Oatmeal cookies Juice	**LUNCH** Instant hummus, spread on pita bread Oranges
	SNACK Trail mix
DINNER Instant brown rice Stir-fried tofu (use tofu in aseptic packages; it doesn't require refrigeration and travels well), with carrots, zucchini, and peanuts	**DINNER** Instant curried vegetable soup Instant rice, with spicy black beans (made from dried black-bean mix) Lemonade (made from mix)
OVER THE EVENING CAMPFIRE Hot chocolate (soymilk and cocoa mix) Toasted kosher marshmallows	**OVER THE EVENING CAMPFIRE** Chamomile tea Peanut butter cookies

easy to transport. Backpackers can use instant, powdered soymilk, which is lightweight and mixes with cold water. Bring along your own cocoa mix by mixing together a quarter cup unsweetened cocoa powder, a quarter cup of sugar, and a half cup instant soymilk powder. Add a half teaspoon of cinnamon for an authentic cup of Mexican hot chocolate. Use one-fourth cup of the mix for every six ounces of hot water.

Good camping breakfasts include instant oatmeal or cold cereal with milk or soymilk. Bear Mush is a whole wheat version of Cream of Wheat. It cooks quickly and makes a good, hot camping breakfast. Pancakes made from a mix are a good breakfast, too.

BUSINESS TRAVEL

Business travel can present the toughest vegetarian challenge. Business travelers may find themselves limited to an airport hotel with few restaurant options. If it is a busy, meeting-packed trip, the traveler may not have the luxury of meandering through town looking for great vegetarian eateries.

Business travelers may choose to rely on room service for some meals. Lacto-ovo vegetarians will generally find plenty to choose from on these menus, but vegans may find it difficult to come up with something healthy, tasty, and satisfying. Most room-service menus aren't loaded with vegan options. But they are loaded with vegan *ingredients*, and if the hotel staff is at all accommodating, they will be happy to put something special together for you.

For example, a room-service menu might list mushrooms braised in wine as an appetizer, asparagus with hollandaise sauce as a side dish, and pasta with seafood as an entrée. Omit the hollandaise sauce and the seafood, and you have a potential vegan feast. Just ask the kitchen staff to provide you with a dish of pasta topped with braised asparagus and mushrooms.

Appetizers tend to be the best category. You might find baked potato skins stuffed with refried beans, nachos with guacamole, or vegetables in wine sauce. Ask the kitchen to hold the sour cream and cheese on these items and then put several together to make a meal.

Breakfast menus usually offer hot cereal, such as oatmeal; fruit platters; and a variety of baked goods, such as English muffins and bagels with jams. In a pinch, some vegans enjoy granola or other ready-to-eat cereal with fruit juice poured over it instead of milk.

EMERGENCY STASH

We are encouraged by the increasing availability of vegetarian foods in restaurants and stores, but we have to admit that when we travel, even on business, we still bring our own stash of some vegan essentials. They include the following:

• Soymilk travels well in the small aseptic cartons and instantly solves the problem of breakfast. We can order hot or cold cereal from room service or the coffee shop and have something to pour over it and to use in our coffee.

• Instant hummus can save many a meal when you are stuck in your hotel room and simply can't find anything suitable on the room-service menu or in the coffee shop. With some bread and a salad from room service, it makes a great meal. Because it is dehydrated, it's easy to transport. For long trips, when you are having trouble finding healthy meals, hummus is a great way to give your menus a dose of calcium.

• Instant cups of soup are a terrific choice when you want something hot and you want it fast. There are a number of vegetarian varieties, and some are fat free. You can tote a little hot pot with you to heat water in your room or you can order hot tea from room service and use part of the water to make your soup.

• Low-fat cookies, fruit, and vegan desserts are hard to come by in restaurants, so if you want a sweet now and then, it pays to bring your own. We usually cart along a box of fig bars or vanilla wafers. Vegans should check product labels to make sure the brand they buy doesn't contain whey, eggs, or milk.

Banquets

If your vegetarian travels land you at a banquet table—which most typically happens to business travelers—it may be easier than you think to get a vegetarian meal. It isn't fair to expect the chef to whip up a special entrée for you at the last minute. It *is* perfectly reasonable to corner one of the waiters and ask him or her to remove the meat from your plate and replace it with an extra baked potato or scoop of rice.

You also have the option of calling the hotel ahead of time and arranging for a special vegetarian meal. Many vegetarians find that this isn't the best idea, though. A lot of caterers still haven't got the hang of vegetarian entrées; more often than not, your vegetarian platter will be a stunning array of steamed or braised vegetables—and nothing else. Often, you will get a better meal if you opt for the regular dinner without the meat.

The Friendly Skies

Nearly every airline offers vegetarian meals, though you need to remember to order them ahead of time (do it through your travel agent or just call the airline reservations number). Most of the airlines aim toward vegan offerings in order to please all vegetarian customers.

While some of the hot entrées are now surprisingly good, it seems that airline food service has generally had the most trouble with snacks and breakfasts. We've had wonderful curries and stir-fries and pasta primavera for our main meals, but have been disappointed with scant breakfasts of fruit while our fellow passengers enjoy more satisfying hot entrées. One airline serves half of a peanut-butter-and-jelly sandwich for its vegetarian version of a "light snack." We've learned that it's best to bring our own snacks for long trips.

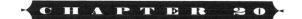

VEGETARIAN LIFESTYLE

◆◆◆

We knew one self-righteous vegetarian who, entertaining us for dinner, ignominiously relegated his wife and daughter, still flesh-eaters, to the kitchen to eat while we were served, with our host, in the dining room. This hardhearted purist had much to learn about right living, although he was on the track to right diet.

—HELEN NEARING,
Good Food for the Simple Life, 1980

◆

You must make your own ideas and style patently clear, or you may end up with a party that, however fashionable or smooth, has nothing to do with you.

—MARTHA STEWART,
Entertaining with Style, 1982

◆

The world is an increasingly kind place to vegetarians, but challenges still abound. There are some suspicious attitudes toward meatless eating out there. And not everyone understands what a meatless meal is, so that the hapless vegetarian might often be faced with a piece of broiled fish prepared by a well-meaning friend (who made it especially for you because he knew you were a vegetarian!). A vegan is even more likely to be faced with challenging situations.

If you travel in traditional circles at all—and most of us do from time to time—you will be faced with meal-related problems. Here are some pointers to help you navigate your way through them.

VEGETARIAN ETIQUETTE AWAY FROM HOME

When a vegetarian is invited to dine at the home of a nonvegetarian there are two big questions. First, is it fair to expect the host to accommodate your vegetarian needs? Second, if your host doesn't know you are vegetarian, should you tell him or her in advance?

Although etiquette provides hard and fast rules for many things, when it comes to these sticky vegetarian situations, the experts differ in their opinions. Elizabeth Post suggests that you do not inform your hosts that you are vegetarian. Instead, she recommends that you bring a dish of your own to be heated up so that your host doesn't feel obligated to prepare something special. She also recommends that you take a little of whatever meat is being served and simply leave it there.

More to our liking is Charlotte Ford's approach. She notes that it is irritating for a host to spend time preparing a dish that the

◆◆◆

guests won't eat and that it is wasteful and conspicuous for the guest to put something on his or her plate and just play with it. Rather, she recommends telling your host in advance. He or she can then choose to make a different entrée or to make more of a side dish.

While we aren't etiquette experts, it seems that some good common sense will dictate how to handle these situations. When people entertain, they aren't running a restaurant. On the other hand, every host wants his or her guests to have an enjoyable meal. Anyone would make an effort to avoid serving food to guests that they dislike or can't eat. So informing your host that you are vegetarian is actually the considerate thing to do. Do offer to bring a vegetarian dish to share with other guests, since your host may not be at all familiar with vegetarian cooking. This is always the best route for vegans especially. Or tell your host that you are very happy to make a meal of any side dishes of salad, rice, vegetables, and rolls.

Although the experts might disagree, we also think it is perfectly reasonable to request a special dish at weddings and other catered events. You don't need to make a big issue of it and don't even need to make your request known ahead of time. When you arrive at the event, just ask a server if he or she can replace the meat with an extra potato or larger serving of rice.

VEGETARIAN ETIQUETTE AT HOME

What about entertaining meat-eating friends in your own home? Some vegetarians believe that they are obligated to offer meat to their guests in order to be polite. Of course, this decision is completely up to you. But don't feel that you are expected to do so. It is reasonable for you to expect your guests to eat what is normally served in your home. Now, this may sound like a direct contradiction to what we said above. If we expect our guests to eat what we usually do, then why shouldn't a host expect us to eat meat in his house? The difference is one of values. You choose to avoid certain foods for some deeply held reason, whether it be concern for the environment, for animal welfare, or for health. It's safe to say that your guests don't have any particular health or ethical-related reasons to avoid pasta or rice pilaf or whatever vegetarian dish you choose to serve. So as long as you serve guests something that they are comfortable eating, it's fine to stick to the principles you always follow in your home.

Since we ourselves choose to be vegetarians partly for ethical reasons, we don't ever serve meat—or dairy or eggs, for that matter—in our home. Unfortunately, some guests will think that it is acceptable to bring their own meat into the home of a vegetarian. Be firm about the fact that you don't allow meat in your house, if that is what you choose. Most people have certain behaviors that they will not allow in their home. Guests are always obligated to respect and honor the rules in someone else's home, whether they involve alcohol, cigarettes, eating meat, or other behaviors.

What to Serve

No matter how many wonderful dishes you prepare for yourself, your family, or vegetarian friends, when nonvegetarians are arriving for dinner, you may find that you just can't think of a single thing to make. Feeding nonvegetarians is a special challenge for many of us. We want the food to be good because we always want to please our guests with a delicious dinner. And, of course, there is much more at stake here for those of us who would like to coax others toward a more vegetarian lifestyle. We want to create the very best positive impression for vegetarianism by serving exceptionally good food.

In choosing your menu, it's a good idea to "know thy guest." Your friends who are world travelers and lovers of new experiences will be thrilled to try a spicy vegetable curry or a savory Indonesian tempeh stew. But when Uncle Dave, who has never eaten a meatless meal in his life, comes for dinner, it's a good idea to put away the sprouts, sea vegetables, and sesame tahini.

We've learned the hard way that many dishes that get rave reviews at vegetarian potlucks just don't cut it at church covered-dish suppers or family barbecues. So, know when to be exotic and when to be basic in your meal planning. For the unadventurous eaters in your circle of family and friends, base dishes on familiar ingredients. Pasta with tomato sauce or pasta primavera, vegetable lasagna, homemade pizza, and cream of potato or broccoli soup are good bets.

To win people over to the glories of vegetarian cooking, pull out all the stops when company is coming. Roasted red peppers, Greek olives, sun-dried tomatoes, and fresh herbs turn the simplest grain or pasta dishes into delightful gourmet entrées.

Be elegant rather than earthy. Many omnivores have a stereotypical view that a vegetarian diet is all brown rice and sprouts consumed by barefoot people sitting cross-legged on the floor. Show them it just isn't so. Bring out the candles, the fresh flowers, the good wine. Dare to be different, but in a way that will absolutely wow your guests. Toss a few edible flower blossoms into the salad. Serve watermelon sorbet for dessert.

Of course, no matter what you do, you won't be able to please everybody all of the time. Some people turn their noses up at vegetarianism just on principle. If that's the case, you might suggest ordering in or having dinner at your favorite Chinese restaurant, where all of you can eat what you please.

Some Sticky Situations

Some people just don't get it. Vegetarians choose meatless diets for many reasons and are usually happy with that choice. Most of us never feel deprived or find ourselves lusting after steaks or Big Macs. In fact, many vegetarians find that once meat is out of their life, it becomes downright repugnant. So why are others so obsessed with our diet?

These obsessions fall into a few different categories. First is the well-meaning friend or relative who can't stand to have you miss out on some meat dish that he finds especially wonderful.—"Oh, you have to taste this; just try one bite." Or "I know you are a vegetarian, but if you are going to Texas, your vacation won't be complete if you don't try some authentic barbecue."

In her newspaper column, Judith Martin

(aka Miss Manners) suggests a polite and effective response. No matter how many times someone cajoles you to try a bite of their lobster thermidor or filet mignon, just respond with a polite "no, thank you." It may take ten or twelve no-thank-yous, but, eventually, even Uncle Bob the cattle rancher should get the picture.

Perhaps even more irritating are the vegetarian baiters. These people seem to be personally affronted by vegetarianism and will harangue you with jokes and comments about vegetarian foods and ask nonsensical questions such as "How do you know plants don't feel pain when you eat them?" It's interesting to speculate about why some people take such offense at the whole idea of a vegetarian diet, especially if you yourself have been quietly eating your rice pilaf and not bothering anyone with slaughterhouse horror tales. Assuming that they don't make their living as a butcher or a hog farmer, there is seemingly no reason for their disdain.

Of course, one reason might be that they know you are right. Most people are aware at least of the harmful health effects of meat eating, about the horrors of factory farming, and perhaps the effects of cattle grazing on rain forests. But they might feel unwilling or unable to do anything about changing their own diet and may find your commitment to vegetarianism to be intimidating or threatening. Just being around you might make them feel guilty about the way they eat.

Often, such people will make any attempt to find a chink in your armor. "How can you say it's wrong to eat meat when you wear leather shoes" is a favorite retort of the vegetarian baiters. Vegetarian baiters might approach the issue with anything ranging from hostility to derision. It's probably best to avoid a hostile response of your own and not to get into any ridiculous discussions about the horrors of plant murdering. We generally tell people that we don't know whether plants feel pain or not—but we do know that we need plant foods to survive and we don't need animal foods. So we simply choose to live as responsibly as we can while still maintaining our health. And if someone points out an animal product in your home, you can note that you don't lead a "perfect" lifestyle by any means, but you are attempting to make as many changes in the way you live as you can.

In the Hospital

It seems that the easiest and most likely place in the world to get good healthy vegetarian fare should be the hospital— a place where the total emphasis should be on health. Unfortunately, however, many vegetarian patients find it difficult to get a decent meal when they are hospitalized. Vegans have the hardest time.

While the staff in some hospital dietary departments may be very savvy about vegetarianism, many don't know enough about vegetarian diets. You are more likely to have better luck in larger urban hospitals, but there is still no guarantee that you'll get satisfactory meals. Choose a Seventh-day Adventist hospital if there is one in your area, because these hospitals always serve vegetarian meals. Otherwise, you'll need to do some planning.

If you know that you are going to be hospitalized, make your needs known ahead of time to your physician. He or she is responsible for ordering your diet—not the hospital dietary staff. It is helpful to be as specific as possible about which foods you wish to avoid. You should be able to get lacto-ovo-vegetarian meals with no trouble and even vegan meals. Macrobiotics will have a much more difficult time, and if you eat only organic foods, you will find that you have little choice in the matter during your hospital stay.

Once you are in the hospital, you might remind your physician about your diet the first time you see him or her. It's also a good idea to ask to speak directly to a dietitian to make sure there is no misunderstanding about your meals. This is probably much more important if you are a vegan. If they balk at your refusal to use dairy products, you'll need to reassure them that your diet is healthy. If necessary, explain which foods you eat that provide calcium, vitamin B_{12}, zinc—or whatever nutrients they seem to be concerned about. At any rate, it is reasonable for you to be adamant in refusing to eat animal products if this is what you choose, but be prepared to be flexible about your meals. If the dietary department really doesn't have any vegan entrées available, let them know that you'll be happy to eat rice with steamed vegetables, rolls, and margarine.

At some point in your hospital stay, you may need to be on a special diet. If you have surgery, you may be placed on a clear-liquid diet. This shouldn't be a problem for most vegetarians. Foods allowed on a clear-liquid diet include bouillon, soft drinks, some fruit juices, herb tea, gelatin, and Popsicles. Be sure to tell the dietitian that you only want vegetable bouillon and that you want to skip the gelatin. You might bring your own packet of vegetable bouillon just in case.

MEALS FOR MIXED HOUSEHOLDS

It's wonderful when couples or families decide to go vegetarian together. And it's great when parents can raise their children as vegetarian right from the beginning. But what happens most frequently is that one family member chooses to experiment with a vegetarian diet while others show little interest. Meal planning can be a challenge when you need to serve the needs of both vegetarians and omnivores. In some households, it's everybody for themselves. A more unifying approach, though, is to find menus that can please the whole household with some minor changes.

Think ethnic—Chinese, Italian, Mexican, Middle Eastern, Indian—when you want to plan menus that appeal to both vegetarians and meat eaters. Since many ethnic dishes use meat as a condiment or flavoring in small amounts, rather than as a focal point of the dish, these meals have flexibility: serve them meatless to household vegetarians or add a bit of meat for others. Prepare a simple stir-fried dish of vegetables and rice, and meat eaters can add slivers of chicken or chunks of beef if they choose. A savory pasta primavera—just toss hot pasta with a platter of steamed or sautéed vegetables—can be served with or without Parmesan cheese on top. Cook up a pot of spaghetti along with a tomato sauce thick with mushrooms. Meat eaters have the option of adding some sautéed ground beef. Or prepare a pan of spicy ground beef and one of refried beans and let people make their own burritos according to their preference.

Perhaps this reflects our own bias, but it makes sense that the emphasis will be on meatless meals in mixed households. After all, vegetarians avoid meat, but most meat eaters don't avoid pasta, grains, and vegetables. You should never expect vegetarians to compromise by eating meat once in a while, but nonvegetarians are usually open to eating meatless meals a few times a week. After all, omnivores are rarely ethically opposed to meatless meals or worried about the health effects of such meals.

Meat eaters might be more willing to experiment with vegetarian dishes that have a familiar culinary ring to them. Try corn chowder, rice-a-veggie mix, or sloppy joes from the recipe section at the back of this book. Some dishes lend themselves easily to "vegetarianizing." For example, a favorite chili recipe can become a vegetarian classic when ground beef is replaced with kidney beans, textured vegetable protein, or both. We've had the most success feeding meat eaters with chili made with textured vegetable protein than with any other vegetarian dish. It always seems to satisfy even the most ardent meat devotees. Meals that have a familiar look and taste to them are often more acceptable to family members who are resistant to vegetarian meals.

If your family is particularly resistant, you might ease them into vegetarian meals by preparing their favorite meat-based dishes with just half the meat. In a series of studies at Southern Illinois University, chefs prepared dishes like tuna casserole and macaroni and cheese by decreasing the meat and adding tofu. When the dishes were served to both preschoolers and college students, the tofu dishes were just as readily accepted as the original, meatier versions. In fact, in a number of cases, the preschoolers preferred the dishes with tofu.

Try replacing half the cheese in macaroni-and-cheese sauce with pureed tofu. You might need to add extra salt to offset the blandness of the tofu. Make chili, beef burritos, or sloppy joes with half ground beef and half textured vegetable protein. Chances are very good that family members will not be able to tell the difference. You can gradually accustom them into less and less beef and more and more TVP until they willingly accept vegetarian versions of those dishes.

To those who aren't familiar with tofu, its texture is sometimes unappealing, and thawed frozen tofu, with its chewy texture, is a good way to introduce it. Marinate the tofu chunks in soy sauce, roll them in flour, and then sauté in a small amount of oil. You can use it to replace the chicken in stir-fried dishes.

Often, blended tofu, used to replace melted or soft cheeses, is more acceptable to people than tofu used as a meat replacement. Try blending tofu with a small amount of olive oil, salt, and chopped parsley as a stuffing for Italian shells or the ricotta-cheese layer in lasagna. If you like, you can mix the tofu with some ricotta cheese or add small amounts of Parmesan.

Meat analogues are wonderful transition

foods, as they are created to look and taste like the meats they replace. Chop these into bean dishes or soups from favorite family recipes. We find most of these products are delicious, but, admittedly, some come closer to tasting like their meat counterparts. Some may taste *too* much like meat for some vegetarians. Also, try vegetarian burgers instead of hamburgers and veggie franks instead of beef hot dogs. Sautéed portabello mushrooms are another delicious treat; they are sometimes referred to as "the steak of vegetarians."

THE VEGETARIAN EVANGELIST

Some vegetarians are content to eat the way they please and leave it at that. Others are eager to spread the word about the virtues of meatless eating. If you are an ethical vegetarian, chances are you would like to see others adopt a vegetarian diet, too. In most cases, you don't need to proselytize. A mere mention that you are a vegetarian will prompt a flurry of questions. People will often ask your reasons for eating this way, giving you a perfect opportunity to educate them a little bit about the health and environmental benefits of vegetarianism and the cruelties of factory farming. It's probably best, though, just to touch on the high points, and not to go into a fifteen-minute diatribe on veal calves. If your listeners are at all open or receptive to the discussion, they'll ask for more details.

Don't underestimate the power of being different. For vegetarians, having dinner with other vegetarians is generally more fun. But if you are the only vegetarian in the crowd, people will naturally be curious about you and your diet and will have lots of questions. What a great opportunity to educate people about the virtues of plant diets. If it's a potluck dinner, it may be the first chance they've had to taste vegetarian food.

Nonvegetarians will rarely be receptive to attacks on the way they eat. You'll probably get further in piquing their curiosity and interest in vegetarianism by sharing information only when it is solicited. Preaching and scolding is bound to be a turnoff to most meat eaters and is likely to elicit a response of defensiveness rather than receptivity. If you set an example (perhaps by bringing something really delicious to a dinner) the nonvegetarians are apt to initiate the conversation about vegetarianism.

SUPPORT FOR VEGETARIANS

Some might argue that vegetarians are a true minority group and that our culture is still not vegetarian friendly. It certainly does feel lonely at times to be the only vegetarian in the crowd. Hooking up with other vegetarians can help. Is there a vegetarian society in your area? Many of these groups have monthly informal get-togethers to share potluck meals. Just chatting with other vegetarians can strengthen your resolve to eat meatless. Just as important, your new vegetarian acquaintances can be a great source of information on recipes, where to shop, or how to find a good meatless restaurant. Members of vegetarian groups are likely to share tips on which cookbooks to buy, where to find sea vegetables, how to get kids to eat kale and spouses to try lentil burgers. To find out about vegetarian groups near you, contact the Vegetarian Resource Group (they're listed in the resource guide at the back of the book). If there is no group nearby, you can reach out to other people in your community. Just advertise a vegetarian potluck in the community-events section of your local newspaper and put up signs near natural-foods stores.

You can also get long-distance support by joining a national vegetarian organization. Its membership publications will keep you up-to-date on what is going on in the vegetarian world. Finally, you will find plenty of vegetarian friends through your computer. Most online services offer groups for vegetarians to exchange information and ideas, and the Internet provides mailing lists for vegetarians. (See the resource section for more information on organizations and online services.)

VEGETARIAN LIFESTYLE: IT'S ABOUT MORE THAN JUST MEAT

For some people vegetarianism is a way of eating; for others, it is a whole way of life. Vegans often describe themselves as people who not only do not eat animal products, but who *do not use* animal products.

For those who are unfamiliar with the vegan lifestyle, some of the issues noted below may seem extreme at first glance. Shunning fur coats may make perfect sense, since animals are obviously killed for their fur. But why not use wool? It doesn't hurt a sheep to have its wool sheared, does it? An understanding of these lifestyle choices is gained by understanding the philosophy underlying them.

First, while many vegetarians choose their diet because they don't believe in killing animals for food, others avoid any product that involves the mistreatment of animals. Still others refuse to use any animal products on the principle that it is not our right to use animals in any way. Additionally, the use of animals, even when it might not appear to be inhumane on the surface, always opens up the possibility of abuse.

While the people who make animal products may strive to offer the best treatment possible and, certainly, for economic reasons will keep the animals as healthy as possible, good treatment of animals is not their first objective. Where animals are used for economic gain, they are merchandise. Usually, animal products are produced in large quantities, and individual animals have little identity or worth. It is a safe assumption that where animals are used for economic gain, the potential for abuse and inhumane treatment looms large.

Avoiding Animal Products

Animal products are pervasive in every area of our lives. Sometimes the use of animals is obvious; other times, less obvious. The two biggest sources of animal products are food and personal-care items.

Animal products may lurk in some of the most unlikely foods. Examples include:

- Eggs in baked products

- Whey (from milk) in breads, other baked goods, and products like taco seasoning

- Animal-derived waxes on fruits

- Lactose from milk in vegetable broths

- Romano or Parmesan cheese added to commercial spaghetti sauce

- Lard or beef tallow in baked goods or tortillas

- Gelatin, derived from the hooves and cartilage of horses, in marshmallows, many candies, and gelatin desserts

- Animal products involved in the production of white table sugar, which is sometimes filtered through charred animal bones for purification

- Albumin, from eggs, blood, or cow's milk, in nondairy products

Even products labeled "vegetarian" may not be completely free of animal products. Often vegetarian burgers or frankfurters contain eggs or egg whites as binders. And don't be mollified by the words "cholesterol free" or "made with 100 percent vegetable oil." Products like cheese-flavored chips and other snacks may contain cheese in amounts small enough to earn a cholesterol-free rating, but they still contain some cheese and are not vegan. Cholesterol-free products may also contain egg whites or skim milk.

After food, animal products are most often lurking in clothing and personal-care products. Vegans generally shun the most obvious animal-derived clothing—fur and leather. Alternatives are getting easier to find. Many low-cost shoe chains offer a good variety of nonleather shoes. These are also available through mail order.

As noted previously, vegans are likely to avoid clothing made from wool. They also may not use silk, which comes from silkworms.

Cosmetics, hair-care products, and other personal-care items are also big sources of animal-derived ingredients. Many face creams, shampoos, and hair conditioners contain collagen, which is found in the bones and cartilage of animals. Other ingredients that are often found in these products are lanolin (derived from sheep's wool), mink oil, musk, and animal fats. Most soaps are made with animal fat, listed as "tallow" or "sodium tallowate" on the label. Ground-up fish scales may be used in cosmetics to give them a shimmer.

When we stop eating meat and other animal foods, those by-products become less available, and other ingredients have to be found. So even if you can't avoid all animal products—and nobody can—you can make a significant impact on their use by simply avoiding meat and other animal foods. In addition, avoid animal products when alternatives are easily found. For example, don't wear leather, wool, or silk when cotton and synthetic clothes are so abundant. Avoid personal-care products that contain animal ingredients or are tested on animals whenever you can.

Also, getting by with less can have an impact. One of the ongoing debates among vegans involves the environmental effect of using vinyl shoes instead of leather. Most of us agree that neither one is a particularly good option. The best advice is to learn to get by with fewer shoes, regardless of which type you choose.

It's probably true that none of us can lead a completely vegan lifestyle—but the effect is significant when you avoid animal products in your diet, clothing, and personal-care items.

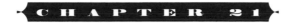

MAKING THE TRANSITION: A PLAN IN NINE STEPS

*Unless we change direction, we are likely
to end up where we are headed.*

—CHINESE PROVERB

◆

*All tastes are acquired tastes, as is easily
seen when one examines the bills of fare of
populations in different parts of the world.*

—EUELL GIBBONS,
Stalking the Wild Asparagus, 1962

◆

We assume that many of you reading this book have a personal interest in vegetarianism but haven't yet taken the plunge toward changing your diet. Admittedly, thoughts of a lifetime of meatless eating can seem daunting to anyone who was raised on a meat-and-potatoes menu. Plus, even the most motivated individual may have to contend with family members who don't relish the change quite as enthusiastically.

It's true that changing your eating style can mean learning new recipes, experimenting with unfamiliar ingredients, and creating new menus. You might even find that some ingredients called for in your new vegetarian cookbooks aren't available where you usually shop. All of this can feel overwhelming at first. It seems the two biggest deterrents to taking the plunge into vegetarianism are lack of time and lack of know-how. You can deal with both of these concerns by taking a reasonably gradual approach to new dietary habits. Give yourself time to try new menu ideas. For your first vegetarian experiments, most or all of what you need can be found at the local grocery store. There is no need to explore natural-foods stores or food co-ops right away—though as you progress in your vegetarian eating plan, you'll eventually want to investigate these places.

Probably the most important way to make a smooth transition to this way of eating is to keep your focus on the positive. Nonvegetarians often think that a vegetarian diet is based on deprivation or a limited way of eating. It is really just the opposite. Even though vegetarians avoid whole categories of foods, the diet of a vegetarian is typically much more interesting than that of a meat eater. You are likely to find that many vegetarian cookbooks draw heavily on the cooking of cultures where plant-based diets are common. So while your vegetarian diet may include familiar staples, such as vegetable soup, macaroni and cheese, and bean burritos, you might also find yourself occasionally making a foray into Indian, Thai, or Mediterranean cuisine.

Some people make the decision to become a vegetarian overnight. It can be the result of a single pivotal event—the scare of a heart attack, the sudden realization that the sweet, fluffy lamb frolicking in the field will be someone's dinner next week, or a television program on the effects of cattle grazing on the rain forests.

But, for most of us, radical diet changes take some getting used to. Although we highly recommend a vegetarian diet for everyone, we also recognize that some of you aren't ready to dive into total vegetarianism immediately. If you can wake up tomorrow morning and be a vegetarian—well, that's great. But for many people it is a gradual process. And when you do it gradually, it is—believe it or not—easy, stress free, and even fun.

Taking one step at a time makes change more manageable. We've outlined a series of nine transition stages to help you achieve your goal. They more or less follow the path that we ourselves took in adopting a vegetarian diet—but they aren't written in stone. They represent *a* way to make the transition to vegetarianism, not *the* way. Feel free to switch them around a little if a different sequence works better for you.

How long should it take you to achieve a vegetarian diet if that's your goal? There is really no answer to that question. While a slow approach is generally easier for some individuals, you also don't want to get too bogged down and lose your motivation to change. There is the danger that you'll make a few changes over the next couple of months and then forget about the whole thing. Some people actually do much better with very comprehensive changes in their diet. Making a sudden shift to a vegetarian diet disrupts old eating behaviors and forces you to seek new ways of eating immediately. Many people thrive on this type of change.

Also, if you are adopting a vegetarian diet to lower your cholesterol, lose weight, or regulate diabetes, then making big changes in your diet fairly quickly can be the best route. For one thing, you might find that you start to feel better right from the start and that you are reaping the benefits of improved health right away. This in itself is motivating and helps you stick with the changes you made. In a community class on weight control that we taught, we advised participants to greatly reduce their meat intake as one step toward lowering fat intake. One woman chose to eliminate meat completely. It made it simpler for her, and she felt the need to make some big changes in the way she was eating. It was the only change she made in her lifestyle, and she lost thirty pounds over six months. As a result, she was by far the most enthused and motivated member of the group.

Six of the following nine stages involve giving up animal flesh. The others focus on dairy and eggs. You may not be interested in eliminating dairy and eggs at this time or ever. But even if this is the case, do try to adopt some of the suggestions in the last three stages of this plan. You'll improve your diet by including more nondairy sources of calcium and by cutting back on cheese, milk, and eggs.

As you consider each phase of change, focus on the wonderful foods that you are adding to your diet, not all of the things you are giving up. And every time you make one of these changes, you can give yourself a pat on the back, because you are doing something good for your own health and having a significant positive impact on the environment and animal welfare.

BECOMING A VEGETARIAN IN NINE EASY STEPS

The first three steps in our transition period involve making changes in your evening meal. People who make an abrupt switch to a vegetarian diet are often overwhelmed at the prospect of coming up with a whole new set of menus. Somehow, most of us have the idea that we eat something different every night of the month. But that isn't true. Most families rely on about ten different dinner entrées and eat only a few choices for breakfast and lunch. They might deviate occasionally and fix something special, but most people count on the same old standbys for their meals. This means that coming up with enough vegetarian meals to get you through the month is less of a challenge than you might think.

The transition plan starts with our "three times three" rule of menu planning to come up with nine new vegetarian entrées for dinner. You'll be amazed at how easy it is to make your evening meals completely meatless when you identify three vegetarian entrées you already eat, three dishes that can be turned into vegetarian entrées with some minor revisions, and three new vegetarian recipes.

This is a good time to reevaluate your beliefs about what constitutes a dinner. Most of us grew up with "four food groups" dinners. Every dinner consisted of a meat, a starch, a vegetable, and, for children, a glass of milk. These guidelines formed our ideas of what a balanced meal is. This causes problems for many new vegetarians, since they often feel compelled to build meals around that same old theme—always including a protein food to take the place of meat. Thus many vegetarians don't feel that a meal is complete without beans, tofu, or another "meat substitute."

These old ideas about meal planning are cumbersome and have no nutritional validity. So toss them out the window. Vegetarian meal planning becomes much easier once you do so. Wonderful vegetarian meals can be as simple as pasta with steamed or sautéed vegetables and a sprinkle of Parmesan cheese if you like. A baked potato topped with steamed vegetables and some whole-grain rolls on the side are a healthy, simple dinner. And for dinners when you really feel like having breakfast, corn flakes and milk or French toast is perfectly fine for a quick meal.

1. Go meatless at dinnertime three nights a week using meals that are already familiar to you and your family.

It is easy to come up with three vegetarian dinner menus if you rely on vegetarian foods you already know and enjoy. Several of the following meals may already be favorites in your household:

Macaroni and cheese

Tomato soup with a salad and bread

Spaghetti with tomato sauce

Vegetable soup

Vegetable chow mein

Cheese pizza

Bean burritos and Spanish rice

Italian stuffed shells or manicotti

Quiche

Split-pea soup

Eggplant Parmesan

Vegetable stir-fry

2. Add three more meatless nights to your schedule by making small changes to favorite recipes that contain meat.

A number of meaty entrées easily lend themselves to vegetarian makeovers:

- Convert your homemade ground-beef chili by replacing the meat with beans and/or textured vegetable protein.

- Replace the meat in tacos or sloppy joes with textured vegetable protein.

- Try tofu stroganoff instead of beef stroganoff. Use the same recipe but replace the beef with chunks of tofu that have been frozen, then defrosted and marinated in soy sauce.

- Omit the ground beef from lasagna and use sliced, sautéed zucchini and eggplant in its place.

- Leave out the chunks of meat from soups, stews, and stir-fried dishes. You can replace them with chunks of tofu, tempeh, or textured vegetable protein— or just add some more vegetables.

3. Find three new vegetarian meals that you enjoy.

You already have six vegetarian menus at your disposal. Now you need to find three new recipes by perusing a few vegetarian cookbooks. You might buy one or two (check our resource section at the back of the book for ideas) or take them out of the library. Browse for dishes that look appealing. Try different recipes until you find just three that you enjoy and are comfortable preparing. Some choices from the recipes in the back of this book that are especially easy to prepare are Mediterranean chickpeas, corn chowder, pilaf with carrots and raisins, and minted couscous salad.

Once you have added three new dishes to your dinner menu repertoire, you'll be ready to declare all of your dinners meatless. As easy as this, from these first three steps, you will have nine vegetarian dinner entrées to choose from. That's enough for most people to go meatless every night of the week without getting tired of the same old thing. Of course, these aren't the only meals that you are going to eat for the rest of your life. You'll find yourself expanding and refining your list of meals as time goes on and as you experiment with new foods. This is just enough to get you started so that you know you won't starve and there will always be something good on the table.

4. Go meatless at lunchtime.

Now that your dinners are meatless, turn your attention to lunches. If you eat lunch out, look for restaurants that serve pasta primavera, vegetable soups, baked potatoes, or that have super salad bars. Many sandwich places offer at least one vegetarian choice. If not, ask for grilled cheese with tomatoes or a pita stuffed with vegetables. Fast-food Mexican restaurants are also an option.

For brown-bag lunches try some of the sandwich spreads in the recipe section of this book or even some of our ideas for brown-bag lunches for children (see page 197). You can also buy vegetarian pâtés and spreads at many natural-foods stores. Many of these are pretty fatty, but they'll help you through the transition phase. There are also a growing number of vegetarian deli "meats" on the market.

If you have a microwave at work you can take leftovers from dinner to heat up for lunch or treat yourself to some special items like frozen veggie burgers and vegetarian hot dogs or some of the new vegetarian frozen entrées. Other quick hot lunches include vegetarian instant cups of soup.

Remember that for lacto-ovo vegetarians some old standbys are vegetarian—such as egg salad or cheese. Again, let these foods help you through the transition. Since they are loaded with fat and cholesterol and devoid of fiber, they shouldn't be everyday choices.

5. Focus on breakfast.

Is there still some meat hiding out in your morning meal? You may occasionally eat breakfast meats such as bacon and sausage. Now is the time to omit those foods from your diet. Once you have done so, you will be a lacto-ovo vegetarian.

If you have a long-standing tradition of eggs with bacon or sausage, then some of the meatless, cholesterol-free sausage links or patties can help you make the switch. Begin exploring some healthier ideas, since eggs, even with vegetarian meats, are still a fatty, high-cholesterol breakfast. Try banana pancakes with maple syrup, eggless French toast, or hearty, steaming seven-grain cereal. Unfortunately, most people don't have time for a leisurely weekday breakfast. If you are in a rush in the morning, consider fast, simple breakfasts, like peanut butter or almond butter on toast, bran muffins with jam, or a fruit-and-milk shake.

6. Experiment with new foods.

There is much more to a vegetarian diet than just giving up meat. In fact, what you don't eat represents just a small part of the changes you will make in your diet. What is really different about this new way of eating is the fact that you are learning to enjoy a wide variety of grains, legumes, nut and seed butters, fruits, and vegetables and perhaps experimenting with new flavors in cooking.

Once you are comfortable with enough meatless dishes to get you through the week, you will want to broaden your food horizons a bit. This is a good time to start expanding your repertoire of vegetarian foods. Browsing through vegetarian cookbooks may inspire you to try a few recipes with new ingredients like tahini, rice milk, or even some sea vegetables. If you haven't done so already, take a trip to a natural-foods store or food co-op. Go with a shopping list in hand or just to browse.

Don't be intimidated by the array of unfamiliar products. We have heard tales of people who walked into a food co-op and walked right out again. They just didn't know where to begin among all those strangely labeled

Replacing Meat with Poultry and Fish

You might notice that as a part of our transition plan, we don't suggest that you eliminate red meat and replace it with chicken and fish. There is a reason for that.

Because chicken and fish tend to be lower in fat than red meat, many people have latched on to the idea that a diet based on these two foods is healthier. In fact, some people who limit their flesh intake to these foods call themselves semivegetarians. There is a certain danger in thinking this way. Replacing red meat with chicken and fish is a halfway measure toward improving your health. Poultry has just as much cholesterol as red meat. In fact, even skinless chicken has just as much cholesterol as steak. This is because cholesterol is found in the lean portion of foods, not the fatty parts. Some types of fish even have more cholesterol than red meat. Also, although fish is generally much leaner than red meat or poultry, many kinds of fish are as much as 50 percent fat.

There are other reasons that switching to chicken and fish won't do much to improve your health. We already saw in chapters 6 and 7 that animal protein may raise blood cholesterol, causes excessive calcium to be lost in the urine, and places a burden on the kidneys. These foods are completely devoid of fiber, other complex carbohydrates, and the phytochemicals that are found only in plant foods.

In short, there is relatively little advantage to making a change to chicken and fish. Although some research shows that fish, which is high in omega-3 fatty acids, can lower the risk for heart disease, vegetarians are already at low risk. Also, many kids of fish are high in fat and fish can replace fiber-rich foods in the diet. Finally, people who eliminate red meat and base their meals on poultry and fish can become complacent—feeling that they've brought themselves close enough to a vegetarian pattern of eating and that further changes are unnecessary.

---

items and, even more confusing, those unlabeled items in the bulk-food bins.

Ethnic markets can be just as problematic. We shop in a Korean grocery where the fresh produce is labeled in Korean and most of the help doesn't speak English. It's an adventure, to say the least!

That's the point, of course. Shopping in different types of food stores, whether they be ethnic markets, food co-ops, or gourmet groceries, is truly an adventure. Take some time to wander around and read labels. Buy a few items that look interesting, and have fun experimenting.

7. Experiment with eggless dishes.

Whether they are used as a main ingredient in egg salad or scrambled eggs, a binder in burgers and loaves, or a leavening ingredient in cakes, eggs are such a functional food that they can be difficult to replace. But experienced vegetarian cooks have come up with a variety of ways to replace eggs in all kinds of recipes.

Tofu is a great replacement for hard-boiled or scrambled eggs. Try it diced and mixed with chopped onions and celery, mayonnaise, and a touch of mustard for a standard vegetarian favorite called missing-egg salad. You can also crumble tofu and sauté it with onions, salt, and turmeric for a wonderful scrambled-egg dish. A light sprinkle of nutritional yeast gives both these dishes a more robust flavor.

It's easier to eliminate eggs in baking than you might think. See "Egg Substitutes" on page 313 for some ideas.

8. Explore plant sources of calcium.

Many foods are abundant in calcium. If you wish to eliminate or reduce your milk consumption, you'll feel more confident about your diet if you are already enjoying other calcium-rich foods. Use two to three servings of nondairy foods that are a good source of calcium every day. The choices are varied and include almonds, leafy green vegetables, figs, soymilk, tofu, and beans. (See chapter 7 for some additional ideas.)

Replace the milk that you use on cereal and in baking with soymilk or one of the other nondairy milks. For younger family members, try to find brands that are calcium fortified. There are many brands and flavors of these products, so if you don't like the first one you try, experiment with some others.

Once you are enjoying a variety of calcium-rich foods, you will feel comfortable about eliminating milk, cheese, and other dairy foods from your diet. This may sound like a big deal, but it won't be. If you have been using nondairy sources of calcium and trying nondairy milks, you'll probably find it pretty easy to go dairy free. You might try some of the soy cheeses on the market to help you through this transition. But many are as fatty as cow's-milk cheese, and you'll want to limit these foods in your meals.

The addition of small amounts of nutritional yeast gives "cheesy" flavors to dishes. Sprinkle it on top of popcorn or pasta or mix it with blended tofu and soymilk, thickened with flour to make a cheese sauce.

9. Read labels.

If you are serious about a vegan diet, start reading labels at the grocery store and look for hidden animal ingredients. At first you might feel overwhelmed. It seems as though there are animal ingredients—lard, whey, dried milk, egg whites—in everything from bread to margarine to veggie burgers. But don't be discouraged—you'll quickly become familiar with products that are truly vegan. Eventually you'll have a shopping list of the products you want to eat. You may feel a little compulsive in the process. Vegans read food labels more than any people we know! Just consider it an education.

You also need to decide your own comfort level. Some people are not comfortable with *any* animal products in their diet. You may find that you feel that way, too. Or you may prefer not to cook with dairy or eggs, but a brand of bread that contains whey may be acceptable to you. It's a personal choice. Don't fall into the trap of thinking that you have to defend every food choice you make in order to call yourself a vegetarian, and don't get bogged down in comparing the purity of your vegan diet with others' diets. Vegetarian diets are always a great choice. You've made a responsible decision in adopting one. If it isn't perfectly vegan every minute of the month, you still are eating responsibly, humanely, and healthfully.

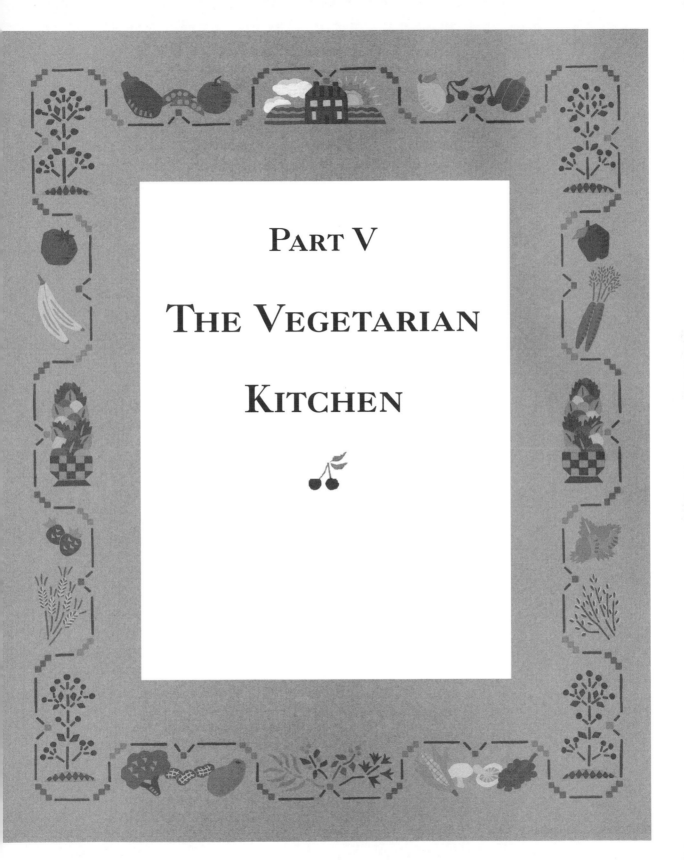

PART V

THE VEGETARIAN

KITCHEN

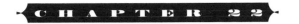
TIPS FOR PLANNING FAST AND EASY VEGETARIAN MEALS

◆◆◆

It's one thing—though nothing small—to turn out a flawless soufflé; it's quite another to come up with an endless variety of appealing, highly nutritious vegetarian meals.

—LAUREL'S KITCHEN, 1976

◆

Some people believe that vegetarian meals require more planning and take more time to cook. On the one hand, this is certainly true. The basics of many vegetarian meals are beans and whole grains, which can take longer to cook than some meats. On the other hand, vegetarian meals are a snap. First, even though whole grains and beans need to cook for a long time, most of the cooking time is unsupervised. While you may need to think ahead a little, you don't need to stand over the stove for hours. Second, other staples that rely on pasta and vegetables cook very quickly. Some of them can be recipes that are old familiar favorites of yours.

In this chapter we outline some steps, timesaving planning tools, and meal ideas that will help even the busiest people to put great vegetarian meals on the table in a jiffy.

SOME GROUND RULES FOR TIMESAVING MEALS

Stock Up

As you expand your culinary horizons, you will most likely find that you are eating more meals based on grains and beans. One advantage of these types of foods is that they have a long shelf life—they can be stored for several months in a cool, dark place—so you can stock up on a variety of them without worrying about food spoilage. Buying in bulk and stocking up on food saves you time on two counts. First, it means much less time spent grocery shopping. Second, the more you have in the house to choose from, the easier it is to toss menus together in just a few minutes.

See our list for the well-stocked pantry in chapter 23. Your own pantry stash may vary from this, depending on the foods you like and your storage limitations.

Cooking in Bulk

Cooking in bulk is a well-known trick for cutting cooking time. If you make enough of your favorite dish for three nights instead of one, you only have to cook dinner two or three times a week. This works especially well for single people, who may find it difficult to get geared up, or may lack the time,

◆◆◆

to cook for themselves every night. If two nights of the same leftovers are too much for you, then freeze extra portions in one-serving containers. Do this a few times, and you'll have a freezer filled with your own homemade, healthy convenience foods.

Recycle Your Meals

This is a more interesting twist on the cooking-in-bulk theme. Instead of serving leftovers as they are, turn them into a completely different dish by making a few small changes. For example, you might cook up a pot of lentils on Sunday night, add some sautéed onions and some curry powder, and serve curried lentils over rice. On Monday night, take half of the lentils, add cooked carrots, thin the mixture with vegetable stock, and serve as a curried lentil soup with a salad and bread. On Tuesday night, take the second half of the leftover lentils, add bread crumbs to form a stiff mixture, and create curried lentil burgers to serve on hamburger buns along with a vegetable.

Along the same lines, you can plan an endless variety of meals by keeping the refrigerator filled with two pots of cooked grains and one or two pots of cooked beans. Don't season them ahead of time; just have them on hand for use throughout the week. For example, keep a pot of brown rice in the refrigerator to serve as a base for chili on Monday, to make rice pudding for breakfast on Tuesday, for a rice pilaf for Wednesday night's supper, and to add to a vegetable soup on Thursday.

The idea of a neatly penned menu with accompanying shopping list taped to the refrigerator door speaks to some of our souls but doesn't work for everyone. Some people are incapable of sitting down on Sunday night and thinking about what they will eat on Wednesday. No matter. It isn't necessary to plan out a week's worth of menus to make this system work. In fact, a more laid-back approach may produce more interesting meals.

Think about foods that lend themselves to many kinds of dishes. Potatoes are one. Five pounds of boiled potatoes can meta-morphose into dishes that are so varied you'll never hear anyone complaining "Potatoes *again?*" You can serve plain boiled potatoes on Monday, cube a few into a lentil curry dish on Tuesday, broil the precooked potatoes with rosemary, olive oil, balsamic vinegar, and herbs for Wednesday's dinner, toss them with mayonnaise for potato salad served with canned vegetarian baked beans on Thursday, and puree them with cow's milk or soymilk to make cream of potato soup on Friday.

If you vary the flavors of dishes enough, they won't get boring even when they are based on the same menu staple.

The End of the Week

By the end of the week you might have an interesting variety of leftovers in the refrigerator—a cup of this and a cup of that. Toss the leftovers together in a pot with some vegetable broth to create end-of-the-week soup, or stir-fry them with a drizzle of soy sauce, or pour them all into a casserole dish and bake them up for "leftover" casserole. That's plenty of menu planning for some people. It's creative, fun, low stress, and it works!

RULES OF THUMB FOR FAST COOKING VEGETARIAN-STYLE

• Once a week, cook up a few pots of grains and beans to keep in the refrigerator for quick meals.

• Have your favorite seasonings on hand. Keep your herb-and-spice rack well stocked, along with plenty of whichever condiments you especially like. Some good choices that give meals a flavor boost are gourmet mustards, balsamic vinegar, herb or raspberry-flavored vinegars, ketchup (it can perk up many a bland bean dish), hot pepper flakes, soy sauce, and hot sauce.

• Keep other flavor boosters on hand. Sunflower seeds and chopped nuts can be added to rice and bean dishes to give them some crunch and a new flavor. Raisins and other chopped dried fruits are also nice additions, especially for spicy soups.

• Keep at least five or six packages of frozen or canned vegetables on hand. If you are really in a hurry, they're much faster to prepare than fresh vegetables, since the canned or frozen variety don't require any washing, trimming, or chopping. And, of course, if you run out of fresh veggies, you don't have to dash to the store or stop on your way home from work. In the wintertime, frozen vegetables are generally more nutritious than the fresh ones that are flown in from warmer parts of the world. Even canned vegetables are more nutritious than is commonly thought.

• Do preparation work ahead of time. You might trim and chop all your vegetables on Sunday afternoon and then store them in airtight containers in the refrigerator. When it's time to make dinner, just give them a quick rinse and toss them into the steamer. Or skip the cooking step and dump them into a salad.

Cook It Fast: Microwaves and Pressure Cookers

The microwave is a favorite for getting food on the table in a hurry. It's especially great for heating leftovers and for cooking foods that ordinarily take a long time such as baked potatoes. It is also wonderful for vegetables—and offers a cooking method that retains nutrients—and dishes such as casseroles. You can also cook whole grains and beans in the microwave, but it won't speed up the cooking time for those dishes.

One of the most useful kitchen helpers for the vegetarian cook is a pressure cooker. Every kitchen had a pressure cooker back in the 1950s, but for a long time they have been out of favor. One reason is that everybody has heard a horror story of the pot exploding, leaving the cook without a meal and scraping potatoes off the ceiling. But the new pressure cookers are perfectly safe and are easy to use. In fact, once you've cooked a batch of beans in one, you'll probably never want to use conventional cooking methods again.

A pressure cooker will produce a nice pot of tender pinto beans in five minutes, potatoes tender enough for mashing in eight minutes, and carrots cooked to a baby's preference for softness in four minutes. For anyone interested in producing great vegetarian meals in the shortest time possible, a pressure cooker is, in our opinion, the most valuable kitchen tool you can have.

Cook It Slow

Paradoxically, another thing that can save you time is a slow cooker. The advantage of these pots (such as the Crock-Pot) is that they will happily simmer along all day while you are working or running errands, so that a savory, hot stew is ready for the table the minute you walk in the door.

You can also fill your Crock-Pot with whole-grain cereal, dried fruit, and water and plug it in before you go to sleep at night. You can wake up to the warming smells of seven-grain cereal with dates—it is a joy to sit down to breakfast without doing more than pouring a glass of juice and popping some bread in the toaster.

Fast Food

Planning, precooking, and using fast-cooking techniques are some ways you can save lots of time. But for those exceptionally busy times, it helps to have a repertoire of meals that can be cooked in twenty minutes. There are endless possibilities for vegetarians. Some of these depend on convenience items, such as packaged mixes, canned foods, and frozen products. While we wouldn't recommend cooking that way all the time, these foods are great to have on hand so that you can have superquick meals one or two times a week. Check local natural-foods stores for some of the vegetarian convenience foods.

Textured vegetable protein. Made from soy protein, TVP is a dried product with a long shelf life; just keep it dry and tightly stored, and it doesn't require any refrigeration. It needs to be rehydrated with hot water before you can use it; once it is rehydrated, it has a texture that is very much like cooked ground beef. Many TVP dishes can be made in under ten minutes. (For information on how to use TVP see page 313.)

Mixes. There are some wonderful mixes on the market now that produce vegetarian meals in minutes. Most of these are powdered bean and grain mixes that require the addition of water and then a few minutes' standing or cooking time.

Quick-cooking grains. Whole grains are almost always the best choice, but they aren't the only good choice. Using processed grains a few times a week will help you to prepare meals quickly. While they aren't quite as nutritious or fiber rich as their whole-grain counterparts, they are still healthful foods that add plenty of good nutrition to your diet. Try couscous, which cooks in just five minutes. Bulgur is another wheat product that is precooked and cracked for faster cooking—it is ready in about fifteen to twenty minutes. White rice cooks in about half the time of brown rice. There is even a Minute Rice version of brown rice on the market that will cook up in ten minutes.

Tofu. This is another product that has saved the life of many a vegetarian cook. It doesn't require any cooking, so you can just flavor it and heat it up. Cubes of tofu sautéed with a few teaspoons of curry powder and spooned into pita bread can be a fast, nutritious meal. Tofu blended with

IDEAS FOR HEALTHY MEALS IN MINUTES

Spaghetti with sauce from a jar

Chili made with canned beans, tomato sauce or stewed tomatoes, and chili powder mix

Commercial veggie burgers

Baked beans and instant brown rice

Bean burritos with canned or instant refried beans

Stir-fried rice with tofu chunks and vegetables

Sloppy joes with TVP and canned sloppy joe sauce

defrosted, chopped frozen spinach and a few tablespoons of soymilk makes a wonderful sauce to toss with hot pasta. Add nutritional yeast or Parmesan cheese for extra flavor. (See "What to Do with Tofu" on page 311 for more tofu cookery ideas.)

THE FRUGAL VEGETARIAN

Chances are, the less you spend for food, the healthier your diet will be. It sounds like a paradox, doesn't it? But it's true. Basic, whole foods, which include whole grains, dried beans, and seasonal fruits and vegetables, are inexpensive, chock-full of nutrients, and, for the most part, low in fat.

Traditional approaches to reducing food costs often ignore the fact that plant sources of protein are dramatically cheaper than animal sources. Vegetarian options, besides being healthier, offer food ideas that are much more interesting. Since economical cooking relies less on overly packaged convenience foods, it will almost always be more environmentally sound cooking, too.

Here are some tips for saving money on

your vegetarian diet. Some of these take more time than others, so choose what will work for you. Do keep in mind that all of these hints will improve the nutritional quality of your diet and most will improve the taste as well.

• Choose foods in their least processed form. Our local grocery store sells dried kidney beans for just half the cost of canned beans.

• Eat in season. The prices of tomatoes, peaches, and lettuce are dear in January—and they just aren't worth it. The taste is far inferior to what you get during the summertime, and so is the nutritional quality.

• Grow it yourself. The advantages of gardening are many. The food is cheap, and it is better than anything you could possibly buy in the store or even at a farmer's market. There are no questions about what was sprayed on the food, since you know everything that went into it. And digging, weeding, and hoeing are fantastic exercise. Gardening is a great "getting in touch with the earth" activity for kids, too, who sometimes haven't the foggiest idea where their food comes from.

• Make it yourself. It is almost always cheaper and better when you make anything from scratch. You'll shave dollars off your grocery bill by making your own eggless mayonnaise, ketchup, barbecue sauce, salad dressing, spaghetti sauce, pancake mix, and bread. You may not have time to do it all, but you might choose just a few items that you use frequently.

• Shop smartly. Some vegetarian items are expensive. Two staples in our house are two of the more costly items on vegetarian menus: soymilk and tofu. Fortunately, some food co-ops sell a powdered soymilk mix that is a little less expensive than the liquid kind. For tofu, try Asian markets. Some markets sell tofu in bulk for just a quarter of the typical supermarket price.

Of course, sometimes it does pay to spend a little bit more. Despite the fact that whole grains require less processing, they generally cost more money. You will nearly always pay more for brown rice compared with white rice and for whole wheat bread compared with white bread. Many whole-grain products are not available in regular grocery stores, and so you will pay more in natural-foods stores or other specialty markets.

We think it is worth paying a little bit more for these healthier products. It's also worthwhile to buy organic produce when you can. It's better for the environment and will give you some peace of mind. In the wintertime, choose frozen vegetables over canned. Canned is usually cheaper, but frozen is healthier and less of a drain on environmental resources.

Finally, don't underestimate the savings that good health brings. Some vegetarian items may cost a bit more, but a vegetarian diet is always cheaper than high-blood-pressure medication, bypass surgery, or the latest weight-loss gimmick.

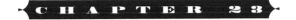

CHAPTER 23

STOCKING THE PANTRY

◆◆◆

*What a wealth of materials we
have to work with.*

—IRMA ROMBAUER, *The Joy of Cooking,* 1975

◆

A key to putting together great vegetarian meals with little fuss is to always have the basics on hand. Of course, what falls into the category "basics" is a personal thing. The following list includes both staples and specialty items. Although many of us have our favorite food items that we eat most often, it's a great idea to keep a good selection of grains, beans, and condiments in the kitchen so that you can experiment with different foods and new recipes when you feel like it. With the growing interest in gourmet cooking and ethnic dishes, an amazing number of the more unusual ingredients are available in large grocery stores. Most of the rest of them can be purchased at natural-foods stores. However, if you can manage a stocking-up trip to a large city that has Asian groceries (check the yellow pages), you'll find that many of the condiments we list here, as well as Asian noodles and sea vegetables, are all much less expensive at these stores, where they are considered staples, not specialty items.

Be certain to buy your herbs and spices from a grocery store that offers them in bulk. They are fresher and much less expensive. You can experiment with just a tiny amount of a new spice until you decide whether it will be a regular part of your cooking.

If the length of this list seems a little off-putting, a quick glance through it will assure you that you probably have a third to a half of these items in your pantry already. And there are others here that you may not be interested in using. This is meant to be a good all-purpose list for those who want to experiment with all types of vegetarian cooking, but you might pick and choose those ingredients that you are most likely to use.

GRAINS

Grains have a long storage life if you keep them cool and dry. Store them in airtight containers away from sunlight, and they will last for several months. To avoid bugs, freeze the grains for twenty-four hours when you first bring them home. If you have the space, grains will definitely stay fresher if you can refrigerate or freeze them. (See page 307 for instructions on cooking grains.)

Amaranth. An ancient Aztec grain with a taste faintly reminiscent of corn. The seeds are yellowish-brown and very tiny; cooked amaranth is often soupy rather than fluffy. Look for amaranth in natural-foods stores. Flavor it with onions and garlic, and try it mixed with other grains.

Barley. A real old-fashioned grain, used by most of our mothers to make hearty, wintertime vegetable soups, with a pleasant taste and a wonderful chewy quality. Hulled barley is the whole grain; it's more nutritious but takes a long time to cook. Pearled barley has the fiber-rich bran portion removed and cooks up in about fifteen minutes. Add barley to soups or stews, or sauté cooked barley with onions and mushrooms.

Buckwheat. A Russian grain called kasha when toasted, with a decidedly strong, earthy flavor that works best when mixed with other, mellower grains. Untoasted buckwheat is milder in flavor.

Cornmeal. Ground, dried corn, used most frequently to make corn bread, muffins, or polenta, a wonderful corn-based Italian porridge whose savory flavor belies the stodgy image of cornmeal. You can also add cornmeal to home-baked wheat breads or other whole-grain breads.

Kamut. An ancient Egyptian wheat. Although it is low fat like other grains, it has a rich, buttery taste that is unrivaled. The texture is chewy and pleasant.

Millet. A tiny, round, yellowish grain widely used in Asia and Africa. Serve millet with chopped onions and fresh or dried herbs such as oregano, rosemary, and basil.

Popcorn. A special type of corn with hard hulls; a great fat-free (if it's air popped) snack food.

Quinoa. Called the Mother Grain by the Incas, a staple in the diet of that civilization.

Serve it with potatoes—probably a traditional dish, since potatoes were also standard fare for the Incas—and gently flavored with herbs.

Rice. Three basic varieties: long-grain rice, fluffy when cooked and nice in pilaf; medium-grain rice, moist and tender right after cooking, but sticky as it cools; and short-grain rice, higher in starch, sticks together when cooked, the traditional rice used in Chinese and Japanese cooking. Within those categories, there are many wonderful types of rice. Here are just a few that you might encounter.

Arborio rice. A very high-starch, short-grain rice used to make risotto, a rich and creamy northern Italian dish. Other types of rice that can be used to make risotto are *vialone nano*, and *canaroli*, but these are much more difficult to find. In a pinch, any short-grain white rice can be used to make risotto, especially when it is made in the pressure cooker.

Basmati rice. An aromatic, long-grain rice imported from India and Pakistan; available as both a brown and a white rice.

Brown rice. The whole rice kernel, with just the outer hull removed, available as long, medium, or short grain and with a nutty flavor and chewy texture.

Japonica rice. A Japanese rice that tends to stick together when cooked; a good choice for Asian dishes.

Jasmine rice. A long-grain, aromatic rice imported from Thailand. Try it in cold salads, since it stays fluffy even after it has cooled.

White rice. Polished or milled rice, with the bran and germ both removed, so it is slightly more tender than brown rice and cooks more quickly. In the United States it is nearly always enriched with B vitamins and iron.

Wild rice. Not a rice at all, belonging to a completely different family of grasses that grow wild in the lakes of upper Michigan and Wisconsin. It is traditionally harvested by hand and is fairly costly. But one cup of wild rice expands to produce four cups of cooked grain.

Wheat berries. The whole kernel of wheat. Ground wheat berries produce whole wheat flour. Whole wheat berries have a nice chewy quality.

LEGUMES

Keep a variety of beans on hand— both canned and dried. In addition to those listed below, you may want to try appaloosas (brown and white speckled), favas, flageolets, and ful medames.

Adzuki beans. Small brownish beans that go well with brown rice or other grains.

Anasazi beans. Pretty maroon-and-white-speckled beans native to the American Southwest and good in Mexican and southwestern dishes.

Black turtle beans. Natives of the Caribbean and Central and South America, wonderful in chili, soups, and spicy dishes.

Black-eyed peas. Brought to the United States by African slaves, a much-loved ingredient in Southern cooking; good in salads or in spicy bean and grain dishes. They cook quickly and don't require soaking.

Brown beans (Swedish beans). Perfect in baked beans with molasses.

Cannellini beans. Small white beans used frequently in Italian cooking. When cooked well, they have a creamy consistency and can be pureed with herbs, garlic, and lemon to make a nice pâté. Or use them in soups or salads.

Chickpeas (garbanzos or cecis). The salad-bar beans; almost round, light brown, very popular in Mediterranean and Indian dishes. Use them in soups, pasta salads, pureed with tahini and lemon to make the Middle Eastern staple hummus, or in a spicy Indian curry.

Cranberry beans. Brownish beans with red spots, a traditional "baked bean" bean. Use them in any favorite baked bean recipe.

Great northern beans. Large white beans with a very mild flavor. Use them for baked beans or bean soups.

Kidney beans. Either white or red, the traditional bean called for in most chili recipes.

Lentils. One of the oldest foods known, used generously in the dishes of the Middle East, the Mediterranean, and India. You'll most likely find brown lentils, but they also come in red and yellow. They cook quickly and don't need to be soaked. Use them in lentil soup, Indian dishes, or salads.

Lima beans (butter beans). Rich, deep flavor, wonderful even with the least amount of seasoning. Use either regular or baby limas in soups and stews.

Navy beans (pea beans). For soups or baked beans.

Pinto beans. Southwestern staple, used in chili or spicy bean stews. They get their name for their pretty look: a pale-beige background with dark-brown speckles.

Soybeans. High-protein, higher-fat beans, with a distinct taste, sometimes described as nutty. They need a longer cooking time than other beans and don't have the mild flavor of most beans. They work very well in barbecued bean dishes or other strongly flavored dishes.

Split peas. Green or yellow, among the fastest cooking of the beans. Cook them in lots of liquid to make a creamy soup, or in less to make a puree or sauce for grains. They are a staple in Indian cooking and take very well to spicy, curried dishes.

NUTS, SEEDS, NUT BUTTERS

Fresh nuts and nut butters can go rancid quickly, so store them in the refrigerator. Nuts (but not nut butters) can also be frozen for longer keeping. Nuts can be added to baked goods or grain dishes.

Almond butter

Almonds

Cashew butter

Cashews

Chestnuts

Coconuts

Hazelnuts (filberts)

Peanut butter

Peanuts

Pecans

Pine nuts (pignoli)

Pumpkin seeds

Sesame seeds

Sunflower seeds

Tahini (sesame seed butter)

Walnuts

SOYFOODS

Soy cheese. An imitation cheese made from soybeans. It is usually not vegan, since most brands contain casein, a milk-derived protein. This is a highly processed product with none of the nutritional benefits of other soy products. We sometimes use small amounts of grated soy cheese in dishes, but don't recommend it for frequent use.

Soymilk. The rich liquid expressed from soaked soybeans, a wonderful alternative to cow's milk.

Soy nuts. Roasted soaked soybeans, great for snacks and salads.

Soy yogurt. A nondairy yogurt available in a variety of flavors.

Tempeh. A cake of fermented soybeans with a rich, earthy, mushroomlike flavor, a traditional Indonesian product; can be crumbled with seasonings into sandwich spreads, baked, or grilled with marinades.

Tofu. The mild tasting, porous curd that results when soymilk is coagulated. (See page 311 for ideas for using tofu.)

TVP. Textured vegetable protein. (See page 313 for ideas for using it.)

Sea Vegetables

You'll find these vegetables in dried form in natural-foods stores and in Asian groceries. Some need to be cooked before they can be eaten. Others just need to be soaked in hot water for a few minutes to soften. Sea vegetables can be cooked in soups, stews, or bean dishes. You can also crumble some dried sea vegetables directly into soups.

Alaria. Soak in boiling water for fifteen minutes, and then remove the tough central rib.

Arame. A great choice if your family isn't already familiar with sea vegetables. It is pre-cooked and has a mild flavor. Crumble it into soups and stews.

Dulse. A deep-red sea vegetable, doesn't require cooking. Add it to soups and stews.

Hijiki. An appearance something like angel-hair pasta. It's very salty, so soak it for fifteen minutes in fresh water and then rinse before cooking. Chopped hijiki can be used in soups, bean dishes, or stews.

Kelp. Usually sold in powdered form, adds a rich, salty, sealike taste to dishes. Sprinkle it over vegetables or grains. We consider it indispensable for our mock tuna salad.

Kombu. Large, flat strips. It's believed that adding strips of this sea vegetable to beans while they are cooking improves their digestibility.

Nori. Sold in dried, flat sheets, used to make vegetarian sushi.

Wakame. Brown leaves with fingerlike protrusions. Soak in water and remove the tough rib in the middle, then slice it into soups.

Dried Fruit

Apples

Apricots

Banana chips

Currants

Dates

Figs

Papayas

Peaches

Raisins

Condiments and Special Ingredients

Agar (agar-agar). A sea vegetable that can be used in place of gelatin in dishes.

Artichokes

Barbecue sauce

Bouillon, vegetable or instant broth

Bragg liquid amino acids. A salty condiment made from amino acids extracted from soybeans. Use it like soy sauce.

Brewer's yeast. A by-product of beer-making, rich in many vitamins and minerals. It can be stirred into juices or mixed into grains, but it is usually used in supplement form.

Capers. Salty, pickled flower buds. Use them in bean and grain salads for a wonderful flavor.

Coconut milk. Look for the reduced-fat variety.

Curry paste. Patak brand. Try the mild ones first.

Extracts. Vanilla, maple, walnut, coconut, lemon.

Fruit spreads, jams, apple butter

Garlic, fresh

Ginger, fresh

Hoison sauce. A sweet Chinese condiment made of soybeans, vinegar, and sweetener.

Hot-pepper sauces. Tabasco or others.

Ketchup

Mayonnaise, eggless. Homemade tofu mayonnaise or Nayonaise tofu mayonnaise.

Mirin. A low-alcohol, fermented Japanese rice wine with a sweet taste that tempers the saltier flavor of some Asian dishes.

Miso. Fermented soybean paste with a wonderful, salty, earthy flavor, an essential condiment in Japanese cooking. Use it in sauces, stews, soups, and grain and bean dishes.

Mustard. Prepared mustard, such as Dijon, and other types.

Nutritional yeast. An inactive yeast (it won't cause bread dough to rise) grown on a nutrient-rich culture so that it is usually rich in vitamins. Look for Red Star brand number T-6635+, which is rich in vitamin B$_{12}$.

Olives. Black, green, oil cured.

Pickles

Pimientos

Salsa

Shiitake mushrooms. Usually sold as dried mushrooms. Soak them in water until they are soft before adding to most recipes. Because their flavor is intense, a few go a long way.

Sun-dried tomatoes. Dehydrated (soak in hot water to soften before adding to dishes) or marinated in olive oil.

Tamari. Real soy sauce fermented and aged by traditional methods, has a much-richer taste than commercial soy sauce.

Umeboshi plum paste. A salty, pickle-flavored paste made of umeboshi plums. Use as a condiment in sauces and marinades.

Wasabi. A very hot Japanese radish, available in powdered or paste form. Use it sparingly in vegetarian sushi and sauces.

Wines. Dry red, sherry, dry white, for sautéing.

Worcestershire sauce. Angostura Lite (vegetarian).

VINEGARS

Apple cidar

Balsamic. A Mediterranean vinegar with a strong taste, more sweet and less acidic than other vinegars.

Herb vinegars. Tarragon and others.

Raspberry. A wonderful choice in home-made oil-and-vinegar dressings.

FLOURS AND OTHER PROCESSED GRAINS

Carob. Produces a mildly sweet flavor that some people compare to cocoa. Use it to replace part of the flour in baked goods or in place of cocoa in brownies and other chocolate desserts.

Oat bran. For muffins or cookies.

Oat flour. For breads, muffins, cookies, cakes.

Rye flour

Soy flour

Wheat bran

Wheat germ

Whole wheat flour. All-purpose whole-grain flour.

Whole wheat bread flour. A higher-gluten flour perfect for bread making.

Whole wheat pastry flour. A lower-gluten flour producing more tender muffins, cakes, and other products not leavened by yeast.

CEREALS

Brown rice cream. Cracked brown rice that cooks up into a creamy rice cereal.

Oats, whole and quick

Ready-to-eat cereals. Best bets—Shredded Wheat and bran flakes.

Seven-grain cereal

OILS

Canola oil

Chili oil

Fat replacers. Just Like Shortenin' and WonderSlim.

Olive oil

Sesame oil. For Asian dishes. Use toasted or roasted sesame oil for best flavor.

Soy margarine

Vegetable oil, pure. Usually soy oil.

PASTA

Asian. Mung-bean noodles, soba noodles (Japanese noodles made from buck-wheat), ramen noodles (thin Chinese curly noodles used in soups), udon (flat whole wheat noodles).

Italian. The traditional semolina pasta, in an endless variety of shapes, some with added vegetables, such as spinach pasta.

Whole grain. Made from whole wheat flour or sometimes other grains, like kamut.

BREADS AND CRACKERS

Graham crackers

Pita

Rice cakes

Tortillas

Whole-grain breads

Whole-grain crackers

QUICK MIXES

Beans, black

Beans, refried

Chili

Falafel

Hummus

Pancake and waffle

Tabouli. A Middle Eastern salad made with bulgur and flavored with lemon and mint.

Tofu burger

CANNED FOODS

We keep canned foods on hand for times when we need dinner in a big hurry. Some products, like canned tomatoes, we use frequently in a wide variety of dishes.

Beans. Chickpeas, black beans, pintos, kidney beans, great northern beans, butter beans.

Beans, chili

Beans, refried

Beans, vegetarian baked

Pumpkin

Spaghetti sauce

Tomatoes, crushed

Tomatoes, stewed

Tomatoes, whole, peeled

Tomato paste

Tomato sauce

MEAT SUBSTITUTES

Seitan. Wheat protein or gluten, produced by kneading bread dough, then rinsing it under water to wash away the starch. The resulting gluten can be baked and used as a tasty and chewy meat substitute. It is sold dried, to be rehydrated, or already prepared in the refrigerator section of health-food stores.

Tofu hot dogs

Veggie burgers

BEVERAGES

Coffee

Grain coffees

Juices

Milk, almond

Milk, rice

Milk, skim

Milk, soy

Take Care. Soy protein beverage.

Tea (regular and herbal)

Vegelicious

BAKING INGREDIENTS

Arrowroot

Baking powder

Baking soda

Egg replacer. Ener-G powdered egg replacer. (Liquid egg substitutes, like Egg Beaters, are *not* egg free.)

SWEETENERS

Barley-malt syrup. Extracted from sprouted, roasted barley. It's only about half as sweet as sugar, but has a pleasant, robust flavor that is nice in baked goods.

Blackstrap molasses. A liquid sweetener produced when sugar is refined. Is more nutritious than light, medium, or dark molasses.

Brown sugar. White refined sugar that has molasses added to it.

Honey. Produced by bees, so not a vegan product. The flavor of honey varies, depending upon the source of the pollen gathered by the bees.

Maple syrup. The concentrated sap of maple trees. It has a distinct flavor that is good in baked products and baked beans.

Sucanat. A brand name for a product made from evaporated and granulated sugarcane juice. Although made from the same plant as white refined sugar, it is a less refined product. Use it in place of granulated sugar, substituting equal amounts of Sucanat for sugar.

White refined sugar. Common table sugar. Many vegans prefer not to use it, since it is sometimes cleaned by running it through charred animal bones.

IN THE FREEZER

Juice

Juice pops

Sorbet

Soybean ice creams

Vegetables and fruits. Berries, frozen bananas, corn, greens, and so on.

HERBS AND SPICES

Keep dried herbs and spices in tightly sealed bottles or bags in a cool, dark cabinet. It's tempting to park your herbs and spices right over the stove where they are convenient, but the constant moist heat will cause their flavors to fizzle quickly.

If you experiment with ethnic dishes, you'll find that the list of herbs and spices you want to use in your dishes will grow and grow. Here is our basic starter list.

Herbs

Basil

Bay

Borage

Chervil

Chives

Cilantro (fresh only; it doesn't dry well)

Dill weed

Mint

Oregano

Parsley

Rosemary

Sage

Savory

Sweet marjoram

Tarragon

Thyme

Thyme, lemon

Spices

Allspice

Aniseed

Caraway seeds

Cardamom

Cayenne pepper

Celery seeds

Chili powder

Cinnamon

Cloves

Coriander powder

Coriander seeds

Cumin

Curry

Garlic powder

Ginger

Mace

Mustard powder

Mustard seeds

Nutmeg

Paprika

Peppercorns (black, green, and white)

Poppy seeds

Turmeric

As you experiment with ethnic cooking you might want to add these herbs and spices to your "basic" list:

Chinese five-spice

Fennel

Fenugreek

Garam masala

Lovage

Saffron

Star anise

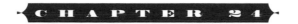
GETTING STARTED WITH VEGETARIAN COOKING

◆◆◆

All this is of course prologue.
The food is the heart of the matter.

—MARTHA STEWART,
Entertaining with Style, 1982

◆

HOW TO COOK GRAINS

When we talk about centering the diet on whole grains, most people think of rice and whole wheat bread. But there is really a wonderful selection of grains available to cooks. Some are old-fashioned favorites, like cornmeal, barley, and oats. Others, such as quinoa, spelt, kamut, and amaranth, are new to many but have actually been around for centuries.

The technique for cooking most grains is basically the same, although the amount of water you use and the cooking time vary.

1. Rinse the grains thoroughly.

2. Toast the grain. Heat a large, heavy skillet, add the rinsed grains, and stir them until the water has evaporated. Continue stirring until the grains begin to pop. (This step is optional. In many cases it makes the grains cook more evenly and enhances the flavor. But because one of the virtues of grains is that they are so easy to prepare, this optional step may seem like too much trouble. If so, feel free to skip it.)

3. Measure the water into a heavy pot with

Grain (1 cup uncooked)	Liquid (cups)	Cooking Time	Yield (cups)
Amaranth	2½	20–25 minutes	3½
Barley (hulled)	3	1½ hours	3½–4
Barley (pearl)	3	50 minutes	3½
Bulgur	2	20 minutes	3
Couscous	2	5 minutes	3
Kamut	3	2 hours	2¾
Millet	2	25 minutes	3
Quinoa	2	15 minutes	3
Wheat berries	3	2 hours	3

TABLE 24.1 COOKING TIMES FOR GRAINS

◆◆◆

TABLE 24.2 GRAIN COOKING TIMES FOR PRESSURE COOKER

Grain (1 cup uncooked)	Liquid (cups)	Time under High Pressure (minutes)	Yield (cups)
Amaranth	1¾	4	2
Barley (hulled)	3	40	3½
Barley (pearl)	3	18	3½
Buckwheat	1¾	3	2
Bulgur	1½	6	3
Kamut	3	40–45	2½
Millet	2–2½	12	3½
Spelt	3	40–45	2½
Triticale	3	35–45	2
Wheat berries	3	35–45	2

a tight-fitting lid and bring it to a boil. You can also use vegetable broth or, for a lightly sweet flavor, half water and half apple juice. Grains will not cook well in tomato sauce, so add any tomato products after cooking is completed.

4. Add the grains, return the mixture to a boil, then lower the heat to simmer. Place the lid on the pan, and cook until all the liquid is absorbed.

5. Most grains will cook best if you add salt after the cooking is completed.

Pressure-Cooking Grains

Because some whole grains take a long time to cook, we recommend using a pressure cooker. The cooking procedure is exactly the same. However, the time needed to cook the grain is much less. In some cases you will use less water, too. When cooking barley, buckwheat, kamut, or oats in the pressure cooker, add several teaspoons of oil to control foaming.

HOW TO COOK BEANS

Beans require a long cooking time, but they are relatively easy to prepare. While they simmer, you don't need to watch the pot, stir them, or otherwise hover.

The first step in preparing dried beans is to rinse them thoroughly. Then to greatly reduce cooking time, most beans (the exceptions are lentils and split peas) should be soaked for several hours. Smaller beans require only about four hours' soaking time; larger ones should be soaked for eight hours or overnight. Use any of the following soaking methods.

Soaking Method 1

1. Place the beans in a large bowl or pot, and add two cups fresh cold water for each cup of dried beans.

2. Place the bowl in the refrigerator and allow the beans to soak for four to eight hours.

3. Drain the beans thoroughly.

Beans (1 cup uncooked)	Cooking Time (hours)		Yield (cups)
	SOAKED	UNSOAKED	
Adzuki	1–1½	2–3	2
Anasazi	2	2½–3	2
Black	1½–2	2–3	2
Black-eyed peas	½	1	2
Cannellini	1–1½	2	2
Chickpeas	2	3½–4	2½
Cranberry	2	2–3	2½
Great northern	1½–2	2–3	2
Kidney	1½–2	2–3	2
Lentils*		½–¾	2
Lima	¾–1	1½	2
Navy	1½–2	2½–3	2
Pinto	1½–2	2–3	2
Soybeans	2–3	3–4	2½
Split peas*		¾	2

*Soaking not required.

Soaking Method 2

If you suffer from gas when you eat beans, try this soaking technique.

1. Place the rinsed beans in a large pot with three cups of water for each cup of dried beans. Bring the mixture to a boil, and boil for two minutes. Drain the beans.

2. Add fresh water, again using three cups water for each cup of beans. Let the beans soak for six or more hours in the refrigerator.

3. Drain the beans.

Soaking Method 3

If you forget to soak your beans try this quick-soak method.

1. Cover the beans with water and bring the mixture to a boil.

2. Remove from heat, cover, and let stand at room temperature for one hour.

Cooking Dried Beans

Be sure to drain the beans well after you have soaked them. Then place them in a large, heavy pot with three cups water for each cup of soaked beans or four cups water for each cup unsoaked beans.

Bring the water to a boil. Reduce the heat, cover the pot, and simmer the beans until they are tender. Use the cooking chart in table 24.3 for approximate cooking times for different varieties of beans.

TABLE 24.4 COOKING TIMES FOR BEANS IN A PRESSURE COOKER

Beans (1 cup uncooked)	Time under High Pressure (minutes)		Yield (cups)
	SOAKED	UNSOAKED	
Adzuki	5–9	14–20	2
Anasazi	4–7	20–22	2
Black	9–11	20–25	2
Black-eyed peas*		9–11	2
Cannellini	9–12	22–25	2
Chickpeas	10–12	30–40	2½
Cranberry	9–12	30–35	2¼
Great northern	8–12	25–30	2¼
Kidney	10–12	20–25	2
Lentils*		7–10	2
Lima	5–7	12–15	2½
Navy	6–8	15–25	2
Pinto	4–6	22–25	2¼
Soybeans	9–12	25–35	2¼
Split peas*		8–10	2

*Soaking not required.

Pressure-Cooking Beans

Because beans take such a long time to cook, a pressure cooker is the best way to prepare them. If you eat a lot of beans and prefer to make them from scratch, you will definitely want to invest in one of these pots. Follow these steps for pressure cooking beans:

1. Use three cups of water for each cup soaked beans or four cups water for each cup of unsoaked beans.

2. If you are using a jiggle-top pressure cooker, add one tablespoon oil for each cup of dried beans.

3. Lock the lid into place and bring the beans and water to high pressure.

4. Cook at high pressure for the time indicated in table 24.4.

5. Release the pressure quickly, according to the directions for your cooker.

6. Test the beans and return them to high pressure for a few minutes if they aren't quite done.

Fast Bean Cookery

Fill your freezer with beans that have been soaked six to eight hours, and you can have bean dishes in a jiffy. First, wash and soak the beans overnight as instructed in soaking method 1, above. Then drain the beans and freeze them in whatever portions you like (two or four cups per container are usually useful). When the beans freeze, the water that they absorbed while soaking expands and breaks down the cellulose in the beans. After the beans are defrosted, they'll cook up on top of the stove in twenty minutes or so.

WHAT TO DO WITH TOFU

Tofu is still a foreign food to many Westerners. If you haven't yet tried it, you are in for a pleasant surprise. Once people experiment with tofu, it quickly becomes a staple in most vegetarian kitchens simply because it is so easy to use, so delicious, and so versatile.

Tofu is much revered in other parts of the world. It has been a staple in Chinese cooking since around 200 B.C. and is still used every day in most households throughout Asia. It is made fresh daily in small tofu shops and sold by street vendors.

Tofu has two distinctive features that make it one of the most versatile foods on earth. First, it is relatively bland. It doesn't compete with other flavors and doesn't contribute any strong flavors of its own to a dish. Second, it is a spongy, porous food that absorbs flavors and sauces well. This means that it takes on the flavor of any other ingredients you cook it with. That's why tofu is at home in a spicy chili or taco but also works as the main ingredient in such sweet, creamy desserts as chocolate cream pie or a strawberry shake.

Tofu is produced from soymilk in much the same way that cheese is created from milk. A curdling agent is added to the tofu—usually a salt such as calcium sulfate—which causes large curds to form. The curds are sub-sequently pressed into a solid block of tofu.

Tofu is a wonderfully nutritious product. When it is made with a calcium salt, it is an excellent source of calcium. In addition, like all soy products, tofu is rich in high-quality protein. It's also a good source of iron and other minerals and vitamins. Although it is free of cholesterol and is low in saturated fat, tofu tends to be fairly high in total fat. However, it is usually lower in fat than the meat and dairy products it replaces in recipes. A number of brands of tofu available now are reduced in fat. Generally, firm tofu tends to be higher in fat than soft tofu.

There are a variety of types of tofu on the market. The kind of dish you are preparing will dictate to some extent which tofu you use. *Firm* tofu works well when you want to marinate chunks of tofu, stir-fry large pieces of it, cook it on the grill, or crumble it into scrambled tofu. *Soft* tofu is a much more delicate product with a higher water content. You can blend this type of tofu to produce a creamy substance that works well in sauces, dressings, fruit shakes, cream pies, dips, cheese-type fillings for pasta, or salad dressings. *Silken* tofu is very soft and custardy, more delicate than the other two kinds of tofu, and especially nice in shakes and desserts.

Tofu is a wonderful food for everyone. Because of its soft consistency and mild taste, pureed tofu can be a good choice for feeding babies. It is also a good food for the many older people who may have trouble chewing tough or crunchy foods.

Generally a recipe will tell you what type of tofu to use. If not, you can usually determine which is best just by thinking about the kind of dish you are making. If you want the tofu in chunks or large pieces, use firm. If you are blending it into a creamy product, choose soft or silken.

You can also create a tofu with a wonderful chewy texture by freezing firm tofu. Just freeze it right in its tub of water. Tofu that has been frozen and then defrosted takes on a caramel color and has a spongy, chewy texture that is very pleasant in stews and on top of the grill, or simply baked in a sauce in the oven.

In addition to regular firm, soft, and silken tofu, there are a number of baked and flavored tofu products available. These are fun and easy to use in a variety of dishes.

Tofu is available in water tubs, vacuum packs, or aseptic brick packages. It is usually found in the produce section of the supermarket, although it can also be located in the dairy case. You can sometimes find bulk tofu in food co-ops or in Asian markets. Unless it is aseptically packaged, tofu should be kept cold. Once you open the package, rinse the tofu, cover it with fresh water daily, and use it within a week. You can freeze tofu for up to five months.

Our resource section in the back of the book lists a number of excellent cookbooks that will introduce you to the versatility of tofu and get you started using this wonderful, nutritious food. With a little imagination and experimentation, you can use tofu in your cooking without a recipe. Try some of these ideas to introduce tofu to those in your household:

• Marinate tofu chunks in tamari or any sauce of your choice and add them to soups and stews.

• Mash tofu with cottage cheese and fresh herbs to make a dip or a sandwich spread.

• Mash tofu with bread crumbs, chopped onions, celery, and your favorite seasonings to create your own tofu burger recipe.

• Defrost frozen tofu, marinate it in barbecue sauce, and char it on the grill. Serve it in crusty rolls with sliced tomatoes and onions.

• Sauté some crumbled firm tofu with chopped onion and add a package of taco seasoning and tomato sauce to create a tasty, cholesterol-free filling for tacos.

• Blend dried onion soup mix into soft or silken tofu to make an onion dip.

• Blend soft tofu with fresh lemon juice, salt, and some fresh herbs for a baked potato topping.

• Blend soft tofu with melted chocolate chips to make a pie filling or a fluffy dessert.

• Replace all or part of the cream in creamed soups with blended silken tofu.

• Replace all or part of the cooked egg in egg salad with diced tofu. Add a little prepared mustard to the mix to perk up the flavor.

• Use blended soft tofu wherever you want to reduce the fat in a creamy dish. Try it instead of ricotta cheese in stuffed shells or lasagna. Use it in creamy ranch or Thousand Island dressing in place of mayonnaise.

What to Do with TVP

"TVP," which stands for textured vegetable protein, is actually a brand name of ADM. The generic name for this product is textured soy protein, or TSP. However, "TVP" is the commonly used term, so we'll use it here to avoid confusion. This is a wonderful food made from soy protein. It is rich in high-quality protein, fiber, calcium, iron, and zinc.

TVP is available as a dried, granular product. When boiling water is added to it, it takes on a tender, chewy consistency that is very similar to ground beef. TVP is also sold in chunks and is sometimes available as a product flavored to taste like beef or chicken. However, most TVP sold in grocery stores or natural-foods stores is the unflavored, granular variety. You can find it in the bulk-food section of many larger grocery stores and in food co-ops and natural-foods stores. Both unflavored and flavored TVP is also sold by mail (see the resource section at the back of this book).

To use TVP, pour seven-eighths cup boiling water over one cup of dry TVP. Let it sit for a few minutes. Chunk-style TVP requires one full cup of water for each cup TVP and may need to be simmered or microwaved to fully rehydrate.

By itself, TVP has a rather strong flavor. It needs the addition of other strong flavors for the best effect in recipes. Studies show that TVP works best in dishes that are flavored with tomato sauce. For that reason, it is a natural to replace the ground beef in chili, tacos, spaghetti sauce, stuffed peppers, stuffed cabbage, and sloppy joes. Just rehydrate the TVP and use it to replace an equal amount of ground beef in those dishes, using your favorite recipe.

Flavored TVP chunks are wonderful in stir-fried dishes, soups, stews, and curries.

Egg Substitutes

You may find that it is no trouble to forgo your scrambled eggs or omelette in the morning. But when it comes to replacing eggs in baked products and other recipes, even the most creative cooks can be challenged. Eggs have two important functions in recipes. First, because the protein in eggs coagulates upon heating, they help to thicken mixtures and hold them together. For example, most meat loaf recipes contain eggs to bind the rest of the ingredients together.

Second, eggs help to leaven baked goods, which makes them lighter and fuller. Eggs also add some moisture to these baked goods.

For vegans or others who prefer to cook without eggs there are a number of ingredients that can take on these roles in most dishes.

In Baked Goods

In baked goods, eggs leaven and add some moisture. Of course they aren't the only leavening agent. Baked goods also contain baking powder, baking soda, or yeast to make products rise and stay light. Try the following in place of eggs in your baking.

Flaxseed. This is one of the best egg replacers we know for baked goods. Grind three level tablespoons of flaxseed in a blender until it is a very fine powder. This will take several minutes. Then add a half cup cold water and blend until the mixture is frothy and viscous. It will have the same texture as well-beaten whole eggs. This is equal to about two large eggs. Add the mixture to your batter when your recipe calls for eggs. You can refrigerate the mixture for several days. One nice bonus of using flaxseed: egg yolks raise your blood cholesterol, but flaxseed contains lecithin, which actually lowers blood cholesterol.

Soy flour. This is another excellent egg substitute for baking. Soy flour has properties not found in other flours that help it to provide some egglike functions in baked goods. For each egg in a recipe, substitute one heaping tablespoon of soy flour and one tablespoon of water. This works well in cakes, muffins, or cookies that call for one, two, or three eggs.

Liquid. Here's the easiest idea. In some recipes that don't require a great deal of leavening and that call for only one egg, such as a pancake recipe, it is usually fine to leave the egg out. Be sure to add two or three additional tablespoons of liquid to the batter.

Mashed fruits. Use one-fourth cup mashed banana, applesauce, or pureed prunes to replace the moisture of one egg and make a product somewhat tender. Of course, the fruit will change the flavor and will also give you slightly heavier baked goods, since the fruit doesn't provide leavening. When using fruit to replace the egg in baked goods, try adding an extra half teaspoon of baking powder for each egg omitted from the recipe.

Flour–baking powder mixture. Try this mixture to replace one egg in baked goods: two tablespoons white flour, one-half tablespoon vegetable oil, two tablespoons water, one-half teaspoon baking powder. Mix them together and add this to the batter when an egg is called for.

Commercial egg replacer. This is a powdered mixture of potato starch, tapioca flour, and leavening agents. We've used it with varying degrees of success. In some baked goods, the end result is fairly dry, but in others it works pretty well. You'll need to experiment a bit to find out how it works best for you.

For Binding

In vegetarian cooking, you might find that you need something to help hold together the ingredients in a veggie burger mixture or in a bean and grain loaf. Try one of the following. Of course, the binder you use will depend a lot on the type of dish you are making since each of these adds a different flavor to the recipe.

- Tomato paste, thinned just a bit with water (not too much water, or it will lose its capacity to hold the recipe together)

- Tahini, mixed with a little bit of tomato paste (also adds a nice flavor)

- Four ounces of soft tofu pureed with one to two tablespoons of white flour

- Thickened white cream sauce made from flour, margarine, and soymilk

- Mashed potatoes

- Mashed banana (It may not work too well in your average bean loaf, but it can give a surprisingly interesting flavor to a vegetarian burger, especially a spicy one.)

• Flour, matzo meal, or quick oats (Use sparingly; they can give your burger or loaf a heavy, dense quality.)

• Moistened bread crumbs

GOING DAIRY FREE

Many of the new vegetarian products on the market make it easier than ever to go dairy free. Nondairy milks are perfect for your morning cereal, shakes, baking, cream sauces, or a refreshing beverage. These milks can do just about anything that cow's milk can do in cooking; they make eliminating milk from your diet a cinch. Soymilks are the most popular, but there are also wonderful milks made from almonds and rice. We have mentioned two nonsoy beverages that we highly recommend because they are so nutritious. These are Vegelicious, which contains honey, and Take Care, which is completely vegan.

You can find nondairy cheese in most natural-foods stores and many supermarkets. These are generally made from soy, although some made from almonds are available also. Unfortunately, many of these cheeses contain casein, which comes from cow's milk, so they are not completely dairy free for those who prefer not to use any dairy products or who have allergies to milk protein.

Tofu is also a great cheese imitator. Soft tofu, blended and flavored with salt and a little fresh parsley, is perfect in place of ricotta cheese in stuffed shells or lasagna. Blend tofu with fresh lemon juice to make a sour-cream substitute, or whip it with sugar and a dash of lemon to make a substitute for whipped cream.

If you are a reformed cheese-aholic and really miss the flavor of cheese, try some of the recipes in *The Uncheese Cookbook* (see the resource section at the back of the book) for instructions to make scores of vegan cheese-like dishes.

FATS IN COOKING

Vegetarian meals tend to be lower in fat than nonvegetarian ones, since meat and dairy products are big contributors of fat to the diet. But plenty of vegetarian recipes are too fatty. If you fry in oils, pile margarine onto your toast and muffins, and eat lots of sweets and prepared processed foods, you might end up with too much fat. Even though plant foods contain no cholesterol and tend to be much lower in saturated fat, too much of any kind of fat is to be avoided.

Consider these cooking techniques to reduce fat:

• Use nonfat cooking methods. That means baking, steaming, or simmering foods whenever possible.

• Invest in a few nonstick pots and pans so that you don't need to add fat to keep foods from sticking.

• Braise foods instead of sautéing them in oil. Cook onions, garlic, and other vegetables in a small amount of vegetable stock, wine, or sherry.

• Try fat-free salad dressings.

• Season vegetables with herb-flavored vinegar or melt a tiny bit of margarine with some Dijon mustard and a few squeezes of fresh lemon juice.

• Create thick, creamy soups by pureeing a bit of mashed potato or instant potato flakes into the broth. Or make a fat-free white sauce by mixing a tablespoon of white flour with two tablespoons of vegetable stock. Cook it over low heat, stirring vigorously, for one minute. Then add a half cup of vegetable stock, stirring to avoid lumps, and bring to a boil. Turn the heat down and simmer for a few minutes until the sauce is thick. Add this to soups to give them a creamy consistency. You can also add a creamy texture to soups by pureeing soft tofu into them.

• Reduce the fat in baked goods by a third or so until you find out just how low you can get the fat content and still have a light, tasty product.

• Try one of the new fat substitutes designed for baking. These are a combination of pureed dried fruits, and they can substitute for as much as half the fat in cookies, cakes, and muffins. Two good choices are Just Like Shortenin' or WonderSlim, both available in natural-foods stores.

For more fat-defying tips, see chapter 17. Although it's a good idea to reduce the fat in your diet, don't make the mistake of thinking that your meals have to be fat free.

Occasionally, we use small amounts of olive oil for sautéing for the special flavor it adds. Sometimes we'll sauté onions and garlic in a teaspoon or two of olive oil and then add vegetable stock to sauté the rest of the vegetables in a recipe.

COOKING WITH SWEETENERS

Although sugar is not nearly the evil that many make it out to be, most of us could stand to eat a little less of it. It is added liberally to processed foods and, of course, is generously dumped into baked goods. It offers calories without much additional nutrition and is especially harmful to dental health. So we don't recommend making sweets a frequent part of your menus. But, if you choose, it is fine to include them once in a while, especially if you use them as a way to get some more nutritious ingredients into your meals, as in zucchini bread or banana-oatmeal cookies.

We've included white sugar in some of our dessert recipes because it is readily available and inexpensive. Although we have no objection to the occasional use of white sugar, you may feel otherwise. Feel free to substitute whichever sweeteners you prefer.

Be aware, however, that sugar travels under many guises. In chapter 23, we listed a number of different sweeteners that can be used in recipes. Although some, like blackstrap molasses, can add some nutrients to your recipes, most are just different forms of sugar. Other than taste, there is no advantage to using maple syrup over white refined sugar. Your body doesn't much care

TABLE 24.5 SUBSTITUTES FOR 1 CUP SUGAR

$\frac{2}{3}$ cup fructose

$\frac{3}{4}$ cup honey (reduce the liquid in the recipe by $\frac{1}{4}$ cup for each $\frac{3}{4}$ cup honey used)

$\frac{3}{4}$ cup maple syrup (reduce the liquid in the recipe by 3 to 4 tablespoons)

$1\frac{1}{4}$ cups molasses (reduce the liquid in the recipe by 6 tablespoons; use molasses for only half the sugar in a recipe and use sugar for the other half)

1 cup Sucanat

1 cup barley malt syrup (reduce the liquid in the recipe by $\frac{1}{2}$ cup)

1 cup brown rice syrup (reduce the liquid in the recipe by $\frac{1}{2}$ cup)

that the maple syrup is "natural" while the sugar is refined. It treats it all the same.

When making substitutions in recipes, keep in mind that changing the sweetener can sometimes change the end result. Substituting honey for sugar will cause cakes and cookies to bake faster and turn browner. It is also sweeter. When you substitute a liquid sweetener for sugar, you will need to reduce the amount of other liquids in the recipe accordingly.

If you like to cook and experiment, you might want to dabble a bit in revising recipes to see if you can reduce the sugar. If your family and friends enjoy foods that are more subtly sweet, you can sometimes reduce the sugar content of a recipe by a quarter to a third and still get good results. Remember, though, that sugar does more than sweeten. It also makes baked goods more tender, so that your less-sweet cakes and muffins may seem heavier and coarser.

You also might try using less sugar and adding more natural sources of sweetness, such as mashed banana or applesauce.

Table 24.5 shows how you can substitute various sweeteners for refined white sugar. (Some of these sweeteners are explained more fully in chapter 23.)

VEGETABLE STOCK

Many of our recipes at the end of the book call for vegetable broth, stock, or bouillon. (We use the terms interchangeably.) This is a wonderful way to add more flavor to bean and grain dishes and is a great base for any kind of soup. Vegetable stock can always be used to replace chicken broth in recipes.

You can make your own stock using our recipe on page 324, or you can keep some instant types on hand. Many grocery stores sell vegetable bouillon cubes (look in the soup aisle) and natural-foods stores sell vegetable broth powders, sometimes packaged and sometimes in bulk.

RECIPES

A Word about the Recipes

We think of these as "starter" recipes, meant to introduce you to a variety of foods, ingredients, and meal ideas. There should be enough ideas here to plan at least a couple weeks' worth of breakfasts, brown-bag lunches, and quick dinners. We aimed for fairly easy and fast recipes that would use mostly familiar ingredients, but would introduce you to some new foods and ingredients as well.

Don't be afraid to be creative and to revise these recipes. In some cases we have opted for the most familiar, easy-to-find ingredient—white sugar, for example. But you may not use sugar in your cooking and may wish to substitute something else. Some dishes may be too spicy for you—or not spicy enough. Taste as you cook, and use your own good sense and preferences to create the dishes that are perfect for you and those you cook for.

As you learn more about vegetarian cooking, you will definitely want to explore some new vegetarian cookbooks, perhaps some that we've recommended in the resource section.

BREAKFAST

◆ BANANA FRENCH TOAST ◆

This unusual recipe for French toast is so healthy and so much fun. The creamy banana batter produces the most delectable French toast we've ever tasted.

2 very ripe bananas
1 cup plain soymilk
8 slices whole wheat bread

In a blender, blend the bananas and soymilk until completely smooth. Pour the mixture into a large bowl. Dip the bread into this mixture and cook on a lightly oiled, hot griddle until just browned on each side.

Serves 4

◆ QUICK COFFEE CAKE ◆

Coffee cake is such a treat for lazy weekend mornings. Mary Clifford's recipe is delicious and, unlike commercial coffee cakes, it is also cholesterol free.

1 cup unsifted all-purpose flour
1 cup unsifted whole wheat flour
¾ cup old-fashioned rolled oats
⅓ cup firmly packed light brown
   sugar
1 tablespoon baking powder
2 teaspoons ground cinnamon
½ teaspoon ground nutmeg
¼ teaspoon ground ginger
Pinch of salt
½ cup margarine
1 cup unsweetened apple juice

Preheat the oven to 350° F. Grease and flour a 9-inch square baking pan.

In a large bowl, combine the flours, ½ cup of the oats, sugar, baking powder, cinnamon, nutmeg, ginger, and salt. Remove ½ cup of the mixture to a cup or small bowl, and add the remaining ¼ cup oats. Cut in 2 tablespoons of the margarine; set the mixture aside.

Cut the remaining margarine into the flour mixture in the large bowl. Stir in the apple juice until well combined. Pour the batter into the prepared pan. Top with the reserved oat mixture.

Bake the cake about 40 minutes, or until a knife inserted in center comes out clean. Let it cool to room temperature.

Serves 6

◆ PUMPKIN-APPLE BREAD ◆

This is a delicious reduced-fat quick bread that is just brimming with the goodness of apples and nutritious pumpkin. Keep it on hand in the freezer for mornings when you need to grab breakfast on the go.

1 cup white flour
1 cup whole wheat pastry flour
1 tablespoon soy flour
1 teaspoon baking soda
1 teaspoon baking powder
⅛ teaspoon salt
½ teaspoon ground cinnamon
¼ teaspoon ground allspice
½ teaspoon ground nutmeg
¼ cup vegetable oil
½ cup sugar
½ cup plain soymilk
¾ cup canned pumpkin
2 sweet apples, such as Delicious,
   finely chopped

Preheat the oven to 350° F.

Mix together the flours, baking soda, baking powder, salt, cinnamon, allspice, and nutmeg in a large bowl. In a separate bowl, beat together the oil and the sugar. Add the soymilk and pumpkin. Stir the dry ingredients into the pumpkin mixture and mix thoroughly. Fold in the apples.

Bake in an oiled loaf pan for 45 minutes.

Serves 10

◆ MUSHROOM PÂTÉ ◆

Make this wonderful, savory pâté with the rich flavor of mushrooms and herbs a day ahead to give the flavors a chance to develop. Serve it with pita wedges, party rye bread, or crackers.

2 tablespoons minced onions
2 cloves garlic, minced
1 tablespoon olive oil
1 pound fresh mushrooms, chopped
2 tablespoons vegetable stock (see page 324)
1 tablespoon white flour
8 ounces (1 cup) soft tofu
½ teaspoon dried oregano
½ teaspoon dried basil
½ teaspoon dried marjoram
1 tablespoon vegetarian Worcestershire sauce
Salt and black pepper to taste

Sauté the onions and garlic in the olive oil for 2 minutes. Add the mushrooms and the vegetable stock. Cover and let the mixture cook until the mushrooms are completely tender. Mix in the flour thoroughly and sauté for an additional 2 minutes, stirring the mixture to keep it from sticking. Place the mushroom mixture and the rest of the ingredients in a food processor and process until they form a smooth pâté. Refrigerate for at least 2 hours. Serve with crackers or spread on bread.

Serves 8

◆ BABA GANOUJ (EGGPLANT PÂTÉ) ◆

Baba ganouj is a traditional Middle Eastern dip, usually served with wedges of pita bread. In Turkey, authentic baba ganouj uses eggplants that have been charred, giving the dish a rich, smoky flavor. You can achieve a similar flavor by adding a drop or two of liquid smoke if you like.

2 medium eggplants
Juice of 1 lemon
¼ cup tahini
3 cloves garlic
¼ cup finely chopped fresh parsley
1 teaspoon salt
¼ cup finely minced green onions
1 tablespoon olive oil
Pinch of cayenne pepper
1 or 2 drops Liquid Smoke (optional)

Wash the eggplants and prick them all over with a fork. Place them on a cookie sheet and bake at 400° F. for about 45 minutes, until they are soft and wrinkled. Cool and then scoop the insides into a food processor. Add the rest of the ingredients and process until smooth. Chill and serve with pita bread wedges.

Makes 2 cups

◆ Sweet-and-Spicy Black-Bean Dip ◆

This dip has the kick of cayenne tempered by a subtle sweetness. Serve it with tortilla chips or with pita wedges.

> 1½ cups cooked or canned black beans
> 1 tablespoon olive oil
> 2 tablespoons vegetarian Worcestershire sauce
> ⅛ teaspoon hot-pepper sauce
> 1 tablespoon sugar
> Salt and black pepper to taste
> 1 medium onion, finely chopped

Place all the ingredients except the onion in a blender and blend until smooth. Stir in the onion. Serve at room temperature.

Makes 1½ cups

◆ Stuffed Mushrooms ◆

This is a wonderful party dish, since you can assemble it the day before and then bake it just before the company arrives. It is deceptively simple because it contains few ingredients, but the flavor is magnificent. We serve the mushrooms as an hors d'oeuvre or as a side dish at Thanksgiving.

> 1 pound fresh mushrooms
> 2 tablespoons minced onions
> 2 tablespoons olive oil
> ½ cup dry bread crumbs
> ½ teaspoon salt
> ¼ teaspoon paprika
> ⅛ teaspoon black pepper

Preheat the oven to 400° F. Remove the stems from the mushroom caps, set aside the caps, and chop the stems finely. Sauté the chopped mushroom stems and minced onions in the olive oil for 5 minutes. Add the bread crumbs, salt, paprika, and pepper, and sauté for about 1 to 2 minutes more. Taste and adjust the seasonings.

Stuff the mushroom caps with this mixture. Place the caps in a nonstick baking pan and bake for 15 to 20 minutes, until the caps are tender.

Serves 8

SOUPS

◆ SPICED LENTIL SOUP ◆

There are probably as many recipes for vegetarian lentil soup as there are vegetarians. This one turns up the spices a bit to create an especially flavorful dish.

> 1 onion, coarsely chopped
> 2 tablespoons olive oil
> 2 carrots, diced
> 2 stalks celery, diced
> 1 green bell pepper, seeded and cut into chunks
> 1 small potato, peeled and diced
> 1 teaspoon ground cumin
> 1 teaspoon chili powder
> ¾ teaspoon ground allspice
> 1 bay leaf
> 1½ cups dried lentils
> 6 cups vegetable stock (see page 324)
> Salt and black pepper to taste

Sauté the onion in the olive oil in a large pot over medium heat until tender. Add the carrots, celery, and green pepper and sauté for 3 minutes, stirring the vegetables. Add the diced potato, cumin, chili powder, and allspice, and sauté for 1 minute. Add the bay leaf, lentils, and vegetable stock. Bring the soup to a boil, and boil for 1 minute.

Lower the heat, cover, and simmer the soup for 1 hour, or until the lentils are tender. Remove the bay leaf. Season with salt and pepper and adjust the spices. Serve with toasted pita bread and a salad.

Serves 6

◆ CREAM OF BROCCOLI SOUP ◆

This soup has a luscious richness with much less fat than is usually found in cream soups. With chunks of potato, it is almost a stew and is so wonderful on those cold, blustery winter evenings.

> 2 teaspoons olive oil
> 1 medium onion, coarsely chopped
> 4 medium potatoes, coarsely diced
> 2 cups vegetable stock (see page 324)
> 1 teaspoon dried thyme
> 2 cups soymilk
> 3 tablespoons white flour
> 2 stalks broccoli, cut into large chunks
> Salt and black pepper to taste

In a large pot, heat the olive oil over medium heat. Sauté the onion for 2 minutes. Add the diced potatoes, the vegetable stock, and the thyme. Allow the mixture to simmer until the potatoes are tender, about 20 minutes.

In a blender, blend together the soymilk and flour. Add the broccoli in several additions and process until it is minced. Pour the broccoli-soymilk mixture into the potatoes and onions.

Bring the soup to a boil. Immediately lower the heat and simmer for 10 minutes. Add salt and pepper and more thyme to taste.

Serves 8

◆ CREAMY CURRIED CARROT SOUP ◆

Silken tofu lends a rich creaminess to a soup that will warm up the coldest winter evening. Serve it with whole wheat rolls and a tossed salad.

6 carrots, thinly sliced
2 cups vegetable stock
  (see page 324)
1 cup chopped onions
2 teaspoons curry powder
8 ounces (1 cup) soft silken tofu
Salt to taste

Combine the carrots, vegetable stock, onions, and curry powder in a medium saucepan. Bring the mixture to a simmer over medium heat, and continue to simmer for 20 minutes, or until the carrots are very tender. Transfer the mixture to a blender (or use a hand blender) and blend until smooth. Add the tofu and blend until the ingredients are mixed and creamy. Return the soup to the saucepan and heat. Add salt to taste.

Serves 4

◆ CORN CHOWDER ◆

This is such a comforting soup, with old-fashioned flavor and appeal. With bread and an additional vegetable, it makes a very filling meal.

1 large onion, coarsely chopped
1 clove garlic, minced
1 green bell pepper, coarsely
  chopped
½ cup chopped celery
1 tablespoon olive oil
6 medium potatoes, diced
2 cups vegetable stock
  (see page 324)
2½ cups frozen or fresh corn
  kernels
2 cups soymilk
½ teaspoon dried sage
½ teaspoon dried rosemary
½ teaspoon dried basil
Salt and black pepper to taste

Sauté the onion, garlic, green pepper, and celery in the olive oil for 2 minutes. Add the potatoes and vegetable stock and simmer over low heat until the potatoes are tender. Add the corn kernels, soymilk, and herbs and simmer for an additional 5 minutes. Season with salt and pepper.

Serves 6

♦ VEGETABLE STOCK ♦

A good vegetable stock forms the basis for many wonderful vegetarian dishes. This one is adapted from a recipe developed by Chef Jay Brinkley and dietitian Mary Clifford for a vegetarian cooking class offered at Community Hospital of Roanoke Valley in Roanoke, Virginia. Simmer the stock until it cooks down to a rich, concentrated broth, strain it, then freeze it in ice-cube trays and store the cubes in resealable plastic bags so you always have some on hand. Save the vegetables and puree them with soymilk and additional herbs, such as basil or marjoram, to make a savory cream of vegetable soup.

> 1 teaspoon olive oil
> 1 large onion, chopped
> 2 stalks celery, chopped
> ½ cup fresh mushrooms, chopped
> 3 potatoes, peeled and diced
> 3 carrots, peeled and chopped
> 1 leek, sliced
> 6 sprigs parsley
> 1 bay leaf
> 2 sprigs fresh thyme, or 1 teaspoon
>   dried thyme
> 8 cups cold water

In a large saucepan, heat the oil over medium heat. Add the onion, celery, and mushrooms and sauté for 2 minutes. Add the potatoes, carrots, leek, parsley, bay leaf, and thyme. Sauté the mixture for 5 minutes. Add the water and bring the soup to a boil. Reduce the heat to low and simmer for at least 2 hours. Strain the stock, reserving the vegetables for another use.

Makes approximately 1 quart stock

ENTRÉES

♦ PILAF WITH CARROTS AND RAISINS ♦

The sweetness of maple syrup and raisins is in pleasant contrast to the spicy Indian flavors in this dish. With a salad or a cooked vegetable on the side, this makes a full meal.

> 4 tablespoons maple syrup
> 3 cups vegetable stock (see
>   preceding recipe)
> 1¼ cups thinly sliced carrots
> 2 tablespoons raisins
> 1 tablespoon vegetable oil
> 1½ cups basmati rice
> ½ teaspoon salt
> ¼ teaspoon ground cardamom
> ¼ teaspoon ground cinnamon
> ¼ teaspoon ground nutmeg
> Freshly grated nutmeg

Mix together the maple syrup and vegetable stock in a medium saucepan. Cook over low heat for 2 to 3 minutes.

In a large skillet, sauté the carrots and raisins in the oil for 10 minutes. Add the rice to the carrot mixture, and stir to coat the grains with the oil. Stir in the syrup and stock and the remaining ingredients except the freshly grated nutmeg. Heat the mixture to boiling; reduce the heat. Simmer, covered, for 35 to 40 minutes, until all the stock is absorbed. Serve sprinkled with freshly grated nutmeg.

Serves 4

♦ BROWN RICE ROYALE ♦

The wonderful flavors of mushrooms and leeks turn this simple dish into something very special. Once the rice is cooked, it takes just 10 minutes to put this meal together.

> 2 cups vegetable stock
>   (see page 324)
> 1 cup brown rice
> 3 cups sliced fresh mushrooms
> ½ cup thinly sliced leeks
> 1 tablespoon olive oil
> 1 teaspoon dried thyme
> Salt and black pepper to taste

Bring the vegetable stock to a boil in a medium saucepan. Add the rice, then return the mixture to a boil. Lower the heat, cover, and simmer until the stock is absorbed and the rice is done, about 40 minutes.

In a large skillet, sauté the mushrooms and leeks in the olive oil over medium heat until tender, about 10 minutes. Add the rice and thyme. Stir until the mixture is thoroughly heated. Season with salt and pepper to taste.

Serves 4

♦ RICE-A-VEGGIE ♦

> 2 cups water
> 1 cup rice-a-veggie quick mix
>   (recipe follows)
> 1 tablespoon margarine

Bring the water to a boil in a medium saucepan. Add the rice mix and the margarine. Lower the heat to simmer and cover the pot. Simmer until all the water is absorbed, about 15 minutes for white rice or 35 minutes for brown.

Serves 6

◆ RICE-A-VEGGIE QUICK MIX ◆

Keep your own mix for seasoned rice on hand to create fast dinners that taste better than anything you can buy in a box.

> 4 cups white or brown rice
> ½ cup dried parsley flakes
> ¾ tablespoon vegetable broth
>   powder
> 1 tablespoon plus 1 teaspoon onion
>   powder
> ½ teaspoon garlic powder
> ¼ teaspoon dried thyme

Mix the ingredients together thoroughly and store in an airtight container.

◆ MINTED COUSCOUS SALAD ◆

In this dish, the traditional Mediterranean flavors of lemon and mint create a refreshing and slightly exotic salad with a minimum of fuss.

> 1 cup uncooked couscous
> 1 cup boiling water
> 2 tablespoons olive oil
> 1 medium carrot, cut into
>   julienne strips
> 1 medium zucchini, cut into
>   julienne strips
> ½ teaspoon ground ginger
> 2 teaspoons dried mint
> ½ cup sliced almonds (optional)
> ½ cup raisins, soaked in 1 cup
>   warm water
> 3 tablespoons fresh lemon juice
> Salt and black pepper to taste

Place the couscous in a bowl and pour the boiling water over it. Let it soak until all the water is absorbed, about 10 minutes.

Heat the olive oil in a large skillet and add the carrot, zucchini, ginger, and mint. Sauté, stirring frequently, for about 5 minutes.

Mix together the couscous, almonds, if using, and vegetables in a bowl. Drain the raisins and add them to the couscous mixture. Toss with lemon juice, and add salt and pepper to taste. Serve at room temperature.

Serves 4

◆ POLENTA ◆

Polenta is a type of cornmeal mush or porridge. It is a traditional dish in northern Italy and is wonderful as a base for vegetables and tomato sauce or as a crust for a savory vegetable pie. Cornmeal tends to lump when it is mixed into water. The following method, which reduces lumps, comes from Lorna Sass's book *Recipes from an Ecological Kitchen*.

8 cups water
2½ cups yellow cornmeal
1 teaspoon salt

Mix together 3 cups of the water and the cornmeal in a bowl, or shake them to mix in a jar.

In a large saucepan, bring the remaining 5 cups of water and the salt to a boil. When the water begins to boil, add the cornmeal batter, stirring vigorously as you pour it in. Reduce the heat and continue to stir and simmer for about 30 minutes, until the polenta is thick and thoroughly cooked.

Makes about 10 cups

◆ POLENTA WITH RATATOUILLE ◆

Spicy vegetables are a perfect accompaniment to the mild taste of polenta.

1 large onion, coarsely chopped
3 cloves garlic, minced
3 tablespoons olive oil
1 small eggplant
1 28-ounce can crushed tomatoes
1 teaspoon dried basil
1 teaspoon dried marjoram
½ teaspoon dried oregano
2 medium zucchini squash, diced
2 large green bell peppers, diced
2 fresh tomatoes, cut into chunks
2 tablespoons dry red wine
Salt and black pepper to taste
¼ cup chopped fresh parsley
1 recipe polenta (see preceding recipe)

Sauté the onion and garlic in the olive oil in a large skillet over medium heat until the onion is transparent. Add the eggplant, crushed tomatoes, basil, marjoram, and oregano. Cover and simmer for 10 minutes. Add the zucchini and peppers and cover and simmer for an additional 10 minutes. Add the fresh tomatoes, wine, salt, and pepper, and simmer for 10 minutes more or so, until all the vegetables are tender. Stir in the fresh parsley and serve over the polenta.

Serves 6

◆ Quinoa, Corn, and Potatoes ◆

Quinoa grew high in the Andes Mountains of what is now Peru and was a staple in the diet of the Incas. They probably paired this quick-cooking grain with potatoes, which also grew well in the cooler climate of the mountains. Here we've added another Latin American staple, corn, to create a dish of lovely complementary flavors and superior nutrition.

1 large onion, coarsely chopped
3 cloves garlic, minced
1 tablespoon olive oil
2 cups diced potatoes (new, waxy potatoes are best)
1½ cups vegetable stock (see page 324)
1 cup uncooked quinoa, rinsed
1½ cups fresh or frozen corn kernels
½ teaspoon dried oregano
½ teaspoon dried tarragon
Salt to taste

Sauté the onion and garlic in the oil in a large skillet over medium heat for 2 minutes. Add the potatoes and sauté for an additional minute. Pour in the vegetable stock, quinoa, corn, oregano, and tarragon. Bring the mixture to a boil. Lower the heat, cover the pan, and simmer for 20 minutes, or until all the stock has been absorbed, and add the salt.

Serves 6

◆ Apricot–Walnut– Wheat Berry Salad ◆

This is a beautiful main-dish salad. The sweetness of orange juice and dried apricots is a perfect complement to the heartiness of the grains in this dish.

3 cups cooked wheat berries
3 cups cooked brown rice
1 teaspoon grated orange zest
4 tablespoons orange juice concentrate
1 tablespoon white wine
1 tablespoon white wine vinegar
4 tablespoons vegetable stock (see page 324)
2 tablespoons vegetable oil
1 navel orange, peeled
1 small head cauliflower
¾ cup dried apricots, coarsely chopped
6 green onions, thinly sliced, including some of the green
1 cup chopped walnuts
1 teaspoon dried oregano
Salt and black pepper to taste

Mix together the wheat berries and rice in a large bowl. Combine the orange zest, orange juice concentrate, wine, wine vinegar, stock, and oil in a jar with a tight-fitting lid. Shake to combine and pour over the wheat berries and rice.

Place the orange in a food processor, and process until it is in tiny chunks. Stir into the grains.

Cut the cauliflower into florets, and steam them over boiling water for 5 to 7 minutes, or until just tender. Add the cauliflower, apricots, green onions, walnuts, and oregano to the grains. Add salt and pepper.

Serves 10

♦ MEDITERRANEAN CHICKPEAS ♦

Chickpeas, tomatoes, lemon, and garlic are all flavors that sing of sunny days along the Mediterranean Sea. They come together in this easy dish for a fast supper.

    2 medium onions, chopped
    3 cloves garlic, minced
    1 tablespoon olive oil
    3 cups cooked chickpeas
    1 10-ounce package frozen
       chopped spinach, defrosted
    1 28-ounce can crushed tomatoes
    1 cup chopped fresh tomatoes
    1 teaspoon crushed red pepper
       flakes
    1 teaspoon dried oregano
    Juice of 2 lemons
    Salt and black pepper to taste

Sauté the onions and garlic in the olive oil in a large saucepan over medium heat until the onions are tender. Add the chickpeas, spinach, tomatoes, pepper flakes, and oregano, cover and simmer for 30 minutes. Add the lemon juice, salt, and pepper.

Serves 8

♦ DEVILED BLACK BEANS ♦

The word "deviled" in recipes refers to the addition of mustard. Vegetarian cookbook author Mary Clifford says this recipe is "spicy, spicy, spicy." It also happens to be especially tasty and very easy to make.

    2 teaspoons olive or vegetable oil
    1 teaspoon chili oil or other spicy
       oil
    1 large red onion, thinly sliced
    1¾ cups vegetable stock (see
       page 324) or 1 14½-ounce can
       vegetable stock
    2 cans black beans, drained
    1 4-ounce can mild green chilies,
       diced
    2 teaspoons prepared mustard
    Salt and black pepper to taste
    1 tablespoon cornstarch

In a large, nonstick saucepan, heat the oils over medium heat. Add the onion and sauté until it is very well browned.

Set aside ¼ cup of the stock. Add the remaining stock, beans, chilies, mustard, and salt and pepper to the onion. Heat to boiling.

Stir the cornstarch into the reserved broth. Add the mixture to the beans and cook, stirring, until the sauce is clear and thickened, about 5 minutes. Serve over rice, barley, or other grains.

Serves 4

♦ CHILI WITH CHOCOLATE ♦

Although chocolate conjures up images of sweet desserts for most people, its deep, rich flavor works well in savory dishes as well. The chocolate bean is native to Mexico, and chili dishes there traditionally include a teaspoon or so of this ingredient. Make this chili a day ahead to give the flavors a chance to develop. Refrigerate overnight, and reheat. For a special treat, serve with pink onions.

        3 medium onions, coarsely
            chopped
        1 large green bell pepper, seeded
            and chopped
        2 tablespoons vegetable oil
        1 tablespoon whole mustard seeds
        1 tablespoon chili powder, or more
            to taste
        1 teaspoon whole cumin seeds
        1 teaspoon unsweetened cocoa
        $\frac{1}{4}$ teaspoon ground cinnamon
        1 16-ounce can crushed tomatoes
        2 16-ounce cans pinto or kidney
            beans, with liquid reserved
        1 6-ounce can tomato paste
        Salt to taste
        Pink onions (recipe follows)
        Chopped fresh tomatoes
        Chopped cucumbers
        Sliced green onions

In a large saucepan, sauté the onions and green pepper in the oil over medium heat until the onions are browned. Add the mustard seeds and cook, stirring, for 1 minute. Add the chili powder, cumin seeds, cocoa, cinnamon, tomatoes, beans with their liquid, and tomato paste. Simmer gently for about 40 minutes, uncovered and stirring frequently, until the chili is thick.

Season with salt and serve with pink onions, chopped fresh tomatoes, chopped cucumbers, and sliced green onions.

Serves 6

♦ PINK ONIONS ♦

        2 cups water
        2 tablespoons cider vinegar
        1 large red onion, thinly sliced
        1 tablespoon vegetable oil
        $\frac{1}{2}$ teaspoon whole mustard seeds
        $\frac{1}{4}$ teaspoon whole cumin seeds
        Salt to taste

Place the water and $1\frac{1}{2}$ tablespoons vinegar in a medium saucepan and bring them to a boil. Add the red onion. Return the mixture to a boil, then lower the heat and simmer, uncovered, for 2 to 3 minutes. Drain the onion and let it cool. In a bowl, stir together the onion, the remaining $1\frac{1}{2}$ teaspoons vinegar, vegetable oil, mustard seeds, cumin seeds, and salt. Refrigerate if not using right away but allow the onions to come to room temperature before serving.

◆ White Bean Salad ◆

Beans make beautiful salads. This is a nice one to serve at a picnic or for a light summer supper.

> 2 tablespoons herb-flavored white wine vinegar
> 2 tablespoons olive oil
> ½ teaspoon Dijon mustard
> 1 clove garlic, minced
> ¼ teaspoon dried oregano
> ¼ teaspoon dried basil
> Pinch of freshly grated nutmeg
> 1½ cups cooked navy or great northern beans
> 2 ripe tomatoes, chopped
> ½ red onion, thinly sliced

In a jar, shake together the vinegar, oil, mustard, garlic, oregano, basil, and nutmeg.

In a bowl, mix together the beans, tomatoes, and onion. Pour the dressing over the bean mixture and toss gently to mix. Serve at room temperature.

Serves 4

◆ Betsy's German Potato Salad ◆

Tempeh is a cultured soybean product with a rich, earthy flavor. In Indonesia, it is a dietary staple. Betsy Shipley, co-owner of Betsy's Tempeh Company, offers this tasty way to introduce tempeh to your menus.

> 6 medium potatoes
> 2 tablespoons nutritional yeast
> 2 tablespoons tamari
> 1 tablespoon water
> ½ teaspoon dry mustard
> 8 ounces tempeh, grated
> ½ cup chopped fresh parsley
> ¼ cup minced onions
> ½ cup minced celery
> ¼ cup chopped black olives
> ¼ cup chopped red bell pepper
> ¼ cup olive oil
> ¼ cup wine vinegar
> ¼ teaspoon black pepper

Boil the potatoes until tender, about 20 minutes. Drain and set them aside to cool.

In a small bowl, mix the nutritional yeast, tamari, water, and half of the mustard. Add the tempeh and mix well. Spread the mixture on a cookie sheet and broil until it is light brown, about 5 minutes. Remove the tempeh from the oven and set it aside.

Dice the potatoes into a large bowl. Add the parsley, onions, celery, olives, and red pepper.

In a jar with a tight-fitting lid, combine the oil, vinegar, remaining mustard, and pepper, and shake the jar well to combine. Pour the dressing over the potatoes. Add the tempeh to the potatoes, and toss to mix completely. Serve chilled.

Serves 8

◆ TOFU CORN PUFFS ◆

These light and airy croquettes make wonderful burgers.

½ cup cashews
½ cup water
½ pound tofu
2 tablespoons nutritional yeast
1 small onion, finely chopped
2 cups fresh or frozen defrosted
  corn kernels
¼ teaspoon dried basil
2 cups fresh whole wheat bread
  crumbs
Vegetable oil, for frying

Place the cashews and water in a blender and process until the cashews are completely pureed. Add the tofu and nutritional yeast and blend until all the ingredients are well mixed. Place the mixture in a bowl and stir in the onion, corn, basil, and bread crumbs.

Form the mixture into patties and brown them in a small amount of vegetable oil.

Makes 8 patties

◆ TOFU FRENCH FRIES WITH SPICY PEANUT SAUCE ◆

This dish is adapted from a recipe developed by Spring Creek Natural Foods, a West Virginia–based tofu company. It makes a fun hors d'oeuvre or supper.

2 pounds firm tofu
3 tablespoons vegetable oil
5 tablespoons smooth peanut
  butter
3 tablespoons brown sugar
4 tablespoons tamari
1 teaspoon cayenne pepper
1 teaspoon minced garlic
1 to 2 tablespoons water

Cut the tofu into pieces the size and shape of French fries. Brush the pieces lightly with the oil. Spread in 1 layer on a cookie sheet and place under the broiler. Broil on both sides for about 10 minutes until crispy and golden brown.

In a bowl, mix together the peanut butter, brown sugar, tamari, cayenne, and garlic. Add enough of the water to give the sauce a creamy consistency. Use as a sauce or a dip for the tofu French fries.

Serves 8 as entrée

◆ TOFU WITH SHIITAKE MUSHROOMS ◆

Treat yourself to tofu—the most traditional of Asian foods—in Mary Clifford's recipe, which brings together the best of Asian flavors. Shiitake mushrooms make this dish very special.

1 1.5-ounce package dried shiitake
   mushrooms
1½ cups warm water
1 tablespoon oil
1 small green bell pepper, thinly
   sliced
1 small red bell pepper, thinly sliced
1 green onion, sliced
1 pound firm tofu, sliced
2 tablespoons rice wine vinegar
   (or lemon juice)
¼ teaspoon red pepper flakes
⅛ teaspoon garlic powder
⅛ teaspoon ground ginger
Salt and black pepper to taste
3 tablespoons cornstarch, dissolved
   in ¼ cup teriyaki sauce

In a small bowl, combine the mushrooms and water. Set them aside for 30 minutes.

In a large, nonstick saucepan, heat the oil over medium heat. Add the peppers, green onion, and tofu. Sauté, stirring occasionally, until the peppers are brightly colored and the tofu is lightly browned, about 10 minutes.

Remove the stems from the mushrooms. Add the mushrooms, soaking liquid, and the vinegar, pepper flakes, garlic powder, ginger, salt, and pepper to the tofu. Heat the mixture to boiling.

Stir the cornstarch mixture into the tofu and reheat to boiling, stirring constantly until thickened. Serve over rice.

Serves 4

◆ CURRIED VEGETABLES ◆

This Indian dish takes a little extra time to make but is worth the effort.

5 cloves garlic, minced
2 cups chopped onions
3 tablespoons olive oil
2 tablespoons curry powder
1½ teaspoons turmeric
1 tablespoon ground coriander
1½ teaspoons mustard seeds
Pinch of cloves
Pinch of ground allspice
Pinch of cayenne pepper
1 16-ounce can chickpeas
1 cup sliced carrots
1 cup sliced green bell peppers
1 small head cauliflower, cut into
   florets
3 cups diced potatoes
1¼ cups water
4 cups diced zucchini
4 cups diced fresh tomatoes
2 cups low-sodium vegetable juice,
   such as V-8
¼ cup cider vinegar
2 tablespoons honey
2 tablespoons tamari or soy sauce
2 teaspoons fresh lemon juice
Black pepper to taste

In a 12-quart pot, sauté the garlic and onions in olive oil for 2 minutes. Add the spices and sauté for 30 seconds more. Add the chickpeas, carrots, green peppers, cauliflower, and potatoes and sauté for 30 seconds. Add the water and simmer for 5 minutes, or until all the water is evaporated. Add the remaining ingredients and stir. Cover and simmer for 15 minutes, until the vegetables are tender. Serve over white or brown rice.

Serves 12

♦ VEGETABLE CROQUETTES ♦

These patties are a super way to get a variety of vegetables into those who aren't vegetable lovers. Vary the vegetables to suit your own preferences. This is also a perfect way to use up vegetables that have hung around in the refrigerator just a few days past their prime.

1 pound broccoli, chopped
¼ pound green beans, chopped
2 carrots, chopped
1 onion, finely chopped
2 cloves garlic, minced
2 cups fresh bread crumbs (try sour-dough bread crumbs for an especially nice flavor)
¼ cup unbleached flour
2 tablespoons soymilk
1 teaspoon dried basil
Salt and black pepper to taste
2 tablespoons vegetable oil

Steam the broccoli, green beans, and carrots until tender. Place the steamed vegetables in a food processor with the onion and garlic and puree. Transfer the mixture to a bowl. Mix in the bread crumbs and flour. Stir in the soymilk and basil, and season with salt and pepper. Refrigerate the mixture for at least an hour.

Form the mixture into patties. Heat the oil in a large frying pan and sauté the patties on each side until they are browned. Drain them on paper towels and serve with salsa or ketchup.

Makes 8 patties

♦ OVEN-ROASTED VEGETABLES ♦

These vegetables are pretty arranged on a large platter and garnished with sprigs of fresh rosemary. They make a beautiful edible centerpiece for a dinner party or buffet.

3 medium red-skinned potatoes
2 carrots, thinly sliced
1 small eggplant, peeled and cut into ½-inch chunks
2 medium zucchini, cut into ½-inch chunks
1 red onion, thinly sliced
¼ cup olive oil
2 cloves garlic, minced
1½ tablespoons chopped rosemary leaves
Salt and black pepper to taste

Wash the potatoes and place them in a medium pot. Cover them with water and simmer until the potatoes are just tender, about 30 minutes. Cut them into ½-inch cubes.

Preheat the oven to 450° F. Place all the vegetables in a bowl and toss them with the olive oil, garlic, and rosemary. Add salt and pepper. Spread the vegetables in a single layer on a cookie sheet, and roast them in the oven for 20 minutes, or until almost tender. Turn on the broiler and broil for 1 to 2 minutes, until the edges of vegetables are brown.

Serves 6

♦ POTATO AND SPINACH PUREE ♦

Potatoes are a great way to subdue the strong flavor of spinach for children. You can also use any other leafy green vegetable in this recipe, such as turnip greens, kale, or collards.

> 4 large potatoes
> 2 cloves garlic, minced
> 2 teaspoons olive oil
> 1 pound fresh spinach or other leafy greens, or 1 10-ounce package frozen, defrosted and drained

Wash and peel the potatoes. Cut them into large chunks and simmer them in salted water until they are very tender, about 20 minutes. Drain the potatoes and set them aside.

In a large skillet, sauté the garlic in the olive oil for 2 minutes. Add the spinach and sauté until it is completely wilted and tender. Place the spinach and the potatoes in a food processor and blend to mix and puree completely. Serve immediately, or preheat the oven to 400° F., place mounds of the puree on a cookie sheet (use an ice-cream scoop), and bake for a few minutes until the tops are browned.

Serves 8

♦ CRUNCHY GREEN BEANS ♦

Give this favorite vegetable some pizzazz with the addition of crunchy almonds and water chestnuts.

> 1 pound green beans
> 2 teaspoons margarine, melted
> ¼ cup slivered toasted almonds
> ¼ cup sliced water chestnuts
> Salt and black pepper to taste

Steam the green beans until they are just tender. Toss them with the margarine, almonds, water chestnuts, salt, and pepper.

Serves 6

◆ SUNSHINE CARROTS ◆

Carrots are a favorite with children, especially when you include a touch of something sweet in their preparation.

>   5 medium carrots
>   1 tablespoon sugar
>   1 teaspoon cornstarch
>   ¼ teaspoon ground ginger
>   ¼ teaspoon salt
>   ¼ cup orange juice
>   2 tablespoons margarine

Cut the carrots on the bias in 1-inch chunks. Cook, covered in boiling salted water, until just tender, about 20 minutes, and drain.

In a saucepan, mix the sugar, cornstarch, ginger, and salt. Add the juice. Cook over low heat, stirring until the mixture is thick and bubbly. Boil 1 minute, then stir in the margarine. Toss with the carrots.

Serves 4

◆ SPICY COLLARDS ◆

In their native Africa, collards are often flavored with some type of hot red pepper. Here, we've added a touch of cayenne and ginger.

>   1 pound fresh collards, rinsed and
>   cut into strips
>   2 cups vegetable stock
>   (see page 324)
>   ¾ cup chopped onions
>   1 clove garlic, minced
>   1 tablespoon olive oil
>   1 tablespoon freshly grated ginger
>   ¼ teaspoon cayenne pepper, or
>   more to taste
>   **Salt and black pepper to taste**

Place the collards and stock in a large saucepan and simmer for 30 minutes, until the collards are completely tender.

In a large skillet, sauté the onions and garlic in the olive oil until the onions are transparent. Add the ginger and cayenne and stir for 1 minute. Add the collards and the stock and simmer until most of the liquid has evaporated, about 15 minutes. Season with salt and pepper.

Serves 4

◆ CREAMED GREENS ◆

This is a simple way to lighten the flavor of some of the stronger-tasting greens. Serve it as a side dish or spoon it over rice or baked potatoes for a main course.

> 1½ pounds turnip greens, mustard greens, kale, or collards
> 2 cups Low-Fat White Sauce (see page 340)
> Salt and black pepper to taste

Rinse the greens and tear them into bite-sized pieces. Drop them into simmering water and simmer until tender, about 10 to 15 minutes. Drain and squeeze out any excess water. Mix the white sauce into the greens and season with salt and pepper.

Serves 4

◆ KALE WITH CINNAMON ◆

A hint of cinnamon gives kale an unusual and appealing flavor.

> 1 medium onion, minced
> 1 tablespoon vegetable oil
> 1 clove garlic, minced
> ⅛ teaspoon ground cinnamon
> 1 pound fresh kale, finely chopped
> 1 cup vegetable stock (see page 324)
> 1 teaspoon red wine vinegar
> Salt and black pepper to taste
> Chopped fresh chives

Sauté the onion in the oil for 5 minutes. Add the garlic and cook for an additional 2 minutes. Stir in the cinnamon and add the kale, tossing it to coat with the onion and cinnamon mixture. Add the vegetable stock. Cover and simmer for 15 minutes. Season with vinegar, salt and pepper, and chopped fresh chives.

Serves 4

♦ SAUTEED BROCCOLI WITH GINGER ♦

A simple but traditional Asian stir-fry with the savory flavors of garlic and fresh ginger.

1 clove garlic, minced
½-inch piece fresh gingerroot, peeled and grated
2 teaspoons vegetable oil
1 pound broccoli, cut into florets
1 medium leek, sliced thin (white part only)
2 tablespoons vegetable stock (see page 324)
1 teaspoon tamari

Sauté the garlic and ginger in the oil in a large skillet for 1 minute. Add the broccoli, leek, and stock. Toss together all the ingredients to mix well. Cover the pan and cook for 3 minutes. Remove the cover and continue to sauté, stirring frequently, until the vegetables are just tender, about 10 minutes. Mix in the tamari and serve immediately.

Serves 4

♦ ROASTED PLANTAINS ♦

These large, starchy fruits resemble bananas. When cooked (they can't be eaten raw), they are mildly sweet and may remind you of winter squash. Mary Clifford suggests this especially tasty way to prepare them.

3 large plantains, peeled and cut into chunks
2 large carrots, cut into chunks
1 medium onion, sliced
4 teaspoons olive oil
Salt and black pepper to taste

Preheat the oven to 425° F.

In a large bowl, combine all the ingredients. Transfer them to a greased baking sheet or pan, cover loosely with aluminum foil, and bake the vegetables for 20 minutes. Uncover and bake for 10 to 15 minutes longer, or until the plantains are tender.

Serves 6

Sauces and Dressings

♦ Eggless Mayonnaise ♦

There are commercial eggless mayonnaise products available, but you can also make your own. For the smoothest texture, be sure to use silken tofu.

1 10½-ounce package soft silken tofu
1 tablespoon white vinegar
1 tablespoon fresh lemon juice
½ teaspoon Dijon mustard
1 tablespoon vegetable oil
Pinch of salt

Combine all the ingredients in a blender or food processor and blend until smooth. Refrigerate overnight to allow the flavors to develop. This mayonnaise will keep for up to 2 weeks.

Makes 1¼ cups

♦ Ranch Salad Dressing ♦

Here is a dairy- and egg-free ranch dressing that is quite a bit lower in fat than commercial brands but is still a rich and creamy topping for salads.

1 cup eggless mayonnaise (see preceding recipe)
1 cup plain soymilk
1 tablespoon white vinegar
2 tablespoons finely chopped green onions
¼ teaspoon onion powder
2 teaspoons minced fresh parsley
1 clove garlic, minced
¼ teaspoon paprika
¼ teaspoon salt
¼ teaspoon black pepper
⅛ teaspoon cayenne pepper

Place all the ingredients in a jar with a tight-fitting lid, and shake well to blend.

Makes 2 cups

◆ LOW-FAT WHITE SAUCE ◆

This white sauce is rich and creamy. Serve it over vegetables or blend it with cooked, pureed vegetables to make a savory cream soup or a sauce for grains.

> 1 tablespoon margarine
> 2 tablespoons white flour
> 1 cup plain low-fat soymilk
> Salt and white pepper to taste
> Freshly grated nutmeg

Melt the margarine in a saucepan over low heat. Stir in the flour to make a thick paste, and cook, stirring rapidly, for 1 minute. Pour in the soymilk very slowly, stirring to avoid lumps. Cook and stir with a wooden spoon over low heat for several minutes until the sauce is thick. Season with salt, pepper, and nutmeg.

Makes 1 cup

◆ MUSHROOM GRAVY ◆

This gravy is brimming with sliced mushrooms and tastes wonderful over grains, mashed potatoes, or vegetables.

> 1 cup fresh mushrooms, sliced
> 4 teaspoons olive oil
> 2 tablespoons flour
> 1 cup vegetable stock
>   (see page 324)
> 2 teaspoons vegetarian
>   Worcestershire sauce
> ½ teaspoon dried oregano
> ½ teaspoon dried tarragon

Sauté the mushrooms in 2 teaspoons of the olive oil and set them aside.

In a separate pan, stir the flour into the remaining 2 teaspoons olive oil, and stir over low heat for 1 minute. Slowly add the stock, stirring constantly to avoid lumps. Bring to a boil, stirring constantly.

Remove the gravy from the heat and add the Worcestershire sauce and herbs. Add the sautéed mushrooms.

Makes 1½ cups

SANDWICHES AND SPREADS

Many of these spreads can double as perfect dips for parties.

♦ NOTUNA ♦

This chickpea salad has a texture and taste that is reminiscent of tuna salad. Kelp powder, a sea vegetable, gives this dish a subtle tunalike flavor.

> **4 cups cooked chickpeas, or**
>   **2 16-ounce cans chickpeas,**
>   **well drained**
> **½ cup coarsely chopped celery**
> **½ cup finely chopped onions**
> **2 tablespoons fresh lemon juice**
> **½ cup eggless mayonnaise**
>   **(see page 339)**
> **1 tablespoon dried powdered kelp**
> **Salt and black pepper to taste**

Place the chickpeas in a food processor and process until coarsely chopped. Transfer them to a bowl. Add the rest of the ingredients and mix. Serve stuffed into pita pockets with chopped tomatoes and lettuce.

Makes enough for 6 sandwiches

♦ PEANUT BUTTER–BANANA SPREAD ♦

Here is another reduced-fat peanut-butter spread with a touch of natural sweetness.

> **¼ cup peanut butter**
> **1 large ripe banana**

Place the peanut butter and banana in a blender or food processor and blend until creamy and combined. Serve on crackers or in a sandwich with fruit spread.

Makes 3 sandwiches

◆ HUMMUS ◆

Hummus is a popular dip for parties, usually served with pita wedges. But stuffed into a pita pocket—or spread on whole-grain bread—along with lettuce and sliced tomatoes and cucumbers, it is a wonderful sandwich. You can reduce the tahini in this recipe if you want to reduce the fat content.

2 16-ounce cans chickpeas, drained
¼ cup minced green onions
3 medium cloves garlic, minced
¼ cup finely minced fresh parsley
1½ teaspoons salt
Black pepper to taste
Pinch of cayenne pepper
½ cup tahini
Juice of 2 medium lemons
Dash of tamari or soy sauce

Blend the chickpeas to a thick paste in a food processor. Combine them with the rest of the ingredients and chill thoroughly.

Makes 4½ cups

◆ WHITE-BEAN SPREAD WITH LEMON AND GARLIC ◆

Here is a simple spread made from white beans. This recipe can lead a double life as a sandwich stuffer and a dip.

3 cups cooked navy or cannellini beans
1 tablespoon olive oil
Zest of 1 lemon, grated
Juice of 1 lemon
2 or 3 cloves garlic, minced
Pinch of cayenne pepper
Salt to taste
3 tablespoons chopped chives

In a food processor, process all the ingredients except the chives until completely smooth. Transfer the mixture to a small bowl and mix in the chives.

Makes enough for 6 sandwiches

◆ MISSING-EGG SALAD ◆

Here is a lovely sandwich filling that is somewhat reminiscent of egg salad. Pile it onto whole wheat bread with a sliced tomato and lettuce, or stuff it into a pita pocket.

> 1 pound firm tofu
> 1 tablespoon finely chopped onions
> ¼ cup finely chopped celery
> ¼ cup eggless mayonnaise
>   (see page 339)
> 1 tablespoon dried parsley
> ¼ teaspoon dried dill
> Salt and black pepper to taste
> 1 tablespoon sweet pickle relish
> 1 teaspoon prepared mustard

Cut the tofu into 4 slices and press each one firmly between paper towels to remove excess water. Then mash the tofu coarsely with a fork. Stir in the onions and celery.

Combine the remaining ingredients in a separate bowl and mix into the tofu.

Makes 4 sandwiches

DESSERTS

◆ CHOCOLATE CHIP CAKE ◆

This cake is so easy to make and is always popular. Most of the chocolate chips sink to the bottom, where they form a fudgy layer.

> 1½ cups white flour
> 1 cup sugar
> 1 teaspoon baking soda
> ⅛ teaspoon salt
> 5 tablespoons vegetable oil
> 1 teaspoon vanilla extract
> 1 tablespoon cider vinegar
> 1 cup cold water
> 1 cup semisweet chocolate chips

Preheat the oven to 350° F.

In a large mixing bowl, stir together the flour, sugar, baking soda, and salt. In a separate bowl, stir together the oil, vanilla, vinegar and water. Mix and pour the liquid over the dry ingredients. Stir well to combine.

Pour the batter into an ungreased 8-by-8-inch pan. Sprinkle the chocolate chips over the top. Bake for 35 minutes.

Serves 16

◆ CHOCOLATE CREAM FROSTING ◆

This is an old-fashioned frosting that is easy to make and that turns any cake into a delectable treat.

1¼ cups powdered sugar
2 tablespoons unsweetened cocoa
2 tablespoons margarine, softened
Pinch of salt
2 tablespoons plain or vanilla soymilk
1 teaspoon vanilla extract

Cream together the sugar, cocoa, margarine, and salt. Add the soymilk and vanilla to make a creamy, spreadable consistency.

Makes enough to frost an 8″ × 8″ cake

◆ QUICK WHITE FROSTING ◆

Here is a frosting with endless possibilities. For something different, omit the vanilla and instead add 2 tablespoons of lemon or orange juice or a few tablespoons of apricot-flavored liqueur, and use slightly less soymilk.

4 tablespoons margarine, softened
2 cups sifted powdered sugar
¼ teaspoon salt
1 teaspoon vanilla extract
3 to 4 tablespoons plain soymilk

Cream the margarine and powdered sugar together. Add the salt, vanilla, and soymilk, and mix until completely smooth. Add more powdered sugar or more soymilk to get the consistency you want.

Makes about 1 cup

♦ OATMEAL-BANANA COOKIES ♦

The nutritious goodness of rolled oats and bananas makes these old-fashioned cookies a great choice when you want a sweet snack.

½ cup soy margarine, at room temperature
1 cup firmly packed brown sugar
¼ cup water
1 teaspoon vanilla extract
1 ripe banana, well mashed
½ cup sifted all-purpose flour
½ cup whole wheat flour
1 teaspoon salt
½ teaspoon baking soda
3 cups old-fashioned rolled oats
½ cup walnuts (optional)

Preheat the oven to 350° F.

In a large mixing bowl, cream together the margarine, sugar, water, vanilla, and banana.

In a separate bowl, sift together the flours, salt, and soda. Add the dry ingredients to the creamed mixture and blend well. Stir in the oats, and fold in the walnuts, if using. Drop by teaspoonfuls onto greased cookie sheets, and bake for 12 to 15 minutes.

Makes 3 dozen

♦ PEANUT BUTTER BALLS ♦

Wrap these in wax paper and tuck them into your backpack when you go hiking or camping. They are a high-energy treat and a perfect pick-me-up after strenuous activities.

¼ cup low-fat granola
2 tablespoons brown sugar
¼ cup sunflower seeds
¼ cup raisins
¼ cup finely shredded carrots
¾ cup peanut butter

Mix together the granola, brown sugar, sunflower seeds, raisins, and carrots. Blend in the peanut butter a little at a time to form a smooth mixture. Store the mixture in the refrigerator overnight. Form into balls.

Makes 20 balls

NATIONAL ORGANIZATIONS FOR VEGETARIAN INFORMATION

American Vegan Society, 501 Old Harding Hwy., Malaga, NJ 08328; (609) 694-2887

North American Vegetarian Society, P.O. Box 72, Dolgeville, NY 13329; (518) 568-7970

Physicians Committee for Responsible Medicine, P.O. Box 6322, Washington, DC 20015; (202) 686-2210

Vegetarian Education Network (VE-Net), P.O. Box 3347, West Chester, PA 19381; (717) 529-8638 (promotes the vegetarian perspective in schools and supports young vegetarians)

Vegetarian Nutrition Dietetic Practice Group, c/o American Dietetic Association, 216 W. Jackson Blvd., Suite 800, Chicago, IL 60606-6995; (800) 366-1655

Vegetarian Resource Center, P.O. Box 38-1068, Cambridge, MA 02238-1068; (617) 625-3790

Vegetarian Resource Group, P.O. Box 1463, Baltimore, MD 21203; (410) 366-8343

Vegetarian Society, Inc., P.O. Box 34427, Los Angeles, CA 90034; (310) 281-1907

You can find nutrition counselors by calling the American Dietetic Association's referral service at (800) 877-1600 and asking for a dietitian who specializes in vegetarian nutrition. You can also look for nutritionists in the yellow pages under "Nutrition," "Dietitian," or "Weight Loss." (Even if you don't need to lose weight, this is a good place to find nutritionists.)

COOKBOOKS

There are scores of wonderful cookbooks on vegetarian cooking, and it is difficult to narrow the list down to the twenty or so best ones. We've tried to put together a list that represents different types of cooking for different cooks. The list includes some very basic guides to vegetarian cooking that are great for beginners, as well as a few "specialty" books, and also several books for those who truly enjoy cooking— whether they are new to vegetarianism or not. Among these are our own personal favorites and some that are recommended by the best vegetarian cooks we know.

Elliot, Rose. *The Complete Vegetarian Cuisine*. New York: Pantheon Books, 1988.
> This incredibly beautiful book has color photographs and descriptions of the foods used in vegetarian cooking. The recipes are wonderful for holidays and other special occasions, though they tend to be a bit high in fat for everyday. Many recipes contain eggs or cheese.

Gelles, Carol. *The Complete Whole Grains Cookbook*. New York: Donald Fine, 1989.
> Extensive information is presented about whole grains and their preparation. These basic recipes will help you eat a more grain-centered diet. A few recipes are lacto-ovo.

Goldbeck, Nikki and David. *American Wholefoods Cuisine*. New York: New American Library, 1983.
> The huge collection of recipes here—more than 1,200 of them—covers the whole spectrum of basic vegetarian cooking. Although the approach is lacto-ovo, many recipes are free of animal products. This book is an excellent resource for any vegetarian.

Hagler, Louise, ed. *The Farm Vegetarian Cookbook*. Summertown, Tenn.: Book Publishing Co., 1978.
> Another vegetarian classic and an excellent book for new vegetarians, the book celebrates the cuisine of the best-known vegetarian community in the United States—the Farm, in Summertown, Tennessee. These are home-style recipes with an emphasis on soy products. Included are excellent instructions for making soymilk, tofu, tempeh, and other products. All recipes are vegan.

Madison, Deborah. *The Savory Way*. New York: Bantam, 1990.
> These recipes are slightly more complicated, for wonderful sophisticated vegetarian cuisine.

Moosewood Collective. *Moosewood Restaurant Cooks at Home*. New York: Simon and Schuster, 1994.
> From the renowned restaurant in Ithaca, New

York, that gave us *Moosewood Cookbook* and *Enchanted Broccoli Forest Cookbook*, this new collection of interesting and appealing recipes emphasizes ease of preparation. This is a lacto-ovo cookbook, but there are many vegan choices.

People for the Ethical Treatment of Animals. *The Compassionate Cook*. New York: Warner Books, 1993.

The fun collection of vegan recipes, all very easy to prepare, includes contributions by some of PETA's better-known supporters, such as Linda McCartney and Rue McClanahan.

Robertson, Laurel, Carol Flinders, and Brian Ruppenthal. *The New Laurel's Kitchen*. Berkeley, Calif.: Ten Speed Press, 1986.

This updated, lower-fat version of the original vegetarian classic published in 1976 is a basic guide that relies somewhat heavily on dairy products. But there are plenty of good vegan recipes and excellent information on vegetarian cookery and nutrition. This is a wonderful first cookbook for a new vegetarian.

Sass, Lorna. *Recipes from an Ecological Kitchen*. New York: William Morrow, 1992.

This is our personal recommendation for the best vegetarian cookbook. Every recipe is a winner, and all are vegan. The book includes good instructions for preparing what may be unfamiliar foods to many new vegetarians, and it has a comprehensive glossary of vegan foods. Lorna's specialty is cooking with a pressure cooker, as well as every recipe includes pressure-cooker and standard stove-top instructions. An excellent choice for both new and seasoned vegetarian cooks, this cookbook is also available in soft cover under the title *Lorna Sass' Complete Vegetarian Kitchen* (Hearst Books, 1995).

Wasserman, Debra, and Reed Mangels. *Simply Vegan*. Baltimore, Md.: Vegetarian Resource Group, 1991.

A simple, honest guide to vegan cookery and nutrition, this book will allay all your fears about cooking if you are new to the vegetarian kitchen—or to any kitchen. The recipes have short lists of ingredients and fast and easy instructions. Most of them are quite low in fat. The nutrition section, written by vegetarian dietitian Dr. Reed Mangels, is a clear, concise, well-researched guide to healthy vegan diets.

Seventh-day Adventist Cookbooks

The Seventh-day Adventist church has been producing vegetarian cookbooks for many decades. These are valuable guides to a type of family-style cooking that includes no animal products and that has been perfected over many years of home-style cooking and community cooking demonstrations. A few of these books have become, or are destined to become, classics. The following are the most popular.

Fleming, Diana J., ed. *Country Life*. Sunfield, Mich.: Family Health Publications, 1990.

The recipes are vegan and easy to prepare in this collection from the Country Life chain of Seventh-day Adventist restaurants, including those in France, Korea, and Japan.

Hurd, Frank J. and Rosalie. *Ten Talents*. Collegedale, Tenn.: The College Press.

This pioneering vegan cookbook boasts more than 750 recipes and has sold more than 250,000 copies since its original publication in 1968. This may be the classic Seventh-day Adventist cookbook. These are family-style, vegan recipes.

Specialty Cookbooks

Belsinger, Susan. *Flowers in the Kitchen*. Loveland, Colo.: Interweave Press, 1991.

This book on how to grow and cook with edible flowers is a feast for the eyes as well as the palate. Nearly all the recipes are vegetarian, and the photographs are stunning.

Devi, Yamuna. *The Art of Indian Vegetarian Cooking*. New York: E. P. Dutton, 1987.

A true classic of Indian cooking, this book is the first vegetarian cookbook ever to win the Cordon Bleu's cherished Cookbook of the Year Award. It contains more than five hundred recipes and volumes of information about Indian cooking. Some recipes use dairy products.

Jaffrey, Madhur. *World of the East Vegetarian Cooking*. New York: Knopf, 1981.

This wonderful selection of more than four hundred recipes from the kitchens of India, Bali, Japan, China, and the Middle East is a perfect introduction to vegetarian cooking in other cultures. Many recipes are vegan.

Kushi, Aveline, and Wendy Esko. *Aveline Kushi's Introducing Macrobiotic Cooking*. New York: Japan Publications, 1987.

Two of the best-known macrobiotic cooks present recipes for a macrobiotic diet for those who are new to this way of eating.

Sass, Lorna. *Great Vegetarian Cooking under Pressure*. New York: William Morrow, 1994.

For those who want wonderful vegan food in a jiffy, these recipes—all vegan—are for the pressure cooker.

Shurtleff, William, and Akiko Aoyagi. *The Book of Tofu*. New York: Ballantine, 1988.

This is *the* book on tofu for those who long to know everything there is to know about this wonderful, versatile, ancient food. A true classic, written by the tofu experts, it is packed with helpful and interesting information and recipes.

Stepaniak, Joanne. *The Uncheese Cookbook*. Summertown, Tenn.: Book Publishing Co., 1994.

A wonderful little cookbook for those who shun dairy but miss all those cheesy dishes. Stepaniak works magic with beans, nuts, and various condiments to come up with a whole variety of cheeselike dishes. You won't find fine Brie or Gouda here, just real down-home Cheez Whiz–type fare.

Wasserman, Debra. *The Lowfat Jewish Vegetarian Cookbook*. Baltimore, Md.: Vegetarian Resource Group, 1994.

This book celebrates a cultural cooking tradition that ranges from the most basic home-style dishes to truly festive offerings. It offers low-fat, vegan versions of traditional favorites.

Especially for Low-Fat Cooks

Carroll, Mary, with Hal Straus. *The No-Cholesterol (No Kidding!) Cookbook*. Emmaus, Pa.: Rodale Press, 1991.

Mary Carroll created the recipes used by Dr. Dean Ornish in his study on reversing heart disease. This is an excellent collection of low-fat, no-cholesterol vegan recipes for both beginning and seasoned cooks.

Havala, Suzanne, with recipes by Mary Clifford. *Simple, Low-Fat and Vegetarian*. Baltimore, Md.: Vegetarian Resource Group, 1994.

This guide describes simple changes you can make to cut the fat from your vegetarian diet no matter where you dine—in a restaurant, at an amusement park, on a cruise ship, or at the movies. It includes recipe makeovers to show you how to reduce the fat in your own favorite dishes.

Ornish, Dean. *Eat More, Weigh Less*. New York: HarperCollins, 1993.

This is actually a cookbook preceded by a short discussion of diet and weight control. The emphasis takes you away from the old deprivation approach to dieting and teaches readers how to lose weight while feasting on wonderful low-fat cuisine. Recipes are all vegetarian (some nonfat dairy is used) and were developed by some of the world's best chefs. Many tend to be a bit time-consuming and will appeal most to those who enjoy cooking.

GENERAL VEGETARIAN NUTRITION INFORMATION

Barnard, Neal. *Food for Life*. New York: Harmony Books, 1993.

Dr. Barnard presents evidence for a vegan diet as the optimal eating plan that will dramatically decrease the risk for cancer, heart disease, and other chronic, life-threatening conditions. A twenty-one-day plan to help you adopt a vegan diet and recipes by renowned vegetarian cook Jennifer Raymond make this a comprehensive guide for adults who want practical advice on how to change their diet.

Craig, Winston. *Eating for the Health of It*. Eau Claire, Mich.: Golden Harvest Books, 1993.

We highly recommend this book, which contains sound, reliable vegetarian nutrition information written by a nutrition professor at Andrews University, a Seventh-Day Adventist school. It presents a good overview of nutrition issues and practical advice on meeting nutrient needs on a plant-based diet. A special section on the healing properties of herbs is included.

Klaper, Michael. *Vegan Nutrition: Pure and Simple*. Umatillo, Fla.: Gentle World, 1987.

This easy-to-read guide to planning healthy vegan diets includes guidelines for meal planning, sample menus, and recipes, as well as information on nutrients and vegetarian foods.

Langley, Gil. *Vegan Nutrition: A Survey of Research.* Oxford, Engl.: Vegan Society, Ltd., 1988.

This comprehensive survey presents scientific research supporting the safety of vegan diets for all age groups.

Wasserman, Debra, and Reed Mangels. *Simply Vegan.* Baltimore, Md.: Vegetarian Resource Group, 1991.

We noted this book in our list of recommended cookbooks, but the nutrition section, written by vegetarian nutritionist Dr. Reed Mangels, deserves a separate mention. This is a brief overview of nutrition issues that are especially relevant to vegans. New vegetarians especially will find the information useful.

RATIONALE FOR A VEGETARIAN DIET

Akers, Keith. *A Vegetarian Sourcebook.* Denver, Colo.: Vegetarian Press, 1989.

This book makes the argument for a vegetarian diet from health, ethical, and environmental perspectives and includes an interesting discussion of vegetarianism in the context of the world's major religions.

Lappé, Frances Moore. *Diet for a Small Planet.* New York: Bantam Books, 1982.

Be sure to read the tenth-anniversary edition of this classic book, which corrects some earlier misconceptions. Lappé explores the relationship between food production and use of the earth's resources in this very important work.

Mason, Jim, and Peter Singer. *Animal Factories.* New York: Crown Books, 1980.

This in-depth look at the mass production of animals for food tells how this affects the lives of consumers, farmers, and the animals themselves.

Moran, Victoria. *Compassion: The Ultimate Ethic.* Malaga, N.J.: The American Vegan Society, 1991.

Vegan philosophy, diet, and lifestyle are explored, along with the historical background to vegetarianism and veganism in daily life.

Robbins, John. *Diet for a New America.* Walpole, N.H.: Stillpoint, 1987.

Written by the heir to the Baskin-Robbins ice-cream fortune, this comprehensive book explores the effects of an animal-based diet on animals, the environment, and human health. Along the way, it exposes the impact of the powerful food and agricultural industries on what you eat.

ESPECIALLY FOR YOUNG PEOPLE

Gordon, Jay, with Antonia Barnes Boyle. *Good Food Today, Great Kids Tomorrow.* Studio City, Calif.: Michael Wiese Productions, 1994.

Dr. Gordon is a sort of "pediatrician to the stars," and his patients include the offspring of many Hollywood celebrities. In this book, he gives sound nutrition advice that favors a vegan eating plan and that is presented in a pleasant question-and-answer format. The book includes a series of transition menus (including recipes) that do include small amounts of nonfat dairy foods; they are especially valuable to families who are working toward a vegan diet in a gradual fashion. Despite the use of some dairy, a few menus need to be supplemented with additional calcium-rich foods.

Krizmanic, Judy. *A Teen's Guide to Going Vegetarian.* New York: Viking Children's Books, 1994.

We think every vegetarian teenager should have a copy of this book. It is written specifically for teens and explores the reasons for choosing vegetarianism, then sets young people on the right track toward planning healthy vegetarian diets.

How on Earth! P.O. Box 3347, West Chester, PA 19381

This periodical, published four times a year, on vegetarianism, ecology, and animal rights is written by and for teenagers.

VEGETARIAN RESTAURANT GUIDE

Vegetarian Resource Group. *Vegetarian Journal's Guide to Natural Foods Restaurants in the U.S. and Canada.* Garden City Park, N.Y.: Avery Publishing Group, 1993.

VEGETARIAN MAGAZINES

Vegetarian Gourmet, P.O. Box 7641, Riverton, NJ 08077-7641 (quarterly)

Vegetarian Journal, P.O. Box 1463, Baltimore, MD 21203 (bi-monthly)

Vegetarian Times, P.O. Box 446, Mount Morris, IL 61054 (monthly)

Vegetarian Voice, P.O. 72, Dolgeville, NY 13329

Veggie Life, P.O. Box 57159, Boulder, CO 80323 (quarterly)

ANIMAL RIGHTS/WELFARE ORGANIZATIONS AND PUBLICATIONS

Animal's Agenda, P.O. 25881, Baltimore, MD 21224; (410) 675-4566

This bimonthly magazine features news of the animal rights movement and information on cruelty-free living.

Farm Sanctuary, P.O. Box 150, Watkins Glen, NY 14891, (607) 583-2225

Humane Society of the United States, 2100 L Street, NW, Washington, DC 20037, (202) 452-1100

People for the Ethical Treatment of Animals, P.O. Box 42516, Washington, DC 20015, (202) 726-0156

VEGETARIAN QUANTITY RECIPES

Two organizations that provide quantity vegetarian recipes for use in school cafeterias are the Vegetarian Resource Group and the Physicians Committee for Responsible Medicine. See addresses under "National Organizations Providing Vegetarian Information" at the beginning of this resource section.

VEGETARIAN MATERIALS

Mediterranean Food Pyramid, Oldways Preservation and Exchange Trust, 45 Milk St., Boston, MA 02109, (617) 695-2300

The New Four Food Groups Poster (vegan food guide), Physicians Committee for Responsible Medicine, 5100 Wisconsin Ave, NW, Washington, DC 20016, (202) 686-2210

The Vegetarian Food Pyramid, Health Connection, 55 West Oak Ridge Dr., Hagerstown, MD 21740, (800) 543-8700

Single copies are $1.50 each, or $2.00 for a laminated copy. Posters are $5.95 each, plus $3.50 postage. Bulk prices are available.

ONLINE SERVICES

Each of the online services (American Online, Prodigy, CompuServe, etc.) offers bulletin boards especially for people with interest in a vegetarian diet. Those who have access to the Internet mailing lists can also subscribe to the following vegetarian mailing lists:

VEGAN-L
> To subscribe, address mail to listserv@templevm.bitnet. Your message should read: sub vegan-l <your first and last name> set vegan-l digest.

VEG-COOK
> To subscribe, address mail to: listserv@netcom.com. Your message should read: SUBSCRIBE veg-cook.

VEGGIE
> To subscribe, address mail to veggie-request-@maths.bath.ac.uk. Your message should contain a brief request to subscribe to the mailing list.

VEGLIFE
> To subscribe, address mail to listserv@vtvm1.bitnet. Your message should read: sub veglife<your first and last name> set veglife digest.

MAIL-ORDER VEGETARIAN FOODS

Dixie Diner's Club, P.O. Box 55549, Houston, TX 77255-5549, (713) 688-4993
> The emphasis is on low-fat cookery, with flavored TVP products, condiments, and kitchen gadgets.

Harvest Direct, P.O. Box 4514, Decatur, IL 62525-4514, (800) 835-2867
> This company offers many flavors of TVP, burger mixes, pasta and sauces, soymilk, and cookbooks.

The Mail Order Catalogue, P.O. Box 180, Summertown, TN 38483, (800) 695-2241
> The catalog features nutritional yeast, gluten, tempeh starter, TVP, other food products, and many, many vegetarian books.

REFERENCES

CHAPTER 1. VEGETARIANISM THROUGH THE AGES

1. Bible, Revised Standard Version, Genesis 1:29.
2. S. B. Eaton and M. Shostak, "Fat Tooth Blues," *Natural History*, 95:6–14 (1986).
3. P. Shipman, "The Ancestor That Wasn't," *The Sciences*, 42–48 (1985).
4. S. B. Eaton and D. A. Nelson, "Calcium in Evolutionary Perspective," *Am J Clin Nutr* 54:281S–87S (1991).
5. S. B. Eaton and M. Konner, "Paleolithic Nutrition: A Consideration of Its Nature and Current Implications," *New Engl J Med* 312:283–89 (1985).
6. Shipman, "Ancestor That Wasn't."
7. Eaton and Konner, "Paleolithic Nutrition."
8. R. A. Tannahill, *Food in History* (New York: Stein and Day, 1973).
9. D. A. Roe, "History of Promotion of Vegetable Cereal Diets," *J Nutr* 116:1355–63 (1986).
10. A. Cocchi, *The Pythagorean Diet of Vegetables Only Conducive to the Preservation of Health and the Cure of Disease* (1745).
11. Roe, "History of Promotion."
12. J. Myerson, D. Shealy, and M. B. Stern, eds., *The Journals of Louisa May Alcott* (Boston: Little, Brown, 1989).
13. B. Unti, "The Bible Christians and the Origins of Vegetarianism in North America" (unpublished paper).
14. J. C. Whorton, "Historical Development of Vegetarianism," *Am J Clin Nutr* 59:1103S–9S (1994).
15. Unti, "Bible Christians."
16. E. G. White, *Counsels on Diet and Foods: A Compilation from the Writings of Ellen G. White* (Hagerstown, Md.: Review and Herald Publishing Association, 1938).
17. W. Shurtleff and A. Aoyagi, *History of Soybeans and Soyfoods* (Lafayette, Calif.: Soyfoods Center, forthcoming).
18. Whorton, "Historical Development."
19. Ibid.
20. Shurtleff and Aoyagi, *History of Soybeans.*
21. A. South, "Dr. John Harvey Kellogg: Ideas of a Vegetarian Diet 100 Years Ago," *Vegetarian Journal* 10:14–15 (1991).
22. Unti, "Bible Christians."
23. M. G. Hardinge and H. Crooks, "Non-flesh Dietaries," *J Am Diet Assoc* 43:545–49 (1963).
24. A. Long, "The Well Nourished Vegetarian," *New Scientist*, 330–33 (1981).

CHAPTER 2. DEFINING VEGETARIANISM

1. *The American Vegetarian: Coming of Age in the 90's.* A Study of the Vegetarian Marketplace Conducted for *Vegetarian Times* by Yankelovich, Skelly, and White/Clancy (Shulman, Inc., 1992).
2. Ibid.
3. M. L. Burr and B. K. Butland, "Heart Disease in British Vegetarians," *Am J Clin Nutr* 48:830–32 (1988).
4. M. Kushi and A. Kushi, *Macrobiotic Diet* (Tokyo and New York: Japan Publications, 1989).
5. J. P. Carter et al., "Hypothesis: Dietary Management May Improve Survival from Nutritionally Linked Cancers Based on Analysis of Representative Cases," *J Am Coll Nutr* 12:209–26 (1993); J. H. Weisburger, "A New Nutritional Approach in Cancer Therapy in Light of Mechanistic Understanding of Cancer Causation and Development," *J Am Coll Nutr* 12:205–8 (1993).
6. J. T. Dwyer et al., "Preschoolers on Alternate Life-Style Diets," *J Am Diet Assoc* 72:264–70 (1978); P. C. Dagnelie et al., "High Prevalence of Rickets in Infants on Macrobiotic Diets," *Am J Clin Nutr* 51:202–8 (1990).
7. Kushi and Kushi, *Macrobiotic Diet.*
8. Dagnelie et al., "Rickets in Infants."
9. C. Stahler, "How Many Vegetarians Are There?" *Vegetarian Journal* 13(4):6–9 (1994).

CHAPTER 3. THE WORLD'S HEALTHIEST DIET

1. D. P. Burkitt, A. R. P. Walker, and N. S. Painter, "Dietary Fiber and Disease," *J Am Med Assoc* 229:1068–74 (1974).
2. *Heart and Stroke Facts: 1995 Statistical Supplement* (Dallas, Tex.: American Heart Association, National Center, 1994).
3. R. L. Phillips et al., "Coronary Heart Disease Mortality among Seventh-Day Adventists with Differing Dietary Habits: A Preliminary Report," *Am J*

Clin Nutr 31:S191–98 (1978); M. L. Burr and P. M. Sweetnam, "Vegetarianism, Dietary Fiber, and Mortality," *Am J Clin Nutr* 36:873–77 (1982); M. L. Burr and B. K. Butland, "Heart Disease in British Vegetarians," *Am J Clin Nutr* 48:830–32 (1988); M. Thorogood et al., "Risk of Death from Cancer and Ischaemic Heart Disease in Meat and Non-meat Eaters," *Br Med J* 308:1667–71 (1994); J. Berkel and F. de Waard, "Mortality Pattern and Life Expectancy of Seventh-Day Adventists in the Netherlands," *Int J Epidemiol* 12:455–59 (1983); H. T. Waaler and P. F. Hjort, "Low Mortality among Norwegian Seventh-Day Adventists 1960–1977: A Message on Lifestyle and Health?" *Tidsskr Nor Laegeforen* 101:623–27 (1981); J. Chang-Claude, R. Frentzel-Beyne, and U. Eilber, "Mortality Pattern of German Vegetarians after 11 Years of Follow-up," *Epidemiol* 3:395–401 (1992); T. Hirayama, "Mortality in Japanese with Life-Styles Similar to Seventh-Day Adventists: Strategy for Risk Reduction by Life-Style Modification," *Natl Cancer Inst Monogr* 69:143–53 (1985).

4. *Heart and Stroke Facts*; J. T. Knuiman et al., "Total Cholesterol and High Density Lipoprotein Cholesterol Levels in Populations Differing in Fat and Carbohydrate Intake," *Arteriosclerosis* 7:612–19 (1987).

5. H. Sekimoto et al., "Changes of Serum Total Cholesterol and Triglyceride Levels in Normal Subjects in Japan in the Past Twenty Years," *Jap J Circ J* 47:1351–58 (1983).

6. L. Kushi, E. B. Lenart, and W. C. Willet, "Health Implications of Mediterranean Diets in Light of Contemporary Knowledge. 2. Meat, Wine, Fats, and Oils," *Am J Clin Nutr* 61:1416S–27S (1995).

7. S. Stender et al., "The Influence of Trans Fatty Acids on Health: A Report from the Danish Nutrition Council," *Clin Sci* 88:375–92 (1995).

8. K. Resnicow et al., "Diet and Serum Lipids in Vegan Vegetarians: A Model for Risk Reduction," *J Am Diet Assoc* 91:447–53 (1991).

9. M. Thorogood et al., "Dietary Intake and Plasma Lipid Levels: Lessons from a Study of the Diet of Health Conscious Groups," *Br Med J* 300:1297–1301 (1990); J. T. Knuiman and C. E. West, "The Concentration of Cholesterol in Serum and in Various Serum Lipoproteins in Macrobiotic, Vegetarian and Non-vegetarian Men and Boys," *Atherosclerosis* 43:71–82 (1982); M. L. Burr et al., "Plasma Cholesterol and Blood Pressure in Vegetarians," *J Human Nutr* 35:437–41 (1981); M. Fisher et al., "The Effect of Vegetarian Diets on Plasma Lipid and Platelet Levels," *Arch Intern Med* 146:1193–97 (1986).

10. R. O. West and O. B. Hayes, "Diet and Serum Cholesterol Levels: A Comparision between Vegetarians and Nonvegetarians in a Seventh-Day Adventist Group," *Am J Clin Nutr* 21:853–62 (1968); L. A. Simons et al., "The Influence of a Wide Range of Absorbed Cholesterol on Plasma Cholesterol Levels in Man," *Am J Clin Nutr* 31:1334–39 (1978).

11. Simons et al., "Influence of a Wide Range of Absorbed Cholesterol."

12. R. S. Cooper et al., "The Selective Lipid-Lowering Effect of Vegetarianism on Low Density Lipoproteins in a Cross-over Experiment," *Atherosclerosis* 44:293–305 (1982); O. Lindahl et al., "A Vegan Regimen with Reduced Medication in the Treatment of Hypertension," *Br J Nutr* 52:11–20 (1984).

13. D. Ornish et al., "Can Lifestyle Changes Reverse Coronary Heart Disease?" *Lancet* 336:129–33 (1990).

14. M. Kestin et al., "Cardiovascular Disease Risk Factors in Free-Living Men: Comparison of Two Prudent Diets, One Based on Lactoovovegetarianism and the Other Allowing Lean Mean," *Am J Clin Nutr* 50:280–87 (1989).

15. S. D. Koury and R. E. Hodges, "Soybean Proteins for Human Diets?" *J Am Diabet Assoc* 52:480–84 (1968).

16. J. W. Anderson and B. M. Johnstone, "Meta-analysis of the effects of soy protein intake on serum lipids," *N Engl J Med* 333:276–82 (1995).

17. C. R. Sirtori, R. Even, and M. R. Lovati, "Soybean Protein Diet and Plasma Cholesterol: From Therapy to Molecular Mechanisms," *Ann NY Acad Sci* 676:188–201 (1993).

18. S. R. Glore et al., "Soluble Fiber and Serum Lipids: A Literature Review," *J Am Diet Assoc* 94:425–36 (1994).

19. J. T. Salonen et al., "High Stored Iron Levels Are Associated with Excess Risk of Myocardial Infarction in Eastern Finnich Men," *Circulation* 86:803–11 (1992); J. L. Beard, "Are We at Risk for Heart Disease Because of Normal Iron Status?" *Nutr Rev* 51:112–15 (1993).

20. D. Alexander, M. J. Ball, and J. Mann, "Nutrient Intake and Haematological Status of Vegetarians and Age-Sex Matched Omnivores," *Eur J Clin Nutr* 48:538–46 (1994); B. S. Worthington-Roberts, M. W. Breskin, and E. R. Monsen, "Iron Status of Pre-

menopausal Women in a University Community and Its Relationship to Habitual Dietary Sources of Protein Intake," *Am J Clin Nutr* 47:275–79 (1988).

21. A. Ascherio et al., "Dietary Iron Intake and Risk of Coronary Disease Among Men," *Circulation* 89:969–74 (1994).

22. E. Ernst et al., "Blood Rheology in Vegetarians," *Br J Nutr* 56:555–60 (1986).

23. C. Muir et al., *Cancer Incidence in Five Continents*, IARC Scientific Publication, vol. 5, no. 88 (Lyon: International Agency for Research on Cancer, 1987).

24. NCI, *Cancer Control Objectives for the Nation: 1985–2,000*, NCI Monographs, no. 2 Bethesda, Md.: (National Cancer Institute, 1986).

25. Hirayama, "Mortality"; L. J. Kinlen, C. Hermon, and P. G. Smith, "A Proportionate Study of Cancer Mortality Among Members of a Vegetarian Society," *Br J Cancer* 48:355–61 (1983); J. Chang-Claude and R. Frentzel-Beyne, "Dietary and Lifestyle Determinants of Mortality among German Vegetarians," *Int J Epidemiol* 22:228–36 (1993); M. Kuratsune, M. Ikeda, and T. Hayashi, "Epidemiologic Studies on Possible Health Effects of Intake of Pyrolyzates of Foods, with Reference to Mortality among Japanese Seventh-Day Adventists," *Environmental Health Perspectives:* 67:143–46 (1986); H. Halling and J. Carstensen, "Cancer Incidence among a Group of Swedish Vegetarians," abstract P29:084 in *Cancer Detect Preven* 7:425 (1984).

26. Thorogood et al., "Risk of Death from Cancer and Ischaemic Heart Disease."

27. B. K. Armstrong et al., "Diet and Reproductive Hormones: A Study of Vegetarian and Nonvegetarian Postmenopausal Women," *J Natl Cancer Inst* 67:761–67 (1981); B. R. Goldin et al., "Estrogen Excretion Patterns and Plasma Levels in Vegetarian and Omnivorous Women," *New Engl J Med* 307:1542–47 (1982); H. Adlercreutz et al., "Urinary Estrogen Profile Determination in Young Finnish Vegetarian and Omnivorous Women," *J Steroid Biochem* 24:289–96 (1986); H. Adlercreutz et al., "Diet and Plasma Androgens in Postmenopausal Vegetarian and Omnivorous Women and Postmenopausal Women with Breast Cancer," *Am J Clin Nutr* 49:433–42 (1989); J. C. Barbosa et al., "The Relationship among Adiposity, Diet, and Hormone Concentrations in Vegetarian and Nonvegetarian Postmenopausal Women," *Am J Clin Nutr* 51:798–803 (1990).

28. F. de Waard and D. Trichopoulous, "A Unifying Concept of the Etiology of Breast Cancer," *Int J Cancer* 41:666–69 (1988); A. Sanchez, D. G. Kissinger, and R. L. Phillips, "A Hypothesis on the Etiological Role of Diet on Age of Menarche," *Med Hypothesis* 7:1339–45 (1981); D. G. Kissinger and A. Sanchez, "The Association of Dietary Factors with the Age of Menarche," *Nutr Res* 7:471–79 (1987).

29. A. E. Treolar et al., "Variation of the Human Menstrual Cycle through Reproductive Life," *Int J Fertil* 12:77–126 (1970).

30. D. Y. Jones et al., "Influence of Dietary Fat on Menstrual Cycle and Menses Length," *Human Nutr: Clin Nutr* 41C:341–45 (1987); M. E. Reichman et al., "Effect of Dietary Fat on Length of the Follicular Phase of the Menstrual Cycle in a Controlled Diet Setting," *J Clin Endocrinol Metabol* 74:1171–75 (1992); B. R. Goldin et al., "The Effect of Dietary Fat and Fiber on Serum Estrogen Concentrations in Premenopausal Women under Controlled Dietary Conditions," *Cancer* 74:1125–31 (1994).

31. A. Cassidy, S. Bingham, and K. D. R. Setchell, "Biological Effects of a Diet of Soy Protein Rich in Isoflavones on the Menstrual Cycle of Premenopausal Women," *Am J Clin Nutr* 60:333–40 (1994); M. J. Messina et al., "Soy Intake and Cancer Risk: A Review of the *in Vitro* and *in Vivo* Data," *Nutr Cancer* 21:113-21 (1994).

32. R. L. Phillips and D. A. Snowdon, "Association of Meat and Coffee Use with Cancers of the Large Bowel, Breast, and Prostate among Seventh-Day Adventists: Preliminary Results," *Cancer Res* 43:2403S–8S (1983); O. M. Jensen, "Cancer Risk among Danish Male Seventh-Day Adventists and Other Temperance Society Members," *J Natl Cancer Inst* 70:1011–14 (1983).

33. M. Lipkin et al., "Seventh-Day Adventist Vegetarians Have a Quiescent Proliferative Activity in Colonic Mucosa," *Cancer Lett* 26:139–44 (1985).

34. B. S. Reddy and E. L. Wynder, "Large-Bowel Carcinogenesis: Fecal Constituents of Populations with Diverse Incidence Rates of Colon Cancer," *J Natl Cancer Inst* 50:1437–42 (1973); P. P. Nair et al., "Diet, Nutrition Intake, and Metabolism in Populations at High and Low Risk for Colon Cancer," *Am J Clin Nutr* 40:931–36 (1984); N. Turjman et al., "Diet, Nutrition Intake and Metabolism in Populations at High and

Low Risk for Colon Cancer," *Am J Clin Nutr* 40:937–41 (1984); J. T. Korpela, H. Adlercreutz, and M. J. Turunen, "Fecal Free and Conjugated Bile Acids and Neutral Sterols in Vegetarians, Omnivores, and Patients with Colorectal Cancer," *Scand J Gastroenterol* 23:277–83 (1988).

35. Nair et al., "Diet, Nutrition Intake, and Metabolism"; A. van Faassen et al., "Bile Acids, Neutral Steroids, and Bacteria in Feces as Affected by a Mixed, a Lacto-Ovovegetarian, and a Vegan Diet," *Am J Clin Nutr* 46:962–67 (1987).

36. V. G. Aries et al., "The Effect of a Strict Vegetarian Diet on the Faecal Flora and Faecal Steroid Concentration," *J Pathol* 103:54–56 (1972); M. J. Hill and V. G. Aries, "Faecal Steroid Composition and Its Relationship to Cancer of the Large Bowel," *J Pathol* 104:129–39 (1971); S. M. Finegold et al., "Fecal Microflora in Seventh Day Adventist Populations and Control Subjects," *Am J Clin Nutr* 30:1781–92 (1977); S. M. Finegold, H. R. Attebery, and V. L. Sutter, "Effect of Diet on Human Fecal Flora: Comparison of Japanese and American Diets," *Am J Clin Nutr* 27:1456–69 (1974); S. M. Finegold et al., "Fecal Bacteriology of Colonic Polyp Patients and Control Patients," *Cancer Res* 35:3407–17 (1975).

37. Goldin et al., "Estrogen Excretion"; B. S. Reddy and E. L. Wynder, "Large-Bowel Carcinogenesis: Fecal Constituents of Populations with Diverse Incidence Rates of Colon Cancer," *J Natl Cancer Inst* 50:1437–42 (1973).

38. B. S. Reddy, C. Sharma, and E. Wynder, "Fecal Factors Which Modify the Formation of Fecal Co-mutagens in High- and Low-Risk Population for Colon Cancer," *Cancer Lett* 10:123–32 (1980); B. S. Reddy et al., "Metabolic Epidemiology of Large Bowel Cancer: Fecal Mutagens in High- and Low-Risk Population for Colon Cancer," *Mutat Res* 72:511–22 (1980); U. Kuhnlein, D. Bergstrom, and H. Kuhnlein, "Mutagens in Feces from Vegetarians and Non-vegetarians," *Mutat Res* 85:1–12 (1981); C. J. Nader, J. D. Potter, and R. A. Weller, "Diet and DNA-Modifying Activity in Human Fecal Extracts," *Nutr Rep Int* 23:113–17 (1981).

39. R. L. Phillips et al., "Influence of Selection versus Lifestyle on Risk of Fatal Cancer and Cardiovascular Disease among Seventh-Day Adventists," *Am J Epidemiol* 112:296–314 (1980); R. L. Phillips, "Role of

Lifestyle and Dietary Habits in Risk of Cancer among Seventh-Day Adventists," *Cancer Res* 35:3513–22 (1975).

40. Hirayama, "Mortality."

41. M. C. R. Alvanja et al., "Saturated Fat Intake and Lung Cancer Risk among Nonsmoking Women in Missouri," *J Natl Cancer Inst* 85:1906–16 (1993).

42. G. Z. Colditz, M. J. Stampfer, and W. C. Willett, "Diet and Lung Cancer: A Review of the Epidemiologic Evidence in Humans," *Arch Intern Med* 14:157–60 (1987); R. G. Zeigler et al., "Carotenoid Intakes, Vegetables, and the Risk of Lung Cancer among White Men in New Jersey," *Am J Epidemiol* 123:1080–91 (1986).

43. A. M. Y. Nomura and L. N. Kolonel, "Prostate Cancer: A Current Perspective," *Am J Epidemiol* 13:200–27 (1991).

44. Ibid.; M. L. Slattery et al., "Food-Consumption Trends between Adolescent and Adult Years and Subsequent Risk of Prostate Cancer," *Am J Clin Nutr* 52:752–57 (1990); D. P. Rose, A. P. Boyar, and E. L. Wynder, "International Comparisons of Mortality Rates for Cancer of the Breast, Ovary, Prostate, and Colon, and Per Capita Food Consumption," *Cancer* 58:2363–71 (1986).

45. P. B. Hill and E. L. Wynder, "Effect of a Vegetarian Diet and Dexamethasone on Plasma Prolactin, Testosterone and Dehydroepiandrosterone in Men and Women," *Cancer Lett* 7:273–82 (1979).

46. J. Barone, J. R. Herbert, and M. M. Reddy, "Dietary Fat and Natural-Killer-Cell Activity," *Am J Clin Nutr* 50:861–67 (1989); M. Malter, G. Schriever, and U. Eilber, "Natural Killer Cells, Vitamins, and Other Blood Components of Vegetarian and Omnivorous Men," *Nutr Cancer* 12:271–78 (1989).

47. B. K. Armstrong and R. Doll, "Environmental Factors and Cancer Incidence and Mortality in Different Countries, with Special Reference to Dietary Practices," *Int J Cancer* 15:617–31 (1975); L. N. Kolonel, "Fat and Colon Cancer: How Firm Is the Evidence?" *Am J Clin Nutr* 45:336–41 (1987); M. Jain et al., "A Case-Control Study of Diet and Colo-Rectal Cancer," *Int J Cancer* 26:757–68 (1980); J. D. Potter and A. J. McMichael, "Diet and Cancer of the Colon and Rectum: A Case-Control Study," *J Natl Cancer Inst* 76:557–69 (1986).

48. P. Cruse, M. Lewin, and C. G. Clark, "Dietary

Cholesterol Is Co-carcinogenic for Human Colon Cancer," *Lancet* 1:752–55 (1979).

49. J. L. Lyon and A. W. Sorenson, "Colon Cancer in a Low-Risk Population," *Am J Clin Nutr* 31:227S–30 (1978); R. L. Phillips, D. A. Snowdon, and B. N. Brin, "Cancer in Vegetarians," in *Environmental Aspects of Cancer: The Role of Macro and Micro Components of Foods*, eds. E. L. Wynder et al. (Westport, Conn.: Food and Nutrition Press, 1983); D. M. Klurfield, "Human Nutrition and Health: Implications of Meat with More Muscle and Less Fat," in *Low-Fat Meats* (New York: Academic Press, 1994); D. Kritchevsky, *Meat and Cancer* chapter 4; J. E. Enstrom, "Cancer Mortality among Mormons in California during 1968–75," *J Natl Cancer Inst* 65:1073–82 (1980); R. L. Phillips and D. A. Snowdon, "Dietary Relationships with Fatal Colorectal Cancer among Seventh-Day Adventists," *J Natl Cancer Inst* 74:307–17 (1985).

50. H. V. Kuhnlein, U. Kuhnlein, and P. A. Bell, "The Effect of Short-Term Dietary Modification on Human Fecal Mutagenic Activity," *Mut Res* 113:1-12 (1983).

51. F. T. Hatch, J. S. Felton, and M. G. Knize, "Mutagens Formed in Foods during Cooking," *ISI Atlas of Science: Pharmacology*, 222–27 (1988).

52. D. A. Snowdon, "Animal Product Consumption and Mortality Because of All Causes Combined, Coronary Heart Disease, Stroke, Diabetes, and Cancer in Seventh-Day Adventists," *Am J Clin Nutr* 48:739–48 (1988).

53. P. K. Mills et al., "Bladder Cancer in a Low Risk Population: Results from the Adventist Health Study," *Am J Epidemiol* 133:230–39 (1991).

54. W. C. Willet et al., "Relation of Meat, Fat, and Fiber Intake to the Risk of Colon Cancer in a Prospective Study among Women," *New Engl J Med* 323:1664–72 (1990).

55. E. Giovannucci et al., "A Prospective Study of Dietary Fat and Risk of Prostate Cancer," *J Natl Cancer Inst* 85:1571–79 (1993).

56. B. S. Reddy et al., "Metabolic Epidemiology of Colon Cancer: Effect of Dietary Fiber on Fecal Mutagens and Bile Acids in Healthy Subjects," *Cancer Res* 47:644–48 (1987).

57. Goldin et al., "Effect of Dietary Fat and Fiber"; D. P. Rose et al., "High-Fiber Diet Reduces Serum Estrogen Concentrations in Premenopausal Women," *Am J Clin Nutr* 54:520-25 (1991).

58. R. J. Cahill et al., "Effects of Vitamin Antioxidant Supplementation on Cell Kinetics of Patients with Adenomatous Polyps," *Gut* 34:963–67 (1993).

59. G. van Poppel, "Carotenoids and Cancer: An Update with Emphasis on Human Intervention Studies," *Eur J Cancer* 29A:1335–44 (1993).

60. K. A. Steinmetz and J. D. Potter, "Vegetables, Fruit, and Cancer. I. Epidemiology," *Cancer Causes Control* 2:325–57 (1991).

61. L. B. Page, "Hypertension and Atherosclerosis in Primitive and Acculturating Societies," in *Hypertension Update*, ed. J. C. Hunt (Bloomfield, N.J.: Health Learning Systems, 1980).

62. N. R. Poulter et al., "Migration-Induced Changes in Blood Pressure: A Controlled Longitudinal Study," *Clin Exp Pharmacol Physiol* 12:211–16 (1985).

63. A. N. Donaldson, "The Relation of Protein Foods to Hypertension," *Calif West Med* 24:328–31 (1926).

64. F. Saile, "Uber den Einfluss der vegetarischen Ernahrung auf den Blutdruck," *Med Klin* 26:929–31 (1930).

65. Ibid.; H. A. Schroeder, P. H. Futcher, and M. L. Golden, "Effects of the 'Rice Diet' upon the Blood Pressure of Hypertensive Individuals," *Ann Intern Med* 30:713–32 (1949); J. A. Evans and A. W. Perry, "Use of the Rice Diet in the Management of Hypertensive Cardiovascular Disease," *Lahey Clin Bull* 6:187–92 (1949); F. T. Hatch et al., "Effect of Diet in Essential Hypertension. III. Alterations in Sodium Chloride, Protein and Fat Intake," *Am J Med* 17:499–513 (1954).

66. C. L. Melby, R. M. Lyle, and E. T. Poehlman, "Blood Pressure and Body Mass Index in Elderly Long-Term Vegetarians and Nonvegetarians," *Nutr Rep Int* 37:47–55 (1988); B. Armstrong, A. J. Van Merwyk, and H. Coates, "Blood Pressure in Seventh-Day Adventist Vegetarians," *Am J Epidemiol* 105:444–49 (1977); B. Armstrong et al., "Urinary Sodium and Blood Pressure in Vegetarians," *Am J Clin Nutr* 32:2472–76 (1979); O. Ophir et al., "Low Blood Pressure in Vegetarians: The Possible Role of Potassium," *Am J Clin Nutr* 37:755–62 (1983); A. P. Haines et al., "Haemostatic Variables in Vegetarians and Nonvegetarians," *Thrombosis Res* 19:139–48 (1980); I. L. Rouse, B. K. Armstrong, and L. J. Beilin, "Vegetarian Diet, Lifestyle and Blood Pressure in Two Religious Populations," *Clin Exp Pharmacol Physiol* 9:327–30 (1982).

67. O. Ophir et al., "Low Blood Pressure in Vegetarians."

68. E. Ernst et al., "Blood Rheology."

69. O. Ophir et al., "Low Blood Pressure in Vegetarians."

70. Ibid.; L. J. Beilin et al., "Vegetarian Diet and Blood Pressure Levels: Incidental or Causal Association?" *Am J Clin Nutr* 48:806–10 (1988).

71. B. M. Margetts et al., "Dietary Fat Intake and Blood Pressure: A Double Blind Controlled Trial of Changing Polyunsaturated Fat to Saturated Fat Ratio," *J Hypertens* 2:S201–3 (1984); B. M. Margetts et al., "Blood Pressure and Dietary Polyunsaturated and Saturated Fats: A Controlled Trial," *Clin Sci* 69:165–75 (1985); F. M. Sacks et al., "Effect of Dietary Fats and Carbohydrates on Blood Pressure of Mildly Hypertensive Patients," *Hypertension* 10:452–60 (1987); B. M. Margetts et al., "A Randomized Controlled Trial of the Effect of Dietary Fibre on Blood Pressure," *Clin Sci* 72:343–50 (1987); I. L. Rouse et al., "Blood Pressure Lowering Effect of a Vegetarian Diet: Controlled Trial in Normotensive Subjects," *Lancet* 1:5–10 (1983).

72. L. J. Beilin, "State of the Art Lecture: Diet and Hypertension: Critical Concepts and Controversies," *J Hypertens* 5:S447–57 (1987); F. M. Sacks and E. H. Kass, "Low Blood Pressure in Vegetarians: Effects of Specific Foods and Nutrients," *Am J Clin Nutr* 48:795–800 (1988).

73. B. E. Hazlett, "Historical Perspective: The Discovery of Insulin," in *Clinical Diabetes Mellitus: A Problem Oriented Approach*, ed. John K. Davidson, 2nd ed. (New York: Thieme Medical Publishers; New York, Stuttgart: Georg Thieme Verlag Stuttgart, 1991).

74. W. C. Knowler et al., "Diabetes Mellitus in the Pima Indians: Genetic and Evolutionary Considerations," *Am J Phys Anthropology* 62:107–14 (1983).

75. K. N. West, *Epidemiology of Diabetes and Its Vascular Lesions* (New York: Elsevier/North-Holland, 1978).

76. K. M. West and J. M. Kalbfleisch, "Influence of Nutritional Factors on Prevalence of Diabetes," *Diabetes* 20:99–108 (1971); K. M. West and J. M. Kalbfleisch, "Glucose Tolerance, Nutrition, and Diabetes in Uruguay, Venezuela, Malaya, and East Pakistan," *Diabetes* 15:9–18 (1966).

77. K. Dahl-Jørgensen, G. Joner, and K. F. Hanssen, "Relationship between Cow's Milk Consumption and Incidence of IDDM in Childhood," *Diabetes Care* 14:1081–83 (1991); H. C. Gerstein, "Cow's Milk Exposure and Type I Diabetes Mellitus," *Diabetes Care* 17:13–19 (1993).

78. P. Björntorp, "Abdominal Obesity and the Development of Non-Insulin-Dependent Diabetes Mellitus," *Diabetes Metab Rev* 4:615–22 (1988).

79. J. Hagan and J. Wylie-Rosett, "Lipids: Impact on Dietary Prescription in Diabetes," *J Am Diet Assoc* 89:1104–8 (1989).

80. "Nutrition Recommendations and Principles for People with Diabetes Mellitus," *Diabetes Care* 17:519–22 (1994).

81. G. D'Amico et al., "Effect of Vegetarian Soy Diet on Hyperlipidaemia in Nephrotic Syndrome," *Lancet* 339:1131–34 (1992).

82. R. J. Barnard et al., "Longterm Use of High-Complex-Carbohydrate High-Fiber Diet and Exercise in the Treatment of NIDDM Patients," *Diabetes Care* 6:268–73 (1983); R. J. Barnard et al., "Response of Non-Insulin-Dependent Diabetic Patients to an Intensive Program of Diet and Exercise," *Diabetes Care* 5:370–74 (1982).

83. J. W. Anderson, cited in J. W. Anderson et al., "Metabolic Effects of High-Carbohydrate, High-Fiber Diets for Insulin-Dependent Diabetic Individuals," *Am J Clin Nutr* 54:936–43 (1991).

84. D. A. Snowdon and R. L. Phillips, "Does a Vegetarian Diet Reduce the Occurrence of Diabetes?" *Am J Publ Health* 75:507–12 (1985).

85. Ibid.

86. F. Pi-Sunyer, "Effect of the Composition of the Diet on Energy Intake," *Nutr Rev* 48:94–105 (1990); L. Lissner et al., "Dietary Fat and the Regulation of Energy Intake in Human Subject," *Am J Clin Nutr* 46:886–92 (1987); T. E. Prewitt et al., "Changes in Body Weight, Body Composition, and Energy Intake of Women Fed High- and Low-Fat Diets," *Am J Clin Nutr* 54:304–10 (1991); I. Romieu et al., "Energy Intake and Other Determinants of Relative Weight," *Am J Clin Nutr* 47:406–12 (1988); D. M. Dreon et al., "Dietary Fat: Carbohydrate Ratio and Obesity in Middle-Aged Men," *Am J Clin Nutr* 47:995–1000 (1988); J. P. Flatt, "Dietary Fat, Carbohydrate Balance, and Weight Maintenance," *Annals NY Acad Sci* 122–40 (1993).

87. R. E. Beauchene et al., "Nutrient Intake and Physical Measurements of Aging Vegetarian and Nonvegetarian Women," *J Am Coll Nutr* 1:131 (1982); P. Millet et al., "Nutrient Intake and Vitamin Status of Healthy French Vegetarians and Nonvegetarians," *Am J Clin Nutr* 50:718–27 (1989).

88. K. C. Janelle and S. I. Barr, "Nutrient Intakes and Eating Behavior Scores of Vegetarian and Nonvegetarian Women," *J Am Diet Assoc* 95:180–89 (1995); M. J. Toth and E. T. Poehlman, "Sympathetic Nervous System Activity and Resting Metabolic Rate in Vegetarians," *Metabolism* 43:621–25 (1994).

89. J. K. Ross, D. J. Pusateri, and T. D. Shultz, "Dietary and Hormonal Evaluation of Men at Different Risks for Prostate Cancer: Fiber Intake, Excretion, and Composition, with in Vitro Evidence for an Association between Steroid Hormones and Specific Components," *Am J Clin Nutr* 51:365–70 (1990); T. A. B. Sanders and T. J. A. Key, "Blood Pressure, Plasma Renin Activity and Aldosterone Concentrations in Vegans and Omnivores," *Human Nutr: Appl Nutr* 41A:204-11 (1987).

90. J. P. Bosch et al., "Renal Functional Reserve in Humans: Effect of Protein Intake on Glomerular Filtration Rate," *Am J Med* 75:943–50 (1983).

91. M. J. Wiseman et al., "Dietary Composition and Renal Function in Healthy Subjects," *Nephron* 46:37–42 (1987).

92. P. Kontessis et al., "Renal, Metabolic and Hormonal Responses to Ingestion of Animal and Vegetable Proteins," *Kid Int* 38:136–44 (1990).

93. F. J. Raal et al., "Effect of Moderate Dietary Protein Restriction on the Progression of Overt Diabetic Nephropathy: A 6-Month Prospective Study," *Am J Clin Nutr* 60:579–85 (1994).

94. G. C. Curhan et al., "A Prospective Study of Dietary Calcium and Other Nutrients and the Risk of Symptomatic Kidney Stones," *N Engl J Med* 328:833–38 (1993).

95. J. G. Brockis, A. J. Levitt, and S. M. Cruthers, "The Effects of Vegetable and Animal Protein Diets on Calcium, Urate and Oxalate Excretion," *Br J Urol* 54:590–93 (1982); L. A. Martini et al., "Dietary Habits of Calcium Stone Formers," *Braz J Med Biol Res* 26:805–12 (1993).

96. Curhan et al., "Prospective Study."

97. W. G. Robertson, M. Peacock, and D. H. Marshall, "Prevalence of Urinary Stone Disease in Vegetarians," *Eur Urol* 8:334–39 (1982).

98. B. Fellstrom et al., "The Influence of a High Dietary Intake of Purine-Rich Animal Protein on Urinary Urate Excretion and Supersaturation in Renal Stone Disease," *Clin Sci* 64:399–405 (1983).

99. M. Nikkila, T. Koivula, and H. Jokela, "Urinary Citrate Excretion in Patients with Urolithiasis and Normal Subjects," *Eur Urol* 16:382–85 (1989).

100. F. Pixley et al., "Effect of Vegetarianism on Development of Gall Stones in Women," *Br Med J* 291:11–12 (1985).

101. D. P. Burkitt and M. Tunstall, "Gallstones: Geographical and Chronical Features," *J Trop Med Hyg* 78:140–44 (1975).

102. H. Sarles et al., "Diet and Cholesterol Gallstones—a Study of 101 Patients with Cholelithiasis Compared to 101 Matched Controls," *Am J Dig Dis* 14:531–37 (1969); L. Denbesten, W. E. Connor, and S. Bell, "The Effect of Dietary Cholesterol on the Composition of Human Bile," *Surgery* 73:266–73 (1973); D. A. Smith and M. I. Gee, "A Dietary Survey to Determine the Relationship between Diet and Cholelithiasis," *Am J Clin Nutr* 32:1519–26 (1979); J. Thornton, C. Symes, and K. W. Heaton, "Moderate Alcohol Intake Reduces Bile Cholesterol Saturation and Raises HDL," *Lancet* 2:819–22 (1983).

103. S. Mahfouz-Cercone, J. E. Johnson, and G. U. Liepa, "Effect of Dietary Animal and Vegetable Protein on Gallstone Formation and Biliary Constituents in the Hamster," *Lipids* 19:5–10 (1984); T. Ozben, "Biliary Lipid Composition and Gallstone Formation in Rabbits Fed on Soy Protein, Cholesterol, Casein and Modified Casein," *Biochem J* 263:293–96 (1989).

104. R. Berkow, ed., *Merck Manual of Diagnosis and Therapy*, 14th ed. (Rahway, N.J.: Merck, Sharpe & Dohme Research Laboratories, 1982), p. 794.

105. N. S. Painter and D. P. Burkitt, *Refined Carbohydrate Foods and Disease*, ed. D. P. Burkitt and H. C. Trowell (London: Academic Press, Inc., 1975), p. 99; J. Kyle et al., "Incidence of Diverticulitis," *Scandinavian J Gastro* 2:77–80 (1967).

106. J. S. S. Gear et al., "Symptomless Diverticular Disease and Intake of Dietary Fibre," *Lancet* 1:511–14 (1979).

107. W. H. Aldoori et al., "A Prospective Study of Diet and the Risk of Symptomatic Diverticular Disease in Men," *Am J Clin Nutr* 60:757–64 (1994).

108. K. W. Heaton, "Diet and Diverticulosis: New Leads," *Gut* 26:541–43 (1986).

109. H. Lithell et al., "A Fasting and Vegetarian Diet Treatment Trial on Chronic Inflammatory Disorders," *Acta Derm Venereol* 63:397–403 (1983); L. Skoldstam,

"Fasting and Vegan Diet in Rheumatoid Arthritis," *Scand J Rheumatology* 15:219–23 (1986).

110. J. Kjeldsen-Kragh et al., "Controlled Trial of Fasting and One-Year Vegetarian Diet in Rheumatoid Arthritis" *Lancet* 338:899–902 (1991).

111. R. L. Swank and B. B. Dugan, "Effect of Low Saturated Fat Diet in Early and Late Cases of Multiple Sclerosis," *Lancet* 336:37–39 (1990).

112. G. Fitzgerald et al., "The Effect of Nutritional Counseling on Diet and Plasma FFA Status in Multiple Sclerosis Patients over 3 Years," *Hum Nutr: Appl Nutr* 41A:297–310 (1987).

113. D. A. Evans et al., "Prevalence of Alzheimer's Disease in a Community Population of Older Persons: Higher Than Previously Thought," *J Am Med Assoc* 262:2551–56 (1989).

114. P. Glem, W. L. Beeson, and G. E. Fraser, "The Incidence of Dementia and Intake of Animal Products: Preliminary Findings from the Adventist Health Study," *Neuroepidemiology* 12:28–36 (1993).

115. D. Harman, "Free Radical Theory of Aging: A Hypothesis on Pathogenesis of Senile Dementia of the Alzheimer's Type," *Age* 16:23–30 (1993).

116. R. L. Glass and J. Hayden, "Dental Caries in Seventh-Day Adventist Children," *J Dent Child* 33:22–23 (1966); C. J. Donnelly, "A Comparative Study of Caries Experience in Adventist and Other Children," *Publ Health Report* 76:209–12 (1961); R. Harris; "Biology of Children of Hopewood House," *J Dent Res* 42:1387–98 (1963).

117. Dahl-Jørgensen, Joner, Hanssen, "Cow's Milk Consumption."

118. Gerstein, "Cow's Milk Exposure."

119. D. W. Cramer et al., "Galactose Consumption and Metabolism in Relation to the Risk of Ovarian Cancer," *Lancet* 2:66–71 (1989).

120. Ibid.

121. A. M. Lake, P. F. Whitington, and S. R. Hamilton, "Dietary Protein-Induced Colic Breast-Fed Infants," *J Pediatrics* 101:906–10 (1982); R. R. A. Coombs and S. T. Holgate, "Allergy and Cot Death: With Special Focus on Allergic Sensitivity to Cow's Milk and Anaphylaxis," *Clin Exper Allergy* 20:359–66 (1990).

122. C. A. Ryan et al., "Massive Outbreak of Antimicrobial-Resistant Salmonellosis Traced to Pasturized Milk," *J Am Med Assoc* 258:3269–74 (1987).

123. W. A. Tham and M. M-L. Danielsson-Tham, "Listeria Monocytogenes Isolated from Soft Cheese," *Veterinary Red* 122:539–40 (1988); "'CDC' Traces Listeriosis to Soft Cheeses," *The Nation's Health*, May–June 1992, p. 18.

124. S. J. Fomon et al., "Cow Milk Feeding in Infancy: Gastrointestinal Blood Loss and Iron Nutritional Status," *J Pediatrics* 98:540–45 (1981).

125. L. Hallberg et al., "Calcium and Iron Absorption: Mechanism of Action and Nutritional Importance," *Eur J Clin Nutr* 46:317–27 (1991).

126. J. J. Segall, "Dietary Lactose as a Possible Risk Factor for Ischaemic Heart Disease: Review of Epidemiology," *Intern J Cardio*, 46:197–207 (1994).

127. O. M. Rennert, "Disorders of Galactose Metabolism," *Ann Clin Lab Sci* 7:433–48 (1977).

128. R. Van Heyningen, "Formation of Polyols by the Lens of the Rat with 'Sugar' Cataract," *Nature* 184:194–95 (1959).

129. R. Quan-Ma et al., "Galactitol in the Tissues of a Galactosemic Child," *Am J Dis Child* 112:477–78 (1966); R. Gitzelman, H. C. Curtius, and I. Schneller, "Galactitol and Galactose-1-Phosphate in the Lens of a Galactosemic Infant," *Expl Eye Res* 6:1–3 (1967).

130. H. W. Skalka and J. T. Prchal, "Presenile Cataract Formation and Decreased Activity of Galactosemic Enzymes," *Arch Ophthalmol* 98:269–73 (1980).

131. J. A. Montelone et al., "Cataracts, Galactosiuria, and Galactosemia Due to Galactokinase Deficiency in a Child: Studies of a Kindred," *Am J Med* 50:403–7 (1971); E. Beutler et al., "Galactokinase Deficiency: An Important Cause of Familial Cataracts in Children and Young Adults," *J Lab Clin Med* 76:1006 (1970).

132. K. S. Bhat and C. Gopolan, "Human Cataract and Galactose Metabolism," *Nutr Metab* 17:1–8 (1974).

133. P. F. Jacques et al., "Lactose Intake, Galactose Metabolism and Senile-Cataract," *Nutr Res* 10:225–65 (1990).

CHAPTER 4. MORE REASONS TO GO MEATLESS

1. F. M. Lappé, *Diet for a Small Planet* (New York: Ballantine Books, 1971).

2. D. Pimentel et al., "The Potential for Grass-Fed Livestock: Resource Constraints," *Science* 207:843–48 (1980).

3. J. R. Wright, ed., *The Universal Almanac* (Kansas City, Mo.: Andrews and McMeel, 1990).

4. G. Blix, "Vegetarianism: An Ecological Perspective,"

in *Nutrition 2000 Proceedings* (Loma Linda, Calif.: Andrews University, 1994).

5. D. W. Pimentel et al., "Deforestation: Interdependency of Fuelwood and Agriculture," *Oikos* 46:404–12 (1986).

6. A. B. Durning and H. B. Brough, "Taking Stock: Animal Farming and the Environment," *Worldwatch Paper* 103 (Washington, D.C.: Worldwatch Institute, 1991).

7. Food and Agriculture Organization, *Production Yearbook, 1976* (Rome, 1977).

8. Blix, "Vegetarianism."

9. World Commission on Environment and Development, *Our Common Future: The Brundtland Commission Report* (Oxford: Oxford University Press, 1987).

10. R. Hayes, *Tropical Rainforest Fact Sheet* (San Francisco: Rain Forest Action Network).

11. Blix, "Vegetarianism."

12. D. Pimentel et al., "Water Resources in Food and Energy Production," *BioScience* 32:861–67 (1982).

13. Ibid.

14. Durning and Brough, "Taking Stock."

15. L. R. Brown, *State of the World: A Worldwatch Institute Report on Progress toward a Sustainable Society* (New York: W. W. Norton, 1994).

16. B. Bolin et al., eds., *The Greenhouse Effect, Climatic Change, and Ecosystems,* (Chichester, N.Y.: John Wiley & Sons, 1986).

17. Brown, *State of the World.*

18. Ibid.

19. S. Postel, "Water for Agriculture: Facing the Limits," *Worldwatch Paper* 93 (Washington, D.C.: Worldwatch Institute, 1989).

20. U.S. Department of Agriculture, Economic Research Service, *World Agriculture Supply and Demand Estimates,* WASDE-256 (Washington, D.C.: USDA, July 11, 1991).

21. G. T. Miller, *Living in the Environment: An Introduction to Environmental Science* (Belmont, Calif.: Wadsworth, Inc., 1992).

22. J. Tannenbaum, *Agricultural Animals: Welfare Issues* in *Veterinary Ethics* (Baltimore, Md.: Williams and Wilkins, 1989).

23. M. E. Ensminger, *Poultry Science* (Danville, Ill.: Interstate Publishers, 1992).

24. J. M. Gentle, "Beak Trimming in Poultry," *World's Poultry Science Journal* 42:268–75 (1986).

25. M. J. Gentle et al., "Behavioural Evidence for Persistent Pain Following Partial Beak Amputation in Chickens," *Applied Animal Behaviour Science* 27:149–57 (1990).

26. M. H. Swanson and D. D. Bell, *Force Molting of Chickens; Parts I: Introduction and II. Methods* (Berkeley: University of California Cooperative Extension, 1981).

27. Schmidt, Vleck. *Principles of Dairy Science* (San Francisco: W. H. Freeman, 1974).

28. P. Le Neindre, "Evaluating Housing System for Veal Calves," *J Am Science* 71:1345–54 (1993).

29. *Legislative Policies of the National Grange.*

30. M. E. Ensminger, *The Stockman's Handbook* (Danville, Ill.: Interstate Printers and Publishers, 1983).

31. Tannenbaum, *Agricultural Animals.*

32. R. F. Miller, W. J. van Riet, and J. L. Farley, *Swine Production* (Berkeley: University of California Cooperative Extension Division of Agriculture and Natural Resources, 1987).

33. Tannenbaum, *Agricultural Animals.*

CHAPTER 5. THE POLITICS OF DIET

1. M. Nestle, "Food Lobbies, the Food Pyramid, and U.S. Nutrition Policy," *International J Health Services* 23(3):483–96 (1993).

2. U.S. Department of Agriculture and U.S. Department of Health, Education, and Welfare, *Nutrition and Your Health: Dietary Guidelines for Americans,* Home and Garden Bulletin, no. 232 (Washington, D.C.: U.S. Government Printing Office, 1980).

3. Nestle, "Food Lobbies."

4. National Dairy Council, *The All-American Guide to Calcium-Rich Foods* (NDC, 1990).

5. National Dairy Council, *Super You: A Guide to Getting Fit and Staying Fit* (NDC, 1990).

6. Committee on Diet, Nutrition and Cancer, National Research Council, *Diet, Nutrition and Cancer* (Washington, D.C.: National Academy Press, 1982).

7. E. V. McCollum, *A History of Nutrition* (Boston: Houghton Mifflin, Riverside Press, 1929).

8. N. D. Barnard, L. W. Scherwitz, and D. Ornish, "Adherence and Acceptability of a Low-Fat, Vegetarian Diet among Patients with Cardiac Disease," *J Cardiopulmonary Rehabil* 12:423–31 (1992).

9. W. Insull et al., "Results of a Randomized Feasibility Study of a Low-Fat Diet," *Arch Intern Med* 150:421–27 (1989).

10. R. D. Mattes, "Fat Preference and Adherence to a Reduced-Fat Diet," *Am J Clin Nutr* 57:373–81 (1993).

11. W. S. Browner, J. Westenhouse, and J. A. Tice, "What If Americans Ate Less Fat?" *J Am Med Assoc* 265:3285–91 (1991).

12. D. Ornish et al., "Can Lifestyle Changes Reverse Coronary Heart Disease?" *Lancet* 336:129–33 (1990).

13. Gladwell, "U.S. Rethinks, Redraws the Food Groups," *Washington Post,* Apr. 13, 1991, A1.

14. Ibid.

15. U.S. Department of Agriculture, Human Nutrition Information Service, *USDA's Food Guide Pyramid,* Home and Garden Bulletin no. 249 (Washington, D.C.: U.S. Government Printing Office, 1992); Office of Public Affairs, USDA.

Chapter 6. Protein in Vegetarian Diets

1. K. J. Carpenter, "The History of Enthusiasm for Protein," *J Nutr* 116:1364–70 (1986).

2. J. S. McLester, *Nutrition and Diet in Health and Disease* (New York: W. B. Saunders, 1939), cited in *J Am Diet Assoc* 16:229 (1940).

3. J. H. Kellogg, *The Natural Diet of Man* (Battle Creek, Mich.: Modern Medicine Publishing, 1923; Imlaystown, N.J.: Edenite Society, 1980).

4. World Health Organization, *Diet, Nutrition, and the Prevention of Chronic Diseases,* Technical Report Series, no. 797 (Geneva: World Health Organization, 1990).

5. World Health Organization, *Energy and Protein Requirement: Report of a Joint FAO/WHO/UNU Expert Consultation,* Technical Report Series, no. 724 (Geneva: World Health Organization, 1985).

6. National Research Council, *Recommended Dietary Allowances,* 10th ed. (Washington, D.C.: National Academy Press, 1989).

7. R. J. Williams, "We Abnormal Normals," *Nutr Today* 2:19–28 (1967).

8. Committee on Diet and Health, Food and Nutrition Board, Commission on Life Sciences, National Research Council, *Diet and Health* (Washington, D.C.: National Academy Press, 1989), chapter 3.

9. M. Thorogood, "Dietary Intake and Plasma Lipid Levels: Lessons from a Study of the Diet of Health Conscious Groups," *Br Med J* 300:1297–1301 (1990).

10. Ibid.; B. M. Calkins et al., "Diet, Nutrition Intake, and Metabolism in Populations at High and Low Risk for Colon Cancer," *Am J Clin Nutr* 40:896–905 (1984);
S. K. Rana and T. A. B. Sanders, "Taurine Concentrations in the Diet, Plasma, Urine and Breast Milk of Vegans Compared with Omnivores," *Br J Nutr* 56:17–27 (1986); T. A. B. Sanders and T. J. A. Key, "Blood Pressure, Plasma Renin Activity and Aldosterone Concentrations in Vegans and Omnivores," *Human Nutr: Appl: Nutr* 41A:204–11 (1987); F. A. Tylavsky and J. J. B. Anderson, "Dietary Factors in Bone Health of Elderly Lactoovovegetarian and Omnivorous Women," *Am J Clin Nutr* 48:842–49 (1988); D. J. Pusateri et al., "Dietary and Hormonal Evaluation of Men at Different Risks for Prostate Cancer: Plasma and Fecal Hormone-Nutrient Interrelationships," *Am J Clin Nutr* 51:371–77 (1990).

11. USDA, *Nationwide Food Consumption Survey Continuing Survey of Food Intakes by Individuals. Men 19–50 Years, 1 Day, 1985,* report no. 85–3 (Hyattsville, Md.: Nutrition Monitoring Division, Human Nutrition Information Service, USDA, 1986); USDA, *Nationwide Food Consumption Survey Continuing Survey of Food Intakes by Individuals. Women 19–50 Years and Their Children 1–5 Years, 4 Days, 1985,* report no. 85 (Hyattsville, Md.: Nutrition Monitoring Division, Human Nutrition Information Service, USDA, 1987).

12. J. A. T. Pennington, *Food Values of Portions Commonly Use,* 15th ed. (New York: Harper and Row, 1989).

13. G. Sarwar, R. W. Peace, and H. G. Botting, "Corrected Relative Net Protein Ratio (CRNPR) Method Based on Differences in Rat and Human Requirements for Sulfur Amino Acids," *J Assoc Off Anal Chem* 68:689–93 (1985).

14. *Federal Register.* Food and Drug Administration. 21 CFR, Part 101, et al. Part III. Food Labeling, 1991.

15. Food and Agriculture Organization of the United Nations, *Protein Quality Evaluation, Report of a Joint FAO/WHO Expert Consultation* (Rome: Food and Agricultural Organization of the United Nations, 1990; Geneva: World Health Organization, 1990).

16. Frances Moore Lappé, *Diet for a Small Planet* (New York: Ballantine Books, 1971).

17. Frances Moore Lappé, *Diet for a Small Planet* (New York: Ballantine Books, 1982).

18. S. Havala and J. Dwyer, "Position of the American Dietetic Association: Vegetarian Diets," *J Am Diet Assoc* 93:1317–19 (1993).

19. V. R. Young and P. L. Pellet, "Protein Intake and Requirements with Reference to Diet and Health," *Am J Clin Nutr* 45:1323–43 (1987).

20. J. Bergstrom, P. Frust, and E. Vinnars, "Effect of a Test Meal, without and with Protein, on Muscle and Plasma Free Amino Acids," *Clin Sci* 79:331–37 (1990); E. S. Nasset, "Amino Acid Homeostasis in the Gut Lumen and Its Nutritional Significance," *World Rev Nutr Diet* 14:134–53 (1972).

21. S. Bolourchi, C. M. Friedman, and O. Mickelsen, "Wheat Flour as a Source of Protein for Adult Human Subjects," *Am J Clin Nutr* 21:827–35 (1968).

22. C. Edwards et al., "Utilization of Wheat by Adult Man: Nitrogen Metabolism, Plamsa Amino Acids and Lipids," *Am J Clin Nutr* 24:181–93 (1971); D. M. Hegsted, M. F. Trulson, and F. J. Stare, "Role of Wheat and Wheat Products in the Human Nutrition," *Physiol Rev* 34:221 (1954); A. Begum, N. Radhakrishnan, and S. M. Pereira, "Effect of Amino Acid Composition of Cereal Bread Diets on Growth of Preschool Children," *Am J Clin Nutr* 23:1175 (1970); E. M. Widdowson and R. A. McCance, "Studies on the Nutritive Value of Bread and on the Effect of Variation in the Extraction Rate of Flour on Growth of Undernourished Children," *Med Res Council, London Spec Rept Ser,* no. 287 (1954).

23. C. Lee et al., "Nitrogen Retention of Young Men Fed Rice with or without Supplementary Chicken," *Am J Clin Nutr* 24:318–23 (1971).

24. P. Markadis, "The Nutritive Quality of Potato Protein," part 2 of *Protein Nutritional Quality of Foods and Feeds,* ed. M. Friedman (New York: M. Dekker, 1975); S. K. Kon and A. Kleen, "The Value of Whole Potato Protein in Human Nutrition," *Biochem J* 22:258–61 (1928), and *Am J Clin Nutr* 20:825 (1967).

25. A. Ignatowski, "Changes in Parenchymatous Organs and in the Aorta of Rabbits under the Influence of Animal Protein," *Izvestizy Imperatorskoi Voyenno-Meditsinskoi Akademii* 18:231–44 (St. Petersburg, 1908).

26. K. C. Hayes and E. A. Trautwein, "Taurine," In *Modern Nutrition in Health and Disease,* ed. Maurice E. Shils, James A. Olson, and Moshe Shike, 8th ed. (Philadelphia: Lea and Febiger, 1994).

27. C. S. Irving et al., "New Evidence for Taurine Biosynthesis in Man Obtained from 18 O_2 Inhalation Studies," *Life Sci* 38:491–95 (1986).

28. S. K. Rana and T. A. B. Sanders, "Taurine Concentrations in the Diet, Plasma, Urine and Breast Milk of Vegans Compared with Omnivores," *Br J Nutr* 56:17–27 (1986); S. A. Laidlaw et al., "Plasma and Urine Taurine Levels in Vegans," *Am J Clin Nutr* 47:660–63 (1988).

29. N. E. Vinton et al., "Taurine Concentrations in Plasma and Blood Cells of Patients Undergoing Long-Term Parental Nutrition," *Am J Clin Nutr* 44:398–404 (1986).

30. Rana and Sanders, "Taurine Concentrations"; Laidlaw et al., "Plasma."

31. D. V. Michalk et al., "Development of the Nervous and Cardiovascular Systems in Low-Birth Weight Infants Fed a Taurine-Supplemented Formula," *Eur J Pediatr* 147:296–99 (1988).

32. D. K. Rassin, J. A. Sturman, and G. E. Gaull, "Taurine in Developing Rat Brain," *J Neurochemistry* 28:41–50 (1977).

CHAPTER 7. MEETING CALCIUM NEEDS ON A PLANT-BASED DIET

1. R. K. Montgomery et al., "Lactose Intolerance and the Genetic Regulation of Intestinal-Phlorizin Hydrolase," *FASEB J* 5:2824–32 (1991).

2. J. D. Johnson et al., "Lactose Malabsorption among the Pima Indians in Arizona," *Gastroenterol* 73:1299–1304 (1977).

3. F. J. Simoons, "The Geographic Hypothesis and Lactose Malabsorption," *Dig Dis Sci* 23:963–80 (1989).

4. S. B. Eaton and D. A. Nelson, "Calcium in Evolutionary Perspective," *Am J Clin Nutr* 54:281S–87S (1991).

5. C. M. Schnitzler, "Bone Quality: A Determinant for Certain Risk Factors for Bone Fragility," *Calcif Tissue Int* 53:S27–S31 (1993); R. P. Heaney, "Is There a Role for Bone Quality in Fragility Fractures?" *Calcif Tissue Int* 53:S3–S6 (1993); S. M. Ott, "When Bone Mass Fails to Predict Bone Failure," *Calcif Tissue Int* 53:S7–S13 (1993).

6. R. P. Heaney, "Calcium, Bone Health, and Osteoporosis," in *Bone and Mineral Research, Annual 4: A Yearly Survey of Developments in the Field of Bone and Mineral Metabolism,* ed. W. A. Peck (Elsevier, Amsterdam: Elsevier Science Pub., 1983), 255–301.

7. Committee on Diet and Health, Food and Nutrition Board, Commission on Life Sciences, National Research Council, "Osteoporosis," in *Diet and Health: Implications for Reducing Chronic Disease Risk* (Washington D.C.: National Academy Press, 1989), chapter 23.

8. Osteoporosis Consensus Panel, "Osteoporosis," *J Am Med Assoc* 252:799–802 (1984); S. R. Cummings et al., "Epidemiology of Osteoporosis and Osteoporotic Fractures," *Epidemiol Rev* 7:178–208 (1985).

9. Osteoporosis Consensus Panel, "Osteoporosis."

10. W. S. Pollitzer and J. J. B. Anderson, "Ethnic and Genetic Differences in Bone Mass: A Review with a Hereditary vs. Environmental Perspective," *Am J Clin Nutr* 50:1244–59 (1989); J. J. B. Anderson and J. A. Metz, "Contributions of Dietary Calcium and Physical Activity to Primary Prevention of Osteoporosis in Females," *J Am Coll Nutr* 12:378–83 (1993).

11. A. G. Marsh et al., "Cortical Bone Density of Adult Lacto-Ovo-Vegetarian and Omnivorous Women," *J Am Diet Assoc* 76:148–51 (1980); A. G. Marsh et al., "Vegetarian Lifestyle and Bone Mineral Density," *Am J Clin Nutr* 48:837–41 (1988).

12. F. R. Ellis et al., "Incidence of Osteoporosis in Vegetarians and Omnivores," *Am J Clin Nutr* 25:555–58 (1972); F. R. Ellis, S. Holesh, and T. A. B. Sanders, "Osteoporosis in British Vegetarians and Omnivores," *Am J Clin Nutr* 27:769–70 (1974); T. V. Sanchez et al., "Bone Mineral Density in Elderly Vegetarian and Omnivorous Females," *Proceedings of the 4th International Conference on Bone Mineral Measurements*, ed. R. B. Mazeness (Bethesda, Md.: NIAMMD, 1980), 94–98.

13. J. A. Reed et al., "Comparative Changes in Radial-Bone Density of Elderly Female Lactoovovegetarians and Omnivores," *Am J Clin Nutr* 59:S1197–1202 (1994).

14. L. A. L. Taber and R. A. Cook, "Dietary and Anthropometric Assessment of Adult Omnivores, Fish-Eaters, and Lacto-Ovo-Vegetarians," *J Am Diet Assoc* 76:21–29 (1980); R. E. Beauchene et al., "Nutrient Intake and Physical Measurements of Aging Vegetarian and Nonvegetarian Women," *J Am Coll Nutr* 1:131 (1982); T. D. Shultz and J. E. Leklem, "Dietary Status of Seventh-Day Adventists and Nonvegetarians," *J Am Diet Assoc* 83:27–33 (1983); A. Locong, "Nutritional Status and Dietary Intake of a Selected Sample of Young Adult Vegetarians," *J Can Diet Assoc* 47:101–6 (1986).

15. B. M. Calkins et al., "Diet, Nutrition Intake, and Metabolism in Populations at High and Low Risk for Colon Cancer," *Am J Clin Nutr* 40:896–905 (1984); A. Draper et al., "The Energy and Nutrient Intakes of Different Types of Vegetarian: A Case for Supplements?" *Br J Nutr* 69:3–19 (1993).

16. N. Nnakwe and C. Kies, "Calcium and Phosphorus Utilization by Omnivorous and Lacto-Ovo-Vegetarians Fed Laboratory Controlled Lactoovovegetarian Diets," *Nutr Rep Int* 31:1009–14 (1985).

17. Marsh et al., "Vegetarian Lifestyle."

18. National Research Council, *Recommended Dietary Allowances* (Washington, D.C.: National Academy Press, 1989), chapter 9.

19. J. LeMann, N. D. Adams, and R. W. Gray, "Urinary Calcium Excretion in Human Beings," *New Engl J Med* 301:535–41 (1978); USDA, *Nationwide Food Consumption Survey: Continuing Survey of Food Intakes of Individuals. Women 19–50 years and Their Children 1–5 Years, 4 Days, 1985*, report no. 85-4 (Hyattsville, Md.: Nutrition Monitoring Division, Human Nutrition Information Service, 1987); USDA, *Nationwide Food Consumption Survey: Individuals in 48 States, Year 1977–78*, report no. 1-2 (Hyattsville, Md.: Consumer Nutrition Division, Human Nutrition Information Service, 1984).

20. R. P. Heaney, "Thinking Straight about Calcium," *New Engl J Med* 328:503–5 (1993).

21. R. P. Heaney, P. D. Surille, and R. R. Recker, "Calcium Absorption as a Function of Calcium Intake," *J Lab Clin Med* 85:881–90 (1975).

22. Reed et al., "Comparative Changes."

23. USDA, *Food Consumption Survey: Food Intakes.*

24. B. Dawson-Hughes, P. Jacques, and C. Shipp, "Dietary Calcium Intake and Bone Loss from the Spine in Healthy Postmenopausal Women," *Am J Clin Nutr* 46:685–87 (1987).

25. A. Prentice, "Calcium: The Functional Significance of Trends in Consumption," in *Modern Lifestyles, Lower Energy Intake and Micronutrient Status*, ed. K. Pietrzik (London: Springer-Verlag, 1989).

26. B. J. Abelow, T. R. Holford, and K. L. Insogna, "Cross-Cultural Association between Dietary Animal Protein and Hip Fracture: A Hypothesis," *Calcif Tissue Int* 50:14–18 (1992).

27. H. C. Sherman, "Calcium Requirements of Maintenance in Man," *J Biol Chem* 44:21–27 (1920).

28. A. Wachman and D. S. Bernstein, "Diet and Osteoporosis," *Lancet*, 958–59 (May 4, 1968).

29. J. Lemon, Jr., J. R. Litzow, and E. J. Lennon, "Studies of the Mechanism by Which Chronic Metabolic Acidosis Augments Urinary Calcium Excretion in Man," *J Clin Invest* 46:1318–28 (1967).

30. J. Dwyer et al., "Acid/Alkaline Ash Diets: Time for Assessment and Change," *J Am Diet Assoc* 85:841–45 (1985).

31. T. Remer and F. Manz, "Estimation of the Renal Net

Acid Excretion by Adults Consuming Diets Containing Variable Amounts of Protein," *Am J Clin Nutr* 59:1356–61 (1994).

32. H. M. Linkswiler et al., "Protein-Induced Hypercalciuria," *Federation Proc* 40:2429–33 (1981).

33. S. A. Schuette and H. M. Linkswiler, "Effects of Calcium and P Metabolism in Humans by Adding Meat, Meat Plus Milk, or Purified Proteins Plus Ca and P to a Low Protein Diet," *J Nutr* 112:338–49 (1982).

34. M. Hegsted et al., "Urinary Calcium and Calcium Balance in Young Men as Affected by Level of Protein and Phosphorus Intake," *J Nutr* 111:553–62 (1981).

35. J. E. Kerstetter and L. H. Allen, "Dietary Protein Increases Urinary Calcium," *J Nutr* 120:134–36 (1990).

36. R. P. Heaney and R. R. Recker, "Effects of Nitrogen, Phosphorus, and Caffeine on Calcium Balance in Women," *J Lab Clin Med* 99:46–55 (1982).

37. R. P. Heaney, "Cofactors Influencing the Calcium Requirement—Other Nutrients," *NIH Consensus Development Conference on Optimal Calcium Intake* (program and abstracts from NIH Consensus Development Conference, June 6–8, 1994), 71–77.

38. Kerstetter and Allen, "Dietary Protein."

39. N. A. Breslau et al., "Relationship of Animal Protein-Rich Diet to Kidney Stone Formation and Calcium Metabolism," *J Clin Endocrinol Metabol* 66:140–46 (1988).

40. S. A. Schuette, M. B. Zemel, and H. M. Linkswiler, "Studies on the Mechanisms of Protein-Induced Hypercalciuria in Older Men and Women," *J Nutr* 110:305–15 (1980).

41. R. R. Recker et al., "Bone Gain in Young Adult Women," *J Am Med Assoc* 268:2403–8 (1992).

42. R. P. Heaney, "Protein Intake and the Calcium Economy," *J Am Diet Assoc* 93:1259–60 (1993).

43. C. Shortt and A. Flynn, "Sodium-Calcium Inter-Relationships with Specific Reference to Osteoporosis," *Nutr Res Rev* 3:101–15 (1990); G. A. MacGregor and F. P. Cappuccio, "The Kidney and Essential Hypertension: A Link to Osteoporosis?" *J Hypertension* 11:781–85 (1993).

44. L. D. McBean, T. Forgac, and S. C. Finn, "Osteoporosis: Visions for Care and Prevention—A Conference Report," *J Am Diet Assoc* 94:668–71 (1994).

45. Heaney, "Cofactors"; B. E. C. Nordin et al., "The Nature and Significance of the Relationship between Urinary Sodium and Phosphorus Metabolism," *J Nutr* 123:1615–22 (1993).

46. Intersalt Cooperative Research Group, "Intersalt: An International Study of Electrolyte Excretion and Blood Pressure. Results for a 24 Hour Urinary Sodium and Potassium Excretion," *Br Med J* 297:319–28 (1988).

47. M. J. Barger-Lux and R. P. Heaney, "Caffeine and the Calcium Economy Revisited," *Osteoporosis Int* 5:97–102 (1995).

48. H. H. Draper and C. A. Scythes, "Calcium, Phosphorus and Osteoporosis," *Fed Proc* 40:2434–38 (1981).

49. J. A. T. Pennington, *Bowes and Church's Food Values of Portions Commonly Used*, 15th ed. (New York: Harper and Row, 1989).

50. D. Barltrop, R. H. Mole, and A. Sutton, "Absorption and Endogenous Faecal Excretion of Calcium by Low Birthweight Infants on Feeds with Varying Contents of Calcium and Phosphate," *Arch Dis Child* 52:41–49 (1977); H. Spencer et al., "Effect of Phosphorus on the Absorption of Calcium and on the Calcium Balance," *J Nutr* 108:447–57 (1978).

51. Barger-Lux and Heaney, "Caffeine."

52. G. Wyshak, "Hip Fracture in Elderly and Reproductive History," *J Gerontol* 36:424–27 (1981); N. Kreiger et al., "An Epidemiologic Study of Hip Fracture in Postmenopausal Women," *Am J Epidemiol* 116:141–48 (1982); B. W. Alderman et al., "Reproductive History and Postmenopausal Risk of Hip Fracture and Forearm Fracture," *Am J Epidemiol* 124:262–67 (1986).

53. B. W. Alderman et al., "Reproductive History and Postmenopausal Risk of Hip and Forearm Fracture," *Am J Epidemiol* 124:262–67 (1986).

54. Anderson and Metz, "Contributions"; J. Chalmers and K. C. Ho, "Geographic Variations in Senile Osteoporosis: The Association with Physical Activity," *J Bone Joint Surg* 52B:667–75 (1970).

55. V. S. Schneider, A. Le Blanc, and P. C. Rambaut, "Bone and Mineral Metabolism," in *Space Physiology and Medicine*, ed. A. E. Nicogossian, C. L. Huntoon, and S. L. Pool (Philadelphia: Lea and Febiger, 1989), 214–21.

56. P. C. Jacobson et al., "Bone Density in Women: College Athletes and Older Athletic Women," *J Orthop Res* 2:328–32 (1984).

57. E. A. Krall and B. Dawson-Hughes, "Walking Is Related to Bone Density and Rates of Bone Loss," *Am J Med* 96:20–26 (1994).

58. M. E. Nelson et al., "Effects of High-Intensity Strength Training on Multiple Risk Factors for Osteoporotic Fractures," *J Am Med Assoc* 272:1909–14 (1994).

59. L. Solomon, "Bone Density in Ageing Caucasian and African Populations," *Lancet* 2:1326–30 (1979); P. D. Ross et al., "A Comparison of Hip Fracture Incidence among Native Japanese, Japanese Americans, and American Caucasians," *Am J Epidemiol* 133:801–9 (1991).

60. M. E. Tinetti, M. Speechley, and S. F. Ginter, "Risk Factors for Falls among Elderly Persons Living in the Community," *N Engl J Med* 319:1701–7 (1988); M. C. Nevitt et al., "Risk Factors for Recurrent Nonsyncopal Falls: A Prospective Study," *J Am Med Assoc* 261:2663–68 (1989).

61. D. Hemenway et al., "Risk Factors for Hip Fracture in US Men Aged 40–75 Years," *Am J Publ Health* 84:1843–45 (1994).

62. *Handbook of Human Nutritional Requirements* (Geneva: World Health Organization, 1974).

63. G. Block et al., "Nutrient Sources in the American Diet: Quantitative Data from the NHANES II Survey. I. Vitamins and Minerals," *Am J Epidemiology* 122:13–26 (1985).

64. J. Rattan et al., "A High-Fiber Diet Does not Cause Mineral and Nutrient Deficiencies," *J Clin Gastroenterol* 3:389–93 (1981); H. Spencer et al., "Effect of Oat Bran Muffins on Calcium Absorption and Calcium, Phosphorus, Magnesium and Zinc Balance in Men," *J Nutr* 121:1976–83 (1991); W. van Dokkum, "The Relative Significance of Dietary Fibre for Human Health," *Front Gastrointest Res* 14:135–45 (1988); T. A. Knox et al., "Calcium Absorption in Elderly Subjects on High- and Low-Fiber Diets: Effect of Gastric Acidity," *Am J Clin Nutr* 53:1480–86 (1991); H. H. Sandstead, "Fiber, Phytates, and Mineral Nutrition," *Nutr Rev* 50:30–31 (1992); E. J. Moynahan, "Nutritional Hazards on High-Fibre Diet," *Lancet* (Mar. 19, 1977) 654–55; K. O. O'Brien et al., "High Fiber Diets Slow Bone Turnover in Young Men but Have No Effect on Efficiency of Intestinal Calcium Absorption," *J Nutr* 123:2122–28 (1993).

65. C. M. Weaver et al., "Human Calcium Absorption from Whole-Wheat Products," *J Nutr* 121:1769–75 (1991).

66. R. P. Heaney and C. M. Weaver, "Oxalate: Effect on Calcium Absorbability," *Am J Clin Nutr* 50:830–32 (1989).

67. C. M. Weaver and K. L. Plawecki, "Dietary Calcium: Adequacy of a Vegetarian Diet," *Am J Clin Nutr* 59 (suppl):1238–41 (1994).

68. MacGregor and Cappuccio, "Kidney and Essential Hypertension"; D. A. McCarron et al., "Blood Pressure and Nutrient Intake in the United States," *Science* 224:1392–98 (1984); R. Tesar et al., "Axial and Peripheral Bone Density and Nutrient Intakes of Postmenopausal Vegetarian and Omnivorous Women," *Am J Clin Nutr* 56:699–704 (1992).

69. N. S. Painter and D. P. Burkitt, "Diverticular Disease of the Colon: A Deficiency Disease of Western Civilization," *Br Med J* 11:450–54 (1971); A. R. F. Walker, "Certain Biochemical Findings in Man in Relation to Diet," *Ann NY Acad Sci* 989–1008 (1958).

CHAPTER 8. VITAMINS IN VEGETARIAN DIETS

1. J. A. Halsted, J. Carroll, and S. Robert, "Serum and Tissue Concentration of Vitamin B_{12} in Certain Pathologic States," *N Engl J Med* 260:575–80 (1959).

2. V. Herbert et al., "Are Colon Bacteria a Major Source of Cobalamin Analogues in Human Tissues? 24 Hr Human Stool Contains Only About 5 μg of Cóbalamin But About 100 μg of Apparent Analogue (and 200 μg of Folate)," *Trans Assoc Am Phys* 97:161–71 (1984).

3. V. Herbert and G. Drivas, "Spirulina and Vitamin B_{12}," *J Am Med Assoc* 248:3096–7 (1982); P. C. Dagnelie, W. A. van Staveren, H. van den Berg, "Vitamin B_{12} from Algae Appears Not to be Bioavailable," *Am J Clin Nutr* 53:695–97 (1991); G. J. Davies, M. Crowder, and J. W. T. Dickerson, "Dietary Fibre Intakes of Individuals with Different Eating Patterns," *Human Nutr: Appl Nutr* 39A: 139–48 (1985); P. A. Prasad et al., "Functional Impact of Riboflavin Supplementation in Urban School Children," *Nutr Res* 10:275–81 (1990).

4. I. Chanarin, *The Megaloblastic Anaemias*, 2nd ed. (Oxford: Blackwell, 1979).

5. R. H. Allen et al., "Metabolic Abnormalities in Cobalamin (Vitamin B_{12}) and Folate Deficiency," *FASEB J* 7:1344–53 (1993).

6. T. A. B. Sanders, "The Health and Nutritional Status

of Vegans," *Plant Foods for Man* 2:181–93 (1978); A. M. Immerman, "Vitamin B12 Status on a Vegetarian Diet," *Wld Rev Nutr Diet* 37:38–54 (1981).

7. E. B. Healton et al., "Neurologic Aspects of Cobalamin Deficiency," *Medicine* 70:229–45 (1991).

8. T. A. B. Sanders, F. R. Ellis, and J. W. T. Dickerson, "Haematological Studies on Vegans," *Br J Nutr* 40:9–15 (1978); P. Millet et al., "Nutrient Intake and Vitamin Status of Healthy French Vegetarians and Nonvegetarians," *Am J Clin Nutr* 50:718–27 (1989); A. D. Helman and I. Darnton-Hill, "Vitamin and Iron Status in New Vegetarians," *Am J Clin Nutr* 45:785–89 (1987); F. R. Ellis and V. M. E. Montegriffo, "Veganism, Clinical Findings and Investigations," *Am J Clin Nutr* 23:249–55 (1970); A. Dong and S. C. Scott, "Serum Vitamin B12 and Blood Cell Values in Vegetarians," *Ann Nutr Metab* 26:209–16 (1982); P. Bar-Sella, Y. Rakover, and D. Ratner, "Vitamin B12 and Folate Levels in Long-Term Vegans," *Isr J Med Sci* 26:309–12 (1990).

9. Ellis and Montegriffo, "Veganism."

10. Dong and Scott, "Serum Vitamin B12"; Bar-Sella, Rakover, and Ratner, "Vitamin B12."

11. B. L. Specker et al., "Increased Urinary Methylmalonic Acid Excretion in Breast-Fed Infants of Vegetarian Mothers and Identification of an Acceptable Dietary Source of Vitamin B-12," *Am J Clin Nutr* 47:89–92 (1988).

12. S. M. Grahamn, O. M. Arvela, and G. A. Wise, "Long-Term Neurologic Consequences of Nutritional Vitamin B12 Deficiency in Infants," *J Pediatr* 121:710–14 (1992).

13. Specker et al., "Urinary Methylmalonic Acid Excretion"; A. L. Lubby et al., "Observations on Transfer of Vitamin B12 from Mother to Fetus and Newborn," *Am J Dis Child* 96:532–33 (1958).

14. B. L. Specker et al., "Vitamin B-12: Low Milk Concentrations Are Realted to Low Serum Concentrations in Vegetarian Women and to Methylmalonic Aciduria in Their Infants," *Am J Clin Nutr* 52:1073–76 (1990).

15. V. Herbert, "Recommended Dietary Intakes (RDA) of Vitamin B12 in Humans," *Am J Clin Nutr* 45:671–78 (1987).

16. Herbert, "Colon Bacteria?"; B. K. Armstrong, "Absorption of Vitamin B12 from the Human Colon," *Am J Clin Nutr* 21:298–99 (1968).

17. M. J. Alberts, V. I. Mathan, and S. J. Baker, "Vitamin B12 Synthesis by Human Small Intestinal Bacteria," *Nature* 283:781–82 (1980); C. R. Kapadia, "Free Intrinsic Factor in the Small Intestine in Man," *Gastroenterol* 70:704–6 (1976).

18. M. G. Hardinge et al., "Non Dietary Source of Vitamin B12," abstract in *Fed Proc* 33:665 (1974); M. G. Hardinge et al., "Non Dietary Source of Vitamin B12" (paper presented at Federation proceedings, April 8, 1974).

19. R. L. Mason et al., "Nutrient Intakes of Vegetarian and Nonvegetarian Women," *Tenn Farm Home Science* 1:18–20 (1978); F. A. Tylavsky and J. J. B. Anderson, "Dietary Factors in Bone Health of Elderly Lactoovovegetarian and Omnivorous Women," *Am J Clin Nutr* 48:842–49 (1988); K. C. Janelle and S. I. Barr, "Nutrient Intakes and Eating Behavior Scores of Vegetarian and Nonvegetarian Women," *JADA* 95:180–89 (1995); B. M. Calkins et al., "Diet, Nutrition Intake, and Metabolism in Populations at High and Low Risk for Colon Cancer," *Am J Clin Nutr* 40:896–905 (1984).

20. T. C. Campbell et al., "Questioning Riboflavin Recommendations on the Basis of a Survey in China," *Am J Clin Nutr* 51:436–45 (1990).

21. A. Keys et al., "Physiological and Biochemical Functions in Normal Young Men on a Diet Restricted in Riboflavin," *J Nutr* 27:165–78 (1944); R. D. Williams et al., "Observations on Induced Riboflavin Deficiency and the Riboflavin Requirement of Man," *J Nutr* 25:361–77 (1943); M. K. Horwitt et al., "Correlation of Urinary Excretion of Riboflavin with Dietary Intake and Symptoms of Ariboflavinosis," *J Nutr* 41:247–64 (1950).

22. D. I. Thurnham et al., "A Longitudinal Study on Dietary and Social Influences on Riboflavin Status in Preschool Children in Northeast Thailand," *Southeast Asian J Trop Med Public Health* 2:552–63 (1971); C. J. Bates and H. J. Powers, "Studies on Micronutrient Intakes and Requirements in The Gambia," *J Hum Nutr Diet* 2:117–24 (1989); C. J. Bates et al., "Riboflavin Status in Gambian Pregnant and Lactating Women and Its Implications for Recommended Dietary Allowances," *Am J Clin Nutr* 34:928–35 (1981).

23. R. T. Sterner and W. R. Price, "Restricted Riboflavin: Within-Subject Behavioral Effects in Humans," *Am J Clin Nutr* 26:150–60 (1973); J. A. Tillostson and E. M. Baker, "An Enzymatic Measurement of the

Riboflavin Status in Man," *Am J Clin Nutr* 25:425–31 (1972); P. A. Prasad et al., "Functional Impact of Riboflavin Supplementation."

24. Millet, "Nutrient Intake"; Davies, Crowder, and Dickerson, "Dietary Fibre Intakes"; J. H. Freeland-Graves, P. W. Bodzy, and M. A. Eppright, "Zinc Status of Vegetarians," *J Am Diet Assoc* 77:655–61 (1980).

25. Calkins et al., "Diet, Nutrition Intake, and Metabolism"; Freeland-Graves, Bodzy, and Eppright, "Zinc Status"; M. G. Hardinge and F. J. Stare, "Nutritional Studies of Vegetarians," *Am J Clin Nutr* 2:73–82 (1954); A. Draper et al., "The Energy and Nutrient Intakes of Different Types of Vegetarian: A Case for Supplements," *Br J Nutr* 69:3–19 (1993); T. A. B. Sanders and T. J. A. Key, "Blood Pressure, Plasma Renin Activity and Aldosterone Concentrations in Vegans and Omnivores," *Human Nutr: Appl Nutr* 41A:204–11 (1987).

26. Freeland-Graves, Bodzy, and Eppright, "Zinc Status"; Draper et al., "Energy and Nutrient Intakes"; T. Lloyd et al., "Urinary Hormonal Concentrations and Spinal Bone Densities of Premenopausal Vegetarian and Nonvegetarian Women," *Am J Clin Nutr* 54:1005–10 (1991); T. D. Shultz and J. E. Leklem, "Dietary Status of Seventh-Day Adventists and Nonvegetarians," *J Am Diet Assoc* 83:27–33 (1983).

27. R. D. Reynolds et al., "Nutritional and Medical Status of Lactating Women and Their Infants in the Kathmandu Valley of Nepal," *Am J Clin Nutr* 47:722–28 (1988).

28. J. E. Leklem et al., "Bioavailability of Vitamin B6 from Whole Wheat Bread in Humans," *J Nutr* 110:1819–28 (1980); A. S. Lindberg, J. E. Leklem, and L. T. Miller, "The Effect of Wheat Bran on the Bioavailability of Vitamin B6 in Young Men," *J Nutr* 113:2578–83 (1983).

29. P. R. Trumbo et al., "Bioavailability of Pyridoxine-Beta-Glucoside in Rats and Humans," abstract in *FASEB J* 2:1086 (1988); M. B. Andon et al., "Dietary Intake of Total and Glycosylated Vitamin B-6 and the Vitamin B-6 Nutritional Status of Unsupplemented Lactating Women and Their Infants," *Am J Clin Nutr* 50:1050–58 (1989); T. D. Shultz and J. E. Leklem, "Vitamin B6 Status and Bioavailability in Vegetarian Women," *Am J Clin Nutr* 46:647–51 (1987); M. R. H. Löwik et al., "Effect of Dietary Fiber on the Vitamin B6 Status among Vegetarian and Nonvegetarian Elderly (Dutch Nutrition Surveillance System)," *J Am Coll Nutr* 9:241–49 (1990).

30. Bar-Sella, Rakover, and Ratner, "Vitamin B12"; Lloyd et al., "Urinary Hormonal Concentrations"; Shultz and Leklem, "Dietary Status"; R. Tesar et al., "Axial and Peripheral Bone Density and Nutrient Intakes of Postmenopausal Vegetarian and Omnivorous Women," *Am J Clin Nutr* 56:699–704 (1992); A. B. Pedersen et al., "Menstrual Differences due to Vegetarian and Nonvegetarian Diets," *Am J Clin Nutr* 53:879–85 (1991).

31. G. Brubacher, D. Hornig, and G. Ritzel, "Food Patterns in Modern Society and Their Consequences on Nutrition," *Biblthca Nutr Dieta* 30:90–99 (1981).

32. Draper et al., "Energy and Nutrition Intakes."

33. M. J. Kretsch et al., "Effect of Animal or Plant Protein Composition on the Vitamin B-6 Requirement of Young Women," abstract 52 in *Fed Proc* 21:227 (1982).

34. Löwik et al., "Effect of Dietary Fiber."

35. Draper et al., "Energy and Nutrient Intakes"; E. Carlson et al., "A Comparative Evaluation of Vegan, Vegetarian and Omnivore Diets," *J Plant Foods* 6:89–100 (1985); A. Locong, "Nutritional Status and Dietary Intake of a Selected Sample of Young Adult Vegetarians," *J Can Diet Assoc* 47:101–7 (1986).

36. Helman and Darnton-Hill, "Vitamin and Iron Status"; S. Areekul, K. Churdchu, and V. Pungpapong, "Serum Folate, Vitamin B12 and Vitamin B12 Binding Protein in Vegetarians," *J Med Assoc Thai* 71:253–57 (1987); Ellis and Montegriffo, "Veganism."

37. K. A. Lombard and D. M. Mock, "Biotin Nutritional Status of Vegans, Lactoovovegetarians, and Nonvegetarians," *Am J Clin Nutr* 50:486–90 (1989).

38. M. Glusman, "Syndrome of Burning Feet (Nutritional Melalgia) as Manifestation of Nutritional Deficiency," *Am J Med* 3:211–23 (1947).

39. H. Hemilä, "Does Vitamin C Alleviate the Symptoms of the Common Cold?—a Review of Current Evidence," *Scand J Infect Dis* 26:1–6 (1994).

40. Millet et al., "Nutrient Intake"; Draper et al., "Energy and Nutrient Intakes"; Shultz and Leklem, "Dietary Status"; Carlson et al., "Comparative Evaluation"; L. A. L. Taber and R. A. Cook, "Dietary and Anthropometric Assessment of Adult Omnivores, Fish-Eaters, and Lacto-Ovo-Vegetarians," *J Am Diet Assoc* 76:21–29 (1980); N. E. Hitchcock and R. M. English, "A Comparison of Food Consumption in Lacto-Ovo-Vegetarians and Non-vegetarians," *Food Nutr Notes Rev* 20:141–46 (1963); M. Tayter and K. L. Stanek,

"Anthropometric and Dietary Assessment of Omnivore and Lacto-Ovo-Vegetarian Children," *J Am Diet Assoc* 89:1661–63 (1989).

41. Calkins et al., "Diet, Nutrition Intake, and Metabolism"; Draper et al., "Energy and Nutrient Intakes"; Carlson et al., "Comparative Evaluation."

42. A. W. Norman, "The Vitamin D Endocrine System: Identification of Another Piece of the Puzzle," *Endocrinol* 134:1601A–601C (1994); M. Lipkin et al., "Calcium, Vitamin D, and Colon Cancer," *Cancer Res* 51:3069–70 (1991).

43. L. Y. Matsuoka et al., "Sunscreen Suppresses Cutaneous Vitamin D3 Synthesis," *J Clin Endocrinol Metab* 64:1165–68 (1987).

44. T. L. Clemens et al., "Increased Skin Pigment Reduces Capacity of Skin to Synthesize Vitamin D3," *Lancet* 1:74–76 (1982).

45. B. L. Specker et al., "Sunshine Exposure and Serum 25-Hydroxyvitamin D Concentrations in Exclusively Breast-Fed Infants," *J Pediatric* 107:372–76 (1985).

46. A. R. Webb, L. Kline, and M. F. Holick, "Influence of Season and Latitude on the Cutaneous Synthesis of Vitamin D3: Exposure to Winter Sunlight in Boston and Edmonton Will Not Promote Vitamin D3 Synthesis in Human Skin," *J Clin Endocrinol Metab* 67:373–78 (1988).

47. B. L. Specker, "Do North American Women Need Supplemental Vitamin D during Pregnancy or Lactation?" *Am J Clin Nutr* 59:484S–91S (1994).

48. M. A. Preece et al., "Studies of Vitamin D Deficiency in Man," *Quart J Med* 44:575–79 (1975); S. P. Hunt et al., "Vitamin D Status in Different Subgroups of British Asians," *Br Med J* 2:1351–54 (1976); P. F. Wilmana et al., "Reduction of Circulating 25-Hydroxyvitamin D by Antipyrine," *Br J Clin Pharmac* 8:523–28 (1979); P. Dandona et al., "Persistence of Parathyroid Hypersecretion after Vitamin D Treatment in Asian Vegetarians," *J Clin Endocrinol Metab* 59:535–37 (1984); D. A. Isenberg et al., "Muscle Strength and Pre-osteomalacia in Vegetarian and Asian Women," *Lancet* 1:55 (1982).

49. Wilmana et al., "Reduction of Circulating 25-Hydroxyvitamin D by Antipyrine."

50. J. T. Dwyer et al., "Risk of Nutritional Rickets among Vegetarian Children," *Am J Dis Child* 133:134–40 (1979); I. F. Roberts, R. J. West, and M. J. Dillon, "Malnutrition in Infants Receiving Cult Diets: A Form of Child Abuse," *Br Med J* 1:296–98 (1979); P. C. Dagnelie et al., "High Prevalence of Rickets in Infants on Macrobiotic Diets," *Am J Clin Nutr* 51:202–8 (1990).

51. E. M. E. Poskit, T. J. Cole, and D. E. M. Lawson, "Diet, Sunlight, and 25-Hydroxy Vitamin D in Healthy Children and Adults," *Br Med J* 1:221–23 (1979).

52. B. F. Boyce et al., "Hypercalcemic Osteomalacia due to Aluminum Toxicity," *Lancet* 2:1009–12 (1982); G. Colussi et al., "Vitamin D Treatment: A Hidden Risk Factor for Aluminum Bone Toxicity?" *Nephron* 47:78–80 (1987); J. Moon, A. Davison, and B. Bandy, "Vitamin D and Aluminum Absorption," *Can Med Assoc J* 147:1308–9 (1992).

53. C. H. Jacobus et al., "Hypervitaminosis D Associated with Drinking Milk," *N Engl J Med* 326:1173–77 (1992).

54. Ibid.

55. Ibid.

56. FAO, *Requirements of Vitamin A, Iron, Folate, and Vitamin B12*: Report of a Joint FAO/WHO Expert Consultation, FAO Food and Nutrition Series, no. 23 (Rome: Food and Agriculture Organization, 1988).

57. J. A. Olson, "Recommended Dietary Intakes (RDI) of Vitamin A in Humans," *Am J Clin Nutr* 45:704–16 (1987).

58. R. Abraham et al., "Diets of Asian Pregnant Women in Harrow: Iron and Vitamins," *Human Nutr: Appl Nutr* 41A:164–73 (1987).

59. D. Alexander, M. J. Ball, and J. Mann, "Nutrient Intake and Haematological Status of Vegetarians and Age-Sex Matched Omnivores," *Europ J Clin Nutr* 48:538–46 (1994); S. K. Rana and T. A. B. Sanders, "Taurine Concentrations in the Diet, Plasma, Urine and Breast Milk of Vegans Compared with Omnivores," *Br J Nutr* 56:17–27 (1986).

60. N. I. Krinsky, "Antioxidant Functions of Carotenoids," *Free Rad Biol Med* 7:617–35 (1989); P. Di Mascio, S. Kaiser, and H. Sies, "Lycopene as the Most Efficient Biological Carotenoid Singlet Oxygen Quencher," *Arch Biochem Biophyss* 274:532–38 (1989).

61. H. Gerster, "Anticarcinogenic Effect of Common Carotenoids," *Intern J Vit Nutr Res* 63:93–121 (1993); R. G. Ziegler, "A Review of the Epidemiologic Evidence That Carotenoids Reduce the Risk of Cancer," *J Nutr* 119:116–22 (1989); S. E. Hankinson et al., "Nutrient Intake and Cataract Extraction in

Women: A Prospective Study," *Br Med J* 305:335–39 (1992); P. Knekt et al., "Serum Antioxidant Vitamins and Risk of Cataract," *Br Med J* 305:1392–94 (1992); M. Naruszewica, E. Selinger, and J. Davignon, "Oxidative Modification of Lipoprotein(a) and the effect of β-Carotene," *Metabolism* 41:1215–24 (1992).

62. R. H. Prabhala et al., "The Effects of 13-Cis-Retinoic Acid and Beta-Carotene on Cellular Immunity in Humans," *Cancer* 67:1556–60 (1991).

63. M. S. Micozzi et al., "Carotendemia in Men with Elevated Carotenoid Intake from Food and β-Carotene Supplements," *Am J Clin Nutr* 46:1061–64 (1988).

64. M. J. Stampfer et al., "Vitamin E Consumption and the Risk of Coronary Disease in Women," *N Engl J Med* 328:1444–49 (1993); E. B. Rimm, et al., "Vitamin E Consumption and the Risk of Coronary Heart Disease in Men," *N Engl J Med* 328:1450–56 (1993).

65. H. Hassan et al., "Syndrome in Premature Infants Associated with Low Plasma Vitamin E Levels and High Polyunsaturated Fatty Acid Diet," *Am J Clin Nutr* 19:147–57 (1966).

66. Ellis and Montegriffo, "Veganism"; Lloyd et al., "Urinary Hormonal Concentrations"; T. A. B. Sanders, F. R. Ellis, and J. W. T. Dickerson, "Studies of Vegans: The Fatty Acid Composition of Plasma Choline Phosphoglycerides, Erythrocytes, Adipose Tissue, and Breast Milk, and Some Indicators of Susceptibility to Ischemic Heart Disease in Vegans and Omnivore Controls," *Am J Clin Nutr* 31:805–13 (1978); D. C. Nieman et al., "Dietary Status of Seventh-Day Adventist Vegetarian and Non-vegetarian Elderly Women," *J Am Diet Assoc* 89:1763–69 (1989); A. Pronczuk, Y. Kipervarg, and K. C. Hayes, "Vegetarians Have Higher Plasma Alpha-Tocopherol Relative to Cholesterol Than Do Nonvegetarians," *J Am Coll Nutr* 11:50–55 (1992).

67. Pronczuk, Kipervarg, and Hayes, "Vegetarians"; S. Reddy and T. A. B. Sanders, "Lipoprotein Risk Factors in Vegetarian Women of Indian Descent Are Unrelated to Dietary Intake," *Atherosclerosis* 95:223–29 (1992); T. A. B. Sanders and F. Roshanai, "Platelet Phospholipid Fatty Acid Composition and Function in Vegans Compared with Age- and Sex-Matched Omnivore Controls," *Eur J Clin Nutr* 46:823–31 (1992); E. Kumpusalo et al., "Multivitamin Supplementation of Adult Omnivores and Lactovegetarians:

Circulating Levels of Vitamin A, D, and E, Lipids, Apolipoproteins and Selenium," *Internat J Vit Nutr Res* 60:58–66 (1989).

68. P. Palozza and N. I. Krinsky, "Beta-Caraotene and α-Tocopherol Are Synergistic Antioxidants," *Arch Biochem Biophysic* 297:184–87 (1992).

69. J. W. Suttie et al., "Vitamin K Deficiency from Dietary Vitamin K Restriction in Humans," *Am J Clin Nutr* 47:475–80 (1988).

70. S. J. Hodges et al., "Circulating Levels of Vitamin K1 and K2 Decreased in Elderly Women with Hip Fracture," *J Bone Min Res* 8:1241–45 (1993).

71. P. A. Price, "Vitamin K Nutrition and Postmenopausal Osteoporosis," *J Clin Invest* 91:1266 (1994).

72. *Provisional Table of the Vitamin K Content of Foods*, USDA, Human Nutrition Information Service HNIS/PT-104.

73. A. G. Feller and D. Rudman, "Role of Carnitine in Human Nutrition," *J Nutr* 118:541–47 (1988).

74. A. Etzioni et al., "Systemic Carnitine Deficiency Exacerbated by a Strict Vegetarian Diet," *Arch Dis Child* 59:177–79 (1984).

75. J. Delanghe et al., "Normal Reference Values for Creatine, Creatinine, and Carnitine Are Lower in Vegetarians," *Clin Chem* 35:1802–3 (1989); K. A. Lombard et al., "Carnitine Status of Lactoovovegetarians and Strict Vegetarian Adults and Children," *Am J Clin Nutr* 50:301–6 (1989).

CHAPTER 9. MINERALS IN VEGETARIAN DIETS

1. C. M. McCay, *Notes on the History of Nutrition Research* (Bern: Huber) 138–44, 156–71. E. V. McColum, *A History of Nutrition* (Boston: Houghton Mifflin, 1957), 334–58.

2. E. M. DeMaeyer and M. Adiels-Tegman, "The Prevalence of Anemia in the World," *World Health Stat Q* 38:302–16 (1985).

3. T. H. Bothwell et al., *Iron Metabolism in Man* (Oxford: Blackwell, 1979).

4. J. D. Cook, "Adaptation in Iron Metabolism," *Am J Clin Nutr* 51:301–8 (1990).

5. W. R. Bezwoda et al., "The Relative Dietary Importance of Haem and Non-Haem Iron," *S Afr Med J* 64:552–56 (1983).

6. E. R. Monsen and J. L. Balintfy, "Calculating Dietary Iron Bioavailability: Refinement and Computerization," *J Am Diet Assoc* 80:307–11 (1982).

7. L. Rossander, L. Hallberg, and E. Bjorn-Rasmussen, "Absorption of Iron from Breakfast Meals," *Am J Clin Nutr* 32:2484–89 (1979); P. B. Disler et al., "The Effect of Tea on Iron Absorption," *Gut* 16:193–200 (1975); L. Hallberg and L. Rossander, "Effects of Different Drinks on the Absorption of Non-heme Iron from Composite Meals," *Human Nutr Appl Nutr* 36A:116–23 (1982).

8. T. A. Morck, S. R. Lynch, and J. D. Cook, "Inhibition of Food Iron Absorption by Coffee," *Am J Clin Nutr* 37:416–20 (1983).

9. R. B. S. Narasinga and T. Prabhavathi, "Tannin Content of Foods Commonly Consumed in India and Its Influence on Ionizable Iron," *J Sci Food Agr* 33:89–96 (1982).

10. J. G. Reinhold, F. Ismail-Beigi, and B. Faradji, "Fiber vs Phytate as a Determinant of the Availability of Calcium, Zinc, and Iron of Breadstuffs," *Nutr Rept Int* 12:75–85 (1975); J. D. Cook et al., "Effect of Fiber on Non-heme Iron Absorption," *Gastroenterology* 85:1354–58 (1983).

11. M. Brune, L. Rossander, and L. Hallberg, "Iron Absorption: No Intestinal Adaptation to a High-Phytate-Diet," *Am J Clin Nutr* 49:542–45 (1989).

12. W. van Dokkum, A. Wesstra, and F. A. Schippers, "Physiological Effects of Fibre-Rich Types of Bread," *Br J Nutr* 47:451–60 (1982).

13. D. Soegemberg et al., "Ascorbic Acid Prevents the Dose-Dependent Inhibitory Effects of Polyphenols and Phytates on Nonheme-Iron Absorption," *Am J Clin Nutr* 53:537–41 (1991); L. Hallberg, M. Brune, and L. Rossander, "Iron Absorption in Man: Ascorbic Acid and Dose-Dependent Inhibition by Phytate," *Am J Clin Nutr* 49:140–44 (1989); L. Hallberg and L. Rossander, "Absorption of Iron from Western-Type Lunch and Dinner Meals," *Am J Clin Nutr* 35:502–9 (1982); M. Gillbooly et al., "The Effects of Organic Acids, Phytates, and Polyphenols on the absorption of Iron from Vegetables," *Br J Nutr* 49:311–42 (1983); R. D. Baynes and T. H. Bothwell, "Iron Deficiency," *Annu Rev Nutr* 10:133–48 (1990); D. Ballot et al., "The Effects of Fruit Juices and Fruits on the Absorption of Iron from a Rice Meal," *Br J Nutr* 57:331–43 (1987).

14. FAO, *Requirements of Vitamin A, Iron, Folate, and Vitamin B₁₂: Report of a Joint FAO/WHO Expert Consultation*, FAO Food and Nutrition Series, no. 23 (Rome: Food and Agriculture Organization, 1988).

15. Panel on Dietary Reference Values of the Committee on Medical Aspects of Food Policy, Department of Health, *Dietary Reference Values for Food, Energy and Nutrients for the United Kingdom* (London: Her Majesty's Stationary Office, 1990); I. E. Dreosti, "Recommended Dietary Intakes of Iron, Zinc, and Other Inorganic Nutrients and Their Chemical Form and Bioavailability," *Nutr* 9:542–45 (1993); W. van Dokkum, "Significance of Iron Bioavailability for Iron Recommendations," *Biological Trace Element Res* 35:1–11 (1992); S. V. Apte and P. S. Venkatachalam, "Iron Absorption in Human Volunteers Using High Phytate Cereal Diet," *Ind J Med Res* 50:516–20 (1962).

16. T. A. B. Sanders and R. Purves, "An Anthropometric and Dietary Assessment of the Nutritional Status of Vegan Preschool Children," *J Human Nutr* 35:349–57 (1981).

17. Brune, Rossander, and Hallberg, "Iron Absorption"; L. S. McEndree, C. V. Kies, and H. M. Fox, "Iron Intake and Iron Nutritional Status of Lacto-Ovo-Vegetarian and Omnivore Students Eating in a Lacto-Ovo-Vegetarian Food Service," *Nutr Rep Int* 27:199–206 (1983); B. S. Worthington-Roberts, M. W. Breskin, and E. R. Monsen, "Iron Status of Premenopausal Women in a University Community and Its Relationship to Habitual Dietary Sources of Protein Intake," *Am J Clin Nutr* 47:275–79 (1988); T. A. B. Sanders and T. J. A. Key, "Blood Pressure, Plasma Renin Activity and Aldosterone Concentrations in Vegans and Omnivore Controls," *Human Nutr: Appl Nutr* 41A:204–11 (1987); S. Reddy and T. A. B. Sanders, "Haematological Studies on Premenopausal Indian and Caucasian Vegetarians Compared with Caucasian Omnivores," *Br J Nutr* 64:331–38 (1990); R. Tungtronochitr et al., "Vitamin B₁₂, Folic Acid and Haematological Status of 132 Thai Vegetarians," *Internat J Vit Nutr Res* 63:201–7 (1992); B. M. Anderson, R. S. Gibson, and J. H. Sabry, "The Iron and Zinc Status of Long-Term Vegetarian Women," *Am J Clin Nutr* 34:1042–48 (1981); B. A. Armstrong et al., "Hematological, Vitamin B₁₂, and Folate Studies on Seventh-Day Adventist Vegetarians," *Am J Clin Nutr* 27:712–18 (1974); P. C. Dagnelie et al., "Increased Risk of Vitamin B-12 and Iron Deficiency in Infants on Macrobiotic Diets," *Am J Clin Nutr* 50:818–24 (1989).

18. Brune, Rossander, and Hallberg, "Iron Absorption";

Worthington-Roberts, Breskin, and Monsen, "Iron Status"; A. D. Helman and I. Darnton-Hill, "Vitamin and Iron Status in *New* Vegetarians," *Am J Clin Nutr* 45:785–89 (1987); H. A. M. Brants et al., "Adequacy of a Vegetarian Diet at Old Age (Dutch Nutrition Surveillance System)," *J Am Coll Nutr* 9:292–302 (1990); D. Alexander, M. J. Ball, and J. Mann, "Nutrient Intake and Haematological Status of Vegetarians and Age-sex Matched Omnivores," *Eur J Clin Nutr* 48:538–46 (1994); N-S. Shaw, C-J. Chin, and W-H. Pan, "A Vegetarian Diet Rich in Soybean Products Compromises Iron Status in Young Students," *J Nutr* 125:212–19 (1995).

19. P. Knekt et al., "Body Iron Stores and Risk of Cancer," *Int J Cancer* 56:379–82 (1994); E. Graf and J. W. Eaton, "Suppression of Colonic Cancer by Dietary Phytic Acid," *Nutr Cancer* 19:11–19 (1993); J. T. Salonen et al., "High Stored Iron Levels Are Associated with Excess Risk of Myocardial Infarction in Eastern Finnish Men," *Circulation* 86:803–11 (1992); R. B. Lauffer, "Iron Stores and the International Variation in Mortality from Coronary Artery Disease," *Medical Hypothesis* 35:96–102 (1990).

20. A. Ascherio et al., "Dietary Iron Intake and Risk of Coronary Disease Among Men," *Circulation* 89:969–74 (1994).

21. V. Herbert, "Everyone Should be Tested for Iron Disorders," *J Am Diet Assoc* 92:1502–9 (1992).

22. A. S. Prasad et al., "Zinc Metabolism in Patients with Syndrome of Iron Deficiency Anemia, Hepatospleno-megaly, Dwarfism, and Hypogonadism," *J Lab Clin Med* 61:537–49 (1961).

23. A. Arcasoy, A. O. Cavdar, and E. Babacan, "Decreased Iron and Zinc Absorption in Turkish Children with Iron Deficiency and Geophagia," *Acta Hematol* 60:76–84 (1978).

24. C. Xue-Cun et al., "Low Levels of Zinc in Hair and Blood, Pica, Anorexia and Poor Growth in Chinese Preschool Children," *Am J Clin Nutr* 42:694–700 (1985).

25. K. M. Hambridge et al., "Low Levels of Zinc in Hair, Anorexia, Poor Growth, and Hypogensia in Children," *Pediatr Res* 6:868–74 (1972); P. A. Walravens, N. F. Krebs, and K. M. Hambridge, "Linear Growth of Low Income Preschool Children Receiving a Zinc Supplement," *Am J Clin Nutr* 38:195–201 (1983); R. S. Gibson et al., "A Growth-Limiting Mild Zinc Deficiency Syndrome in Some Southern Ontario Boys with Low Height Percentiles," *Am J Clin Nutr* 45:1266–77 (1989); P. D. S. Vanderkooy and R. S. Gibson, "Food Consumption Patterns of Canadian Preschool Children in Relation to Zinc and Growth Status," *Am J Clin Nutr* 45:609–16 (1987).

26. K. M. Hambridge et al., "Zinc Nutrition of Preschool Children in the Denver Head Start Program," *Am J Clin Nutr* 29:734–38 (1976); N. O. Price, G. E. Bunce, and R. W. Engle, "Copper, Manganese and Zinc Balance in Preadolescent Girls," *Am J Clin Nutr* 23:258–60 (1970).

27. H. H. Sandstead, "Zinc Nutrition in the United States," *Am J Clin Nutr* 26:1251–60 (1973); H. H. Sandstead, "Zinc Interference with Copper Metabolism," JAMA 240. 2188–89 (1978).

28. M. T. Baer and J. C. King, "Tissue Zinc Levels and Zinc Excretion during Experimental Zinc Depletion in Young Men," *Am J Clin Nutr* 39:556–70 (1984); P. E. Johnson et al., "Homeostatic Control of Zinc Metabolism in Men: Zinc Excretion in Men Fed Diets Low in Zinc," *Am J Clin Nutr* 57:557–65 (1993).

29. A. Pecoud, P. Donzel, and J. L. Schelling, "Effect of Foodstuffs on the Absorption of Zinc Sulfate," *Clin Pharmacol Ther* 17:469–73 (1975); J. G. Reinhold et al., "Effects of Purified Phytate and Phytate-Rich Bread Upon Metabolism of Zinc, Calcium, Phosphorus, and Nitrogen in Man," *Lancet* (Feb. 10, 1973), 283–88.

30. B. Navert, B. Sandstrom, and A. Cederblad, "Reduc-tion of the Phytate Content of Bran by Leavening in Bread and Its Effect on Zinc Absorption in Man," *Br J Nutr* 53:47–53 (1985).

31. E. Wisker et al., "Calcium, Magnesium, Zinc, and Iron Balances in Young Women: Effects of Low-Phytate Barley-Fiber Concentrate," *Am J Clin Nutr* 54:553–59 (1991).

32. B. Sandstrom et al., "Zinc Absorption from Composite Meals. I. The Significance of Wheat Extraction Rate, Zinc, Calcium, and Protein Content in Meals Based on Bread," *Am J Clin Nutr* 33:739–45 (1980).

33. Van Dokkum, Westra, and Schippers, "Physiological Effects."

34. E. R. Morris and R. Ellis, "Bioavailability of Dietary Calcium: Effect of Phytate on Adult Men Consuming Non-vegetarian Diets," in *Nutritional Bioavailability of Calcium*, no. 275 (Washington, D.C.: Am. Chem. Soc., 1985), 63–72.

35. H. H. Sandstead, "Availability of Zinc and Its Requirement in Human Subjects," in *Clinical, Biochemical, and Nutritional Aspects of Trace Elements*, ed. A. S. Prasad (New York: Liss, 1982), 83.

36. Alexander, Ball, and Mann, "Nutrient Intake"; K. C. Janelle and S. I. Barr, "Nutrient Intakes and Eating Behavior Scores of Vegetarian and Nonvegetarian Women," *JADA* 95:180–89 (1995); G. J. Davies, M. Crowder, and J. W. T. Dickerson, "Dietary Fibre Intakes of Individuals with Different Eating Patterns," *Human Nutr: Appl Nutr* 39A:139–48 (1985); T. Lloyd et al., "Urinary Hormonal Concentrations and Spinal Bone Densities of Premenopausal Vegetarian and Nonvegetarian Women," *Am J Clin Nutr* 54:1005–10 (1991); J. H. Freeland-Graves, P. W. Bodzy, and M. A. Eppright, "Zinc Status of Vegetarians," *J Am Diet Assoc* 77:655–61 (1980); R. Tesar et al., "Axial and Peripheral Bone Density and Nutrient Intakes of Postmenopausal Vegetarian and Omnivorous Women," *Am J Clin Nutr* 56:699–704 (1992); I-F. Hunt et al., "Bone Mineral Content in Postmenopausal Women: Comparison of Omnivores and Vegetarians," *Am J Clin Nutr* 50:517–23 (1989).

37. Sanders and Purves, "Anthropometric."

38. A. Draper et al., "The Energy and Nutrient Intakes of Different Types of Vegetarian: A Case for Supplements," *Br J Nutr* 69:3–19 (1993); M. Faber et al., "Anthropometric Measurements, Dietary Intake and Biochemical Data of South African Lacto-Ovovegetarians," *S Afr Med J* 69:733–38 (1986); J. C. King, T. Stein, and M. Doyle, "Effect of Vegetarianism on the Zinc Status of Pregnant Women," *Am J Clin Nutr* 34:1049–55 (1981).

39. Anderson, Gibson, and Sabry, "Iron and Zinc"; B. F. Harland and M. Peterson, "Nutritional Status of Lacto-Ovo-Vegetarian Trappist Monks," *J Am Diet Assoc* 72:259-64 (1978); N. Levin, J. Rattan, and T. Gilat, "Mineral Intake and Blood Levels in Vegetarians," *Isr J Med* 22:105–8 (1986); T. S. Srikumar, P. A. Ockerman, and B. Akesson, "Trace Element Status in Vegetarians from Southern India," *Nutr Res* 12:187–98 (1992).

40. J. R. Hunt, L. A. Matthys, and G. I. Lykken, "Reduced Zinc Absorption from a Lacto-Ovo-Vegetarian Diet," abstract in *Am J Clin Nutr* 61:908 (1995); S. Lei et al., "Zinc (Zn) Homeostasis in Young Chinese Women with a Marginal Zn Intake," abstract in *Am J Clin Nutr* 61:908 (1995).

41. P. O. D. Pharoah et al., "Endemic Cretinism," in *Endemic Goiter and Endemic Cretinism*, ed. J. B. Stanbury and B. S. Hetzel (New York: Wiley, 1980), 395–421; T. Ma et al., "The Present Status of Endemic Goiter and Endemic Cretinism in China," *Food Nutr Bull* 4:13–19 (1982).

42. B. E. Brush and J. K. Altland, "Goiter Prevention with Iodized Salt: Results of a Thirty-Year Study," *J Clin Endocrinol Metabol* 12:1380–88 (1952).

43. J. T. Dunn, "Iodized Oil in the Treatment and Prophylaxis of IDD," in *The Prevention and Control of Iodine Deficiency Disorders*, ed. B. S. Hetzel, J. T. Dunn, J. B. Stanbury (Amsterdam: Elsevier, 1987), 127–34.

44. Draper et al., "Energy and Nutrient Intakes"; M. Abdulla et al., "Nutrient Intake and Health Status of Vegans: Chemical Analyses of Diets Using the Duplicate Portion Sampling Technique," *Am J Clin Nutr* 34:2464–77 (1981).

45. Abdulla et al., "Nutrient Intake."

46. M. J. Kuchan and J. A. Milner, "Influence of Intracellular Glutathione on Selenite-Mediated Growth Inhibition of Canine Mammary Tumor Cells," *Cancer Res* 52:1091–95 (1992).

47. J. T. Salonen et al., "Association between Cardiovascular Death and Myocardiology Infarction and Serum Selenium in a Matched-Pair Longitudinal Study," *Lancet* 2:175–79 (1982).

48. G. Gissel-Nielsen et al., "Selenium in Soils and Plants and Its Importance in Livestock and Human Nutrition," *Adv Agronomy* 37:397–464 (1984).

49. S. N. Ganapathy and R. Dhanda, "Selenium Content of Omnivorous and Vegetarian Diets," *Ind J Nutr Dietet* 17:53–59 (1980); R. S. Gibson, B. M. Anderson, and J. H. Sabry, "The Trace Metal Status of a Group of Post-Menopausal Vegetarians," *J Am Diet Assoc* 82:246–50 (1983).

50. Ibid; B. Akesson and P. A. Ockerman, "Selenium Status in Vegans and Lactovegetarians," *Br J Nutr* 53:199–205 (1985); B. Debski et al., "Selenium Content and Glutathione Peroxidase Activity of Milk from Vegetarian and Nonvegetarian Women," *J Nutr* 119:215–20 (1989).

51. K. E. Mason, "A Conspectus of Research on Copper Metabolism and Requirements of Man," *J Nutr* 109:1979–2066 (1979).

52. Janelle and Barr, "Nutrient Intakes"; Draper et al.,

"Energy and Nutrient Intakes"; Gibson, Anderson, and Sabry, "Trace Metal Status."

53. L. M. Klevay et al., "Increased Cholesterol in Plasma in a Young Man during Experimental Copper Depletion," *Metabolism* 33:1112–18 (1984).

54. Abdulla et al., "Nutrient Intake" (1981), I. L. Rouse et al., "Vegetarian Diet, Blood Pressure and Cardiovascular Disease Risk," *Aust NZ J Med* 14:439–43 (1984); M. Abdulla et al., "Nutrient Intake and Health Status of Lactovegetarians: Chemical Analysis of Diets Using Duplicate Portion Sampling Technique," *Am J Clin Nutr* 40:325–38 (1984).

55. Janelle and Barr, "Nutrient Intakes"; L. B. Kramer et al., "Mineral and Trace Element Content of Vegetarian Diets," *J Am Coll Nutr* 3:3–11 (1984).

56. J. J. B. Anderson, "Nutritional Biochemistry of Calcium and Phosphorus," *J Nutr Biochem* 2:300–307 (1991).

57. J. M. Sullivan, R. L. Prewitt, and T. E. Ratts, "Sodium Sensitivity in Normotensive and Borderline Hypertensive Humans," *Am J Med Sci* 295:370–77 (1988).

58. J. A. T. Pennington, "Selected Minerals in Foods Surveys, 1974–1981/1982," *J Am Diet Assoc* 84:771–80 (1984).

59. C. P. Sanchez-Castillo et al., "An Assessment of the Sources of Dietary Salt in a British Population," *Clin Sci* 72:95–102 (1987); C. P. Sanchez-Castillo, W. J. Branch, and W. P. James, "A Test of the Validity of the Lithium-Marker Technique for Monitoring Dietary Sources for Salt in Men," *Clin Sci* 72:87–94 (1987).

60. Freeland-Graves, Bodzy, and Eppright, "Axial and Peripheral Bone Density"; Faber et al., "Anthropometric Measurements"; E. Carlson et al., "A Comparative Evaluation of Vegan, Vegetarian and Omnivore Diets," *J Plant Foods* 6:89–100 (1985).

61. NRC, *Diet and Health: Implications for Reducing Chronic Disease Risk. Report of the Committee on Diet and Health, Food and Nutrition Board* (Washington D.C.: National Academy Press, 1989).

62. B. Armstrong et al., "Urinary Sodium and Blood Pressure in Vegetarians," *Am J Clin Nutr* 32:2472–76 (1979); O. Ophir et al., "Low Blood Pressure in Vegetarians: The Possible Role of Potassium," *Am J Clin Nutr* 37:755–62 (1983).

63. D. S. Bernstein et al., "Prevalence of Osteoporosis in High- and Low-Flouride Areas in North Dakota," *J*

Am Med Assoc 198:499–504 (1966); B. L. Riggs et al., "Effect of the Fluoride/Calcium Regimen on Vertebral Fracture Occurence in Postmenopausal Osteoporosis," *N Engl J Med* 306:446–50 (1982).

64. K. A. V. R. Krishnamachari, "Flourine," in *Trace Elements in Human and Animal Nutrition*, ed. W. Mertz, vol 1 (San Diego, Calif.: Academic Press, 1987), 365–415.

65. J. R. Marier and D. Rose, "The Flouride Content of Some Food and Beverages—a Brief Survey Using a Modified Zr-SPADNS Method," *J Food Sci* 31:941–46 (1966).

66. C. A. Full and F. M. Parkins, "Effect of Cooking Vessel Composition on Flouride," *J Dent Res* 54:192 (1975).

67. R. W. Turnan, J. T. Bilbo, and R. J. Doisy, "Comparison and Effects of Natural and Synthetic Glucose Tolerance Factor in Normal and Genetically Diabetic Mice," *Diabetes* 27:49–56 (1978).

68. R. A. Anderson et al., "Chromium Supplementation of Human Subjects: Effects on Glucose, Insulin, and Lipid Variables," *Metabolism* 32:894–99 (1983).

69. E. G. Offenbacher and F. X. Pi-Sunyer, "Beneficial Effect of Chromium-Rich Yeast on Glucose Tolerance and Blood Lipids in Elderly Subjects," *Diabetes* 29:919–24 (1980).

70. F. H. Nielsen, "Chromium," in *Modern Nutrition in Health and Disease*, ed. Maurice E. Shils, James A. Olson, and Moshe Shike, 8th ed. (Philadelphia: Lea and Febiger, 1994); R. A. Anderson and A. S. Kozlovsky, "Chromium Intake, Absorption, and Excretion of Subjects Consuming Self-Selected Diets," *Am J Clin Nutr* 41:1177–83 (1985).

71. R. Anderson and N. A. Bryden, "Concentration, Insulin Potentiation, and Absorption of Chromium in Beer," *J Agric Food Chem* 31:308–11 (1983).

72. E. G. Offenbacher and F. X. Pi-Sunyer, "Temperature and pH Effects on the Release of Chromium from Stainless Steel into Water and Fruit Juices," *J Agric Food Chem* 31:89–92 (1983).

73. C. N. Rao and B. S. N. Rao, "Absorption and Retention of Magnesium and Some Trace Elements by Man from Typical Indian Diets," *Nutr Metab* 24:244–54 (1980).

74. J. L. Kelsay et al., "Impact of Variation in Carbohydrate Intake on Mineral Utilization by Vegetarians," *Am J Clin Nutr* 48:875–79 (1988).

CHAPTER 11. PREGNANCY AND BREAST-FEEDING

1. Institute of Medicine Subcommittee on Nutritional Status and Weight Gain During Pregnancy, *Nutrition during Pregnancy* (Washington, D.C.: National Academy Press, 1990).

2. J. E. Brown, "Weight Gain during Pregnancy: What Is 'Optimal?'" *Clin Nutr* 7:181 (1988).

3. Ibid.

4. Ibid.

5. J. T. Wyer et al., "Preschoolers on Alternate Life-Style Diets," *J Am Diet Assoc* 72:264–70 (1978); J. T. Dwyer et al., "Size, Obesity, and Leanness in Vegetarian Preschool Children," *J Am Diet Assoc* 77:434–39 (1977).

6. Food and Nutrition Board, National Research Council, *Recommended Dietary Allowances*, 10th ed. (Washington, D.C.: National Academy Press, 1989).

7. E. Carlson et al., "A Comparative Evaluation of Vegan, Vegetarian, and Omnivore Diets," *J Plant Foods* 6:89–100 (1985).

8. D. A. Finely, "Food Choices of Vegetarians and Nonvegetarians during Pregnancy and Lactation," *J Am Diet Assoc* 85, no. 6:678–85 (1985).

9. A. L. Lubby et al., "Observations on Transfer of Vitamin B12 from Mothers to Fetus and Newborn," *Am J Dis Child* 96:532–33 (1958).

10. B. L. Specker et al., "Vitamin B12: Low Milk Concentrations Are Related to Low Serum Concentrations in Vegetarian Women and to Methylmalonic Aciduria in Their Infants," *Am J Clin Nutr* 52:1073–76 (1990).

11. Food and Nutrition Board, NRC, *Recommended Dietary Allowances*.

12. F. R. Ellis, S. Holesh, and T. A. B. Sanders, "Osteoporosis in British Vegetarians and Omnivores," *Am J Clin Nutr* 27:769 (1974).

13. *Recommended Dietary Allowances for Japan* (Tokyo: Ministry of Health and Welfare, 1984).

14. Carlson et al., "Comparative Evaluation."

15. U.S. Preventive Services Task Force, "Routine Iron Supplementation During Pregnancy: Policy Statement," *JAMA* 270:2846 (1993).

16. Carlson et al., "Comparative Evaluation."

17. M. J. Abu-Assal and W. J. Craig, "The Zinc Status of Pregnant Vegetarian Women," *Nutr Rep Intl* 29, no. 2:485–94 (1984).

18. B. M. Anderson, R. S. Gibson, and J. H. Sabry, "The Iron and Zinc Status of Long-Term Vegetarian Women," *Am J Clin Nutr* 34:1042–48 (1981).

19. J. Thomas and F. R. Ellis, "The Health of Vegans during Pregnancy," *Nutr Soc Proc* 36 no. 1:464 (1977); J. P. Carter, T. Furman, and H. R. Hutcheson, "Preeclampsia and Reproductive Performance in a Community of Vegans," *Southern Med J* 80, no. 6:692–97 (1987).

20. Carter, Furman, and Hutcheson, "Preeclampsia."

21. Institute of Medicine Subcommittee on Nutritional Status and Weight Gain During Pregnancy, *Nutrition during Pregnancy*.

22. C. A. Hubel, "Lipid Peroxidation in Pregnancy: New Perspectives on Preeclampsia," *Am J Obstet Gynecol* 161:1025–34 (1989).

23. B. Lonnerdal, "Effects of Maternal Dietary Intake on Human Milk Composition," *J Nutr* 116:499 (1986).

24. "Position of the American Dietetic Association, Vegetarian Diets," *J Am Diet Assoc* 88:351–55 (1988); P. Johnston, "Counseling the Pregnant Vegetarian," *Am J Clin Nutr* 48:901–5 (1988).

25. B. L. Specker et al., "Increased Urinary Methylmalonic Acid Excretion in Breast-Fed Infants of Vegetarian Mothers and Identification of an Acceptable Dietary Source of Vitamin B12," *Am J Clin Nutr* 47:89–92 (1988).

26. B. Debski et al., "Selenium Content and Glutathionine Peroxidase Activity of Milk from Vegetarian and Nonvegetarian Women," *J Nutr* 119:215–20 (1989).

27. W. J. Rogan et al., "Should the Presence of Carcinogens in Breast Milk Discourage Breast Feeding?" *Regulatory Toxicol Pharmacol* 13:228–40 (1991).

28. Wisconsin Division of Health, "Breast Milk Contamination Advisory," press release (Madison: Wisconsin Division of Health, Nov. 28, 1979); D. Axelrod et al., *Report of the Ad Hoc Committee on the Health Implications of PCBs in Mothers' Milk* (Albany: New York State Health Planning Commission, Health Advisory Council, 1977); A. B. Morrison, *Polychlorinated Biphenyls—Committee Report* (Ottawa, Canada: Health and Welfare, 1978).

29. J. Hergenrather et al., "Pollutants in Breast Milk of Vegetarians," *N Engl J Med* 304:792 (1981).

30. P. C. Dagnelie et al., "Nutrients and Contaminants in Human Milk from Mothers on Macrobiotic and Omnivorous Diets," *Eur J Clin Nutr* 46:355–66 (1992).

31. M. Centinkay et al., "Untersuchung uber den Zusammenhang Zwischen Ernahrung und Lebensumstanden stillender Mutter und der Kontamination der Muttermilch mit schwerfluchtigen Organochlorverbindungen," *Akt Ernahr* 9:157–62 (1984).

CHAPTER 12. RIGHT FROM THE START: FEEDING VEGETARIAN INFANTS

1. T. A. B. Sanders and R. Purves, "An Anthropometric and Dietary Assessment of the Nutritional Status of Vegan Preschool Children," *J Hum Nutr* 35:349–57 (1981); J. T. Dwyer et al., "Growth in 'New' Vegetarian Preschool Children Using the Jenss-Bayley Curve Fitting Technique," *Am J Clin Nutr* 37:815–27 (1983); J. T. Dwyer et al., "Size, Obesity and Leanness in Vegetarian Preschool Children," *J Am Diet Assoc* 77:434–37 (1980); J. T. Dwyer, "Preschoolers on Alternate Life-Style Diets," *J Am Diet Assoc* 72:264–70 (1978); M. W. Shull et al., "Velocities of Growth in Vegetarian Preschool Children," *Pediatrics* 60:410–17 (1977).

2. Canadian Pediatric Society, Committee on Nutrition, "Breast Feeding," *Pediatrics* 62:591–601 (1978).

3. Committee on Nutrition, "Soy Protein Formulas: Recommendations for Use in Infant Feeding," *Pediatrics* 72:359 (1983).

4. K. G. Dewey et al., "Growth Patterns of Breastfed and Formula-Fed Infants from 0 to 18 Months: The DARLING Study," *Pediatrics* 89:1035–41 (1992).

5. I. F. Roberts et al., "Malnutrition in Infants Receiving Cult Diets: A Form of Child Abuse," *Br Med J* 1:296–98 (1979); J. R. K. Robson et al., "Zen Macrobiotic Dietary Problems in Infancy," *Pediatrics* 53:326–29 (1974).

6. P. C. Dagnelie and W. A. van Staveren, "Macrobiotic Nutrition and Child Health: Results of a Population-Based, Mixed-Longitudinal Cohort Study in The Netherlands," *Am J Clin Nutr* 59:1187S–96S (1994); P. C. Dagnelie et al., "High Prevalence of Rickets in Infants on Macrobiotic Diets," *Am J Clin Nutr* 51:202–8 (1990).

7. Dagnelie et al., "Rickets in Infants."

8. P. B. Acosta, "Availability of Essential Amino Acids and Nitrogen in Vegan Diets," *Am J Clin Nutr* 48:868–74 (1988).

9. S. L. Groh-Wargo and K. Antonelli, "Normal Nutrition during Infancy," in *Handbook of Pediatric Nutrition*, ed. P. M. Queen and C. E. Lang (Gaithersburg, Md.: Aspen Publishers, 1993), 107–44.

10. A. S. Cunningham, D. B. Jelliffe, and E. F. P. Jelliffe, "Breast-Feeding and Health in the 1980s: A Global Epidemiologic Review," *J Pediatr* 118:659 (1991).

11. Committee on Nutrition, American Academy of Pediatrics, "The Use of Whole Cow's Milk in Infancy," *Pediatrics* 72:253 (1983).

12. E. E. Ziegler et al., "Cow Milk Feeding in Infancy: Further Observations on Blood Loss from the Gastrointestinal Tract," *J Pediatr* 116:11 (1990).

13. Committee on Nutrition, "Whole Cow's Milk."

14. J. Coveney and I. Darnton-Hill, "Goat's Milk and Infant Feeding," *Med J Australia* 143:508–10 (1985).

15. Committee on Nutrition, American Academy of Pediatrics, "Vitamin and Mineral Supplement Needs in Normal Children in the United States," *Pediatrics* 66:1015 (1980); S. J. Fomon et al., "Recommendations for Feeding Normal Infants," *Pediatrics* 63:52 (1979).

16. J. Karjalainen et al., "A Bovine Albumin Peptide as a Possible Trigger of Insulin-Dependent Diabetes Mellitus," *N Engl J Med* 327:302–7 (1992); H. C. Gerstein "Cow's Milk Exposure and Type I Diabetes Mellitus: A Critical Overview of the Clinical Literature," *Diabetes Care* 17:13–19 (1994).

17. S. J. Fomon, "Reflections on Infant Feeding in the 1970's and 1980's," *Am J Clin Nutr* 46:171 (1987).

18. Canadian Pediatric Society, "Soy Protein Formulas"; A. Ashworth and R. G. Feachem, "Interventions for the Control of Diarrhoeal Disease among Young Children: Weaning and Education," *Bull WHO* 63:1115–27 (1985); R. G. Whitehead, "Nutritional Aspects of Human Lactation," *Lancet* 1:167–69 (1983).

19. D. A. Kautter et al., "Clostridium Botulinum Spores in Infant Foods: A Survey," *J Food Protection* 45:1028 (1982).

20. H. A. Sampson, "Food Hypersensitivity," in *Insights in Allergy*, ed. J. A. Grant (St. Louis, Mo.: CV Mosby, 1986).

21. V. L. Olejer, "Food Hypersensitivities," in *Handbook of Pediatric Nutrition*, ed. Queen and Lange, 206–31.

22. L. S. Taitz, "Soy Feeding in Infancy," *Arch Dis Child* 57:814–15 (1982); G. L. Gruskay, "Comparison of Breast, Cow and Soy Feedings in the Prevention of Onset of Allergic Disease," *Clinical Pediatrics*, 21 no. 8:486–91 (1982).

23. J. W. Gerrard et al., "Cow's Milk Allergy: Prevalence

and Manifestations in an Unselected Series of Newborns," *Acta Paediatr Scand* 234S:1 (1973); N-I. M. Kjellman and S. G. O. Johansson, "Soy versus Cow's Milk in Infants with a Biparental History of Atopic Disease: Development of Atopic Disease and Immunoglobulins from Birth to 4 Years of Age," *Clin Allergy* 9:347 (1979); M. S. Brady et al., "Specialized Formulas and Feedings for Infants with Malabsorption or Formula Intolerance," *J Am Diet Assoc* 86:191 (1986).

24. Groh-Wargo and Antonelli, "Normal Nutrition."

25. P. J. Kilshaw and A. J. Cant, "Passage of Maternal Dietary Proteins into Human Breast Milk," *Arch Allergy Appl Immunol* 75:8 (1984).

Chapter 13. Vegetarian Children

1. Centers for Disease Control, *Ten-State Nutrition Survey. 1968–70*, DHEW pub. no. (HSM) 72-8130-34 (Washington, D.C.: U.S. Department of Health, Education and Welfare, Health Services and Mental Health Administration, 1972); Science and Education Administration, *Nationwide Food Consumption Survey, 1977–1978, Preliminary Rep. No. 2, Food and nutrient intakes of individuals in 1 day in the US, Spring 1977* (Hyattsville, Md.: USDA, 1980).

2. J. T. Dwyer et al., "Preschoolers on Alternate Life-Style Diets," *J Am Diet Assoc* 72:264–70 (1978); J. T. Dwyer et al., "Growth in 'New' Vegetarian Preschool Children Using the Jenss-Bayley Curve Fitting Technique," *Am J Clin Nutr* 37:815–27 (1983); P. C. Dagnelie et al., "Nutritional Status of Infants Aged 4 to 18 Months on Macrobiotic Diets and Matched Omnivorous Control Infants: A Population-Based Mixed Longitudinal Study. II. Growth and Psycho-motor Development," *Eur J Clin Nutr* 43:325–38 (1989).

3. M. Kushi and A. Kushi, *Macrobiotic Child Care and Family Health* (Tokyo: Japan Publications, 1986).

4. J. Sabaté et al., "Anthropometric Parameters of Schoolchildren with Different Life-Styles," *Am J Dis Child* 144:1159–63 (1990); J. Sabaté et al., "Attained Height of Lacto-Ovo Vegetarian Children and Adolescents," *Eur J Clin Nutr* 45:51–58 (1991); J. Sabaté, C. Llorca, and A. Sanchez, "Lower Height of Lacto-Ovo Vegetarian Girls at Pre-adolescence: An Indicator of Physical Maturation Today?" *J Am Diet Assoc* 92:1263–64 (1992).

5. Sabaté et al., "Attained Height."

6. T. A. B. Sanders, "Growth and Development of British Vegan Children," *Am J Clin Nutr* 48:822–25 (1988).

7. J. M. O'Connell, M. J. Dibley, J. Siena, et al., "Growth of Vegetarian Children: The Farm Study," *Pediatrics* 84:475–81 (1989).

8. D. Albanes et al., "Adult Stature and Risk of Cancer," *Cancer Res* 48:1658–62 (1988); D. Albanes and P. R. Taylor, "International Differences in Body Height and Weight and Their Relationship to Cancer Incidence," *Nutr Cancer* 14:69–77 (1990).

9. J. T. Dwyer et al., "Nutritional Status of Vegetarian Children," *Am J Clin Nutr* 35:204–16 (1982); W. A. van Staveren et al., "Food Consumption and Height/Weight Status of Dutch Preschool Children on Alternative Diets," *J Am Diet Assoc* 85:1579–84 (1985); M. Tayter and K. L. Stanek, "Anthropometric and Dietary Assessment of Omnivore and Lacto-Ovo Vegetarian Children," *J Am Diet Assoc* 89:1661–63 (1989).

10. Sabaté et al., "Attained Height."

11. Sabaté et al., "Anthropometric Parameters"; Dwyer et al., "Size, Obesity, and Leanness"; Dwyer et al., "Nutritional Status"; Tayter and Stanek, "Anthropometric and Dietary Assessment"; J. Ruys and J. B. Hickie, "Serum Cholesterol and Triglyceride Levels in Australian Adolescent Vegetarians," *Br Med J.* 2:87 (1976).

12. S. Shea et al., "Is There a Relationship between Dietary Fat and Stature or Growth in Children Three to Five Years of Age," *Pediatrics* 92:579–86 (1993).

13. Committee on Nutrition, American Academy of Pediatrics, "Statement on Cholesterol," *Pediatrics* 90:469–73 (1992); National Cholesterol Education Program, "Report of the Expert Panel on Population Strategies for Blood Cholesterol Reduction: Executive Summary," *Arch Intern Med* 151:1071–84 (1991).

14. J. T. Dwyer et al., "Mental Age and I.Q. of Predominantly Vegetarian Children," *J Am Diet Assoc* 76:142–47 (1980).

15. Dwyer et al., "Nutritional Status"; Dwyer et al., "Mental Age and I.Q."

16. V. R. Young and P. L. Pellet, "Plant Proteins in Relation to Human Protein and Amino Acid Nutrition," *Am J Clin Nutr* 59:1203S–12S (1994).

17. Sanders, "Growth and Development"; Dwyer et al., "Nutritional Status"; J. R. Fulton, C. L. Hutton, and

K. R. Stitt, "Preschool Vegetarian Children," *J Am Diet Assoc* 76:360–65 (1980).

18. J. T. Dwyer et al., "Risk of Nutritional Rickets among Vegetarian Children," *Am J Dis Child* 133:134–40 (1979).

19. Food and Nutrition Board, *Recommended Dietary Allowances*, 20th ed. (Washington, D.C.: National Academy of Sciences, 1989); B. L. Specker et al., "Sunshine Exposure and Serum 25-Hydroxyvitamin D Concentrations in Exclusively Breast-Fed Infants," *J Pediatr* 107:372–76 (1985).

20. V. Herbert, "Staging Vitamin B₁₂ Status in Vegetarians," *Am J Clin Nutr* 59:1213S–22S (1994).

21. P. R. Dallman, "Iron," in *Present Knowledge in Nutrition*, ed. M. L. Brown, 6th ed. (Washington, D.C.: International Life Sciences Institute—Nutrition Foundation, 1990), 241–50.

22. T. A. B. Sanders and S. Reddy, "Vegetarian Diets and Children," *Am J Clin Nutr* 59:1176S–81S (1994).

23. H. R. L. Ashraf, C. Schoeppel, and J. A. Nelson, "Use of Tofu in Preschool Meals," *J Am Diet Assoc* 90:1114–16 (1990).

24. J. A. Burghardt, B. L. Devaney, and A. R. Gordon, "The School Nutrition Dietary Assessment Study: Summary and Discussion," *Am J Clin Nutr* 61:252S–57S (1995).

25. W. H. Dietz, "Obesity in Infants, Children and Adolescents in the United States. I. Identification, Natural History, and After Effects," *Nutr Res* 3:43–50 (1983).

26. Testimony of the American Heart Association Concerning National School Lunch Program and School Breakfast Program: Nutrition Objectives for School Meals, before the Food and Nutrition Service, USDA, Dec. 7, 1993.

27. "ADA Comments on Proposed Rule for Meat Alternates Used in Child Nutrition Programs," *J Am Diet Assoc* 86:530–31 (1986).

Chapter 14. Vegetarian Nutrition for Teenagers

1. B. R. Carruth, "Adolescence," in *Present Knowledge in Nutrition*, ed. M. L. Brown et al., 6th ed. (Washington, D.C.: International Life Sciences Institute, 1990).

2. W. H. Dietz, "Obesity in Infants, Children and Adolescents in the United States. I. Identification, Natural History, and After Effects," *Nutr Res* 3:43–50 (1983).

3. Human Nutrition Information Service, USDA, *Nutrient Intake: Individuals in 48 States, Year 1977–78 Nationwide Food Consumption Survey, 1977–1978*, HNIS report no. 1–2, (Washington, D.C.; U.S. Government Printing Office, 1985).

4. G. B. Forbes, "Nutritional Requirements in Adolescence," in *Textbook of Pediatric Nutrition*, ed. R. M. Suskind (New York: Raven Press, 1981).

5. K. L. Mahan and R. H. Rosebrough, "Nutritional Requirements and Nutritional Status Assessment in Adolescence," in *Nutrition in Adolescence*, eds. K. L. Mahan and J. M. Reese (St. Louis, Mo.: Times Mirror/Mosby, 1984).

6. J. Sabaté et al., "Attained Height of Lacto-Ovo Vegetarian Children and Adolescents," *Eur J Clin Nutr* 45:51–58 (1991).

7. D. G. Kissinger and A. Sanchez, "The Association of Dietary Factors with the Age of Menarche," *Nutr Res* 7:471–79 (1987); A. Sanchez, D. G Kissinger, and R. J. Phillips, "A Hypothesis on the Etiologic Role of Diet on Age of Menarche," *Med Hypothesis* 7:139–45 (1981).

8. F. De Waard and D. Tricholpoulous, "A Unifying Concept of the Aetiology of Breast Cancer," *Int J Cancer* 41:666–69 (1988).

9. R. Ross and J. A. Glomset, "The Pathogenesis of Atherosclerosis," *N Engl J Med* 295:369–77 (1976); 295:420–25 (1976).

10. Human Nutrition Information Service, *Nutrient Intake*.

11. B. A. Sloane, C. C. Gibbons, and M. Hegsted, "Evaluation of Zinc and Copper, Nutritional Status and Effects upon Growth of Southern Adolescent Females," *Am J Clin Nutr* 42:235–44 (1985).

12. M. Levine, *How Schools Can Combat Student Eating Disorders: Anorexia Nervosa and Bulimia* (Washington, D.C.: National Education Association, 1987); C. Johnson and M. Connors, *The Etiology and Treatment of Bulimia Nervosa* (New York: Basic Books, 1987).

13. D. M. Huse and A. R. Lucas, "Dietary Patterns in Anorexia Nervosa," *Am J Clin Nutr* 40:251–54 (1984).

14. C. L. Rock and J. Yager, "Nutrition and Eating Disorders: A Primer for Clinicians," *Int J Eating Dis* 6:267–80 (1987); W. D. De Wys, "Taste and Feeding Behavior in Patients with Cancer," in *Nutrition and Cancer*, ed. M. Winick (New York: John Wiley and Sons, 1977).

15. Rock and Yager, "Nutrition and Eating Disorders."

Chapter 15. The Older Vegetarian

1. *The American Vegetarian: Coming of Age in the 90's*. A Study of the Vegetarian Marketplace Conducted for *Vegetarian Times* by Yankelovich, Skelly, and White/Clancy (Shulman, Inc., 1992).

2. R. L. Kane and R. A. Kane, "Long-Term Care: Can Our Society Meet the Needs of the Elderly?" *Ann Rev Public Health* 1:227–53 (1980).

3. U.S. Bureau of the Census, *Current Projections of the Population of the United States by Age, Sex, and Race: 1983–2080* (Washington, D.C.: U.S. Government Printing Office, 1984).

4. *American Vegetarian*.

5. H. A. M. Brants et al., "Adequacy of a Vegetarian Diet at Old Age (Dutch Nutrition Surveillance System)," *J Am Coll Nutr* 9:292–302 (1990).

6. D. C. Nieman et al., "Dietary Status of Seventh-Day Adventist Vegetarian and Non-vegetarian Elderly Women," *J Am Diet Assoc* 89:1763–69 (1989).

7. I. F. Hunt, N. J. Murphy, and C. Henderson, "Food and Nutrient Intake of Seventh-Day Adventist Women," *Am J Clin Nutr* 48:850–51 (1988).

8. G. B. Forbes and J. C. Reind, "Adult Lean Body Mass Declines with Age: Some Longitudinal Observations," *Metabolism* 19 no. 9:653–63 (1970).

9. M. D. Carroll, S. Abraham, and C. M. Dresser, *Dietary Intake Source Data: United States, 1976–1980*, Vital and Health Statistics, Series 11, no. 231, DHHS pub. no. (PHS) 83-1681 (Hyattsville, Md.: National Center for Health Statistics, Public Health Service, U.S. Department of Health and Human Services, 1981).

10. M. B. Kohns, "A Rational Diet for the Elderly," *Am J Clin Nutr* 36:735–36 (1982); B. Shannon and H. Smicklas-Wright, "Nutrition Education in Relation to the Needs of the Elderly," *J Nutr Educ* 11:85–89 (1979).

11. W. W. Campbell et al., "Increased Protein Requirements in Elderly People: New Data a Retrospective Reassessment," *Am J Clin Nutr* 60:501–9 (1994).

12. S. C. Hartz, R. M. Russel, and I. H. Rosenberg, *Nutrition in the Elderly: The Boston Nutritional Status Survey* (London: Smith-Gordon and Company Limited, 1992).

13. E. M. Widdowson, "Physiological Processes of Aging: Are There Special Nutritional Requirements for Elderly People? Do McCay's Findings Apply to Humans?" *Am J Clin Nutr* 55:1246–49 (1992).

14. R. P. Heaney et al., "Calcium Nutrition and Bone Health in the Elderly," *Am J Clin Nutr* 36:986–1013 (1982); M. R. H. Lowik et al., "Marginal Nutritional Status among Institutionalized Elderly Women as Compared to Those Living More Independently (Dutch Nutrition Surveillance System)," *J Am Coll Nutr* 11:673–81 (1992).

15. I. Aksnes, O. Rodland, and D. Aarskog, "Serum Levels of Vitamin D_3 and 25-Hydroxyvitamin D_3 in Elderly and Young Adults," *Bone Miner* 3:351–57 (1988).

16. S. D. Krasinski et al., "Fundic Atrophic Gastritis in an Elderly Population: Effect on Hemoglobin and Several Serum Nutritional Indicators," *J Am Geriatr Soc* 34:800–806 (1986).

17. V. Herbert, "Vitamin B-12 and Elderly People," *Am J Clin Nutr* 59:1093–94 (1994).

18. R. M. Russel, "Vitamin B-12 and Elderly People: Reply to V Herbert," *Am J Clin Nutr* 59:1094–95 (1994).

19. J. Dommisse, "Subtle Vitamin-B_{12} Deficiency and Psychiatry: A Largely Unnoticed but Devastating Relationship?" *Med Hypotheses* 34:131–40 (1991); E. J. Fine and E. D. Soria, "Myths about Vitamin B_{12} Deficiency," *Southern Med J* 84:1475–81 (1991).

20. J. L. Greger, "Potential for Trace Mineral Deficiencies and Toxicities in the Elderly," in *Mineral Homeostasis in the Elderly*, ed. C. W. Bales, vol. 21, *Current Topics in Nutrition and Disease* (New York: Alan R. Liss, 1982).

21. H. A. M. Brants et al., "Adequacy of a Vegetarian Diet at Old Age (Dutch Nutrition Surveillance System)," *J Am Coll Nutr* 9:292–302 (1990); Nieman et al., "Dietary Status."

22. W. A. Boisvert and R. M. Russell, "Riboflavin Requirement of Healthy Elderly: Effect of Carbohydrate and Fat Composition of the Diet," *J Nutr* 123:915–25 (1993).

23. L. R. T. Winters et al., "Riboflavin Requirements and Exercise Adaptation in Older Women," *Am J Clin Nutr* 56:526–32 (1992).

24. Boisvert and Russell, "Riboflavin Requirement."

25. C. E. Ferroli and P. R. Trumbo, "Bioavailability of Vitamin B-6 in Young and Older Men," *Am J Clin Nutr* 60:68–71 (1994).

26. H. A. Schroeder, "Losses of Vitamins and Trace Minerals Resulting from Processing and Preservation of Foods," *Am J Clin Nutr* 24:562–75 (1971).

27. A. Draper et al., "The Energy and Nutrient Intakes of Different Types of Vegetarian: A Case for Supplements," *Br J Nutr* 69:3–19 (1993); T. D. Shultz and J. E. Leklem, "Vitamin B$_6$ Status and Bioavailability in Vegetarian Women," *Am J Clin Nutr* 46:647–51 (1987); M. R. H. Löwik et al., "Effect of Dietary Fiber on the Vitamin B$_6$ Status among Vegetarian and Nonvegetarian Elderly (Dutch Nutrition Surveillance System)," *J Am Coll Nutr* 9:241–49 (1990).

28. M. A. Fiatrarona et al., "High Intensity Strength Training in Nonagenarians: Effects on Skeletal Muscle," *J Am Med Assoc* 263:3029–34 (1990).

29. U.S. Department of Health and Human Services, Public Health Service, Centers for Disease Control, *Physical Functioning of the Aged United States. 1984,* DHHS pub. no. (PHS) 89-1595 (Hyattsville, Md.: DHHS, 1989).

30. W. S. Cain, "Flavoring Foods for a Grayer U.S.," *Food Engineering* 56:103 (1984).

31. S. S. Schiffman, J. Moss, and R. P. Erickson, "Thresholds of Food Odors in the Elderly," *Exp Aging Res* 2:389 (1976).

32. Nieman et al., "Dietary Status."

33. D. A. Snowdon and R. L. Phillips, "Does a Vegetarian Diet Reduce the Occurrence of Diabetes?" *Am J Publ Health* 75:507–12 (1985).

CHAPTER 16. THE VEGETARIAN DIABETIC

1. B. E. Hazlett, "Historical Perspective: The Discovery of Insulin," in *Clinical Diabetes Mellitus: A Problem Oriented Approach*, ed. John K. Davidson, 2nd ed. (New York: Thieme Medical Publishers, 1991; Stuttgart and New York: Georg Thieme Verlag, 1991).

2. K. M. West and J. M. Kalbfleisch, "Influence of Nutritional Factors on Prevalence of Diabetes," *Diabetes* 20:99–108 (1971); K. M. West and J. M. Kalbfleisch, "Glucose Tolerance, Nutrition, and Diabetes in Uruguay, Venezuela, Malaya, and East Pakistan," *Diabetes* 15:9–18 (1966).

3. J. K. Davidson and M. DiGirolamo, "Non-Insulin-Dependent Diabetes Mellitus," in *Clinical Diabetes Mellitus*, ed. Davidson.

4. K. N. West, *Epidemiology of Diabetes and Its Vascular Lesions* (New York: Elsevier/North-Holland, 1978).

5. J. W. Yoon and U. Ray, "Perspectives on the Role of Viruses in Insulin-Dependent Diabetes," *Diabetes Care* 8:39–44 (1985).

6. H. C. Gerstein, "Cow's Milk Exposure and Type I Diabetes Mellitus," *Diabetes Care* 17:13–19 (1993); K. Dahl-Jørgensen, G. Joner, and K. F. Hanssen, "Relationship between Cow's Milk Consumption and Incidence of IDDM in Childhood," *Diabetes Care* 14:1081–83 (1991).

7. I. Libman, T. Songer, and R. LaPorte, "How Many People in the U.S. Have IDDM?" *Diabetes Care* 16:841–42 (1993).

8. T. M. Dokheel, "An Epidemic of Childhood Diabetes in the United States: Evidence from Allegheny County, Pennsylvania," *Diabetes Care* 16:1606–11 (1993).

9. Hazlett, "Historical Perspective."

10. Ibid.

11. West, *Epidemiology.*

12. Ibid.

13. NIH, *Diet and Exercise in Noninsulin-Dependent Diabetes Mellitus*, National Institutes of Health Consensus Development Conference Statement, vol. 6 (Bethesda, Md.: National Institute of Arthritis, Diabetes and Digestive and Kidney Diseases, and the Office of Medical Applications of Research. U.S. Department of Health and Human Services, 1986).

14. J. Hagan and J. Wylie-Rosett, "Lipids: Impact on Dietary Prescription in Diabetes," *J Am Diet Assoc* 89:1104–8 (1989).

15. H. P. Himsworth, "Diet in the Etiology of Human Diabetes," *Proc Royal Soc Med* 42:323:9–12 (1949).

16. Hazlett, "Historical Perspective."

17. Ibid.

18. Ibid.

19. T. Teuscher et al., "Absence of Diabetes in a Rural West African Population with a High Carbohydrate/Cassava Diet," *Lancet* 1: 765–68 (Apr. 4, 1987).

20. H. P. Himsworth, "The Dietetic Factor Determining the Glucose Tolerance and Sensitivity to Insulin in Healthy Men," *Clin Sci* 2:67–94 (1935).

21. American Diabetes Association, "Principles of Nutrition and Dietary Recommendations for Individuals with Diabetes Mellitus: 1979," *Diabetes* 28:1027 (1979).

22. R. J. Barnard et al., "Longterm Use of High-Complex-Carbohydrate High-Fiber Diet and Exercise in the Treatment of NIDDM Patients," *Diabetes Care* 6:268–73 (1983); R. J. Barnard et al., "Response of Non-Insulin-Dependent Diabetic Patients to an Intensive Program of Diet and Exercise," *Diabetes Care* 5:370–74 (1982).

23. E. Hjollund et al., "Increased Insulin Binding to Adipocytes and Monocytes and Increased Insulin Sensitivity of Glucose Transport and Metabolism in Adipocytes from Non-insulin Dependent Diabetics after a Low Fat/High Starch/High-Fiber Diet," *Metabolism* 32:1067–75 (1983).

24. A. Garg et al., "Effects of Varying Carbohydrate Content of Diet in Patients with Non-insulin-dependent Diabetes Mellitus," *J Am Med Assoc* 271:1421–28 (1994).

25. Barnard et al., "Longterm Use"; Barnard et al., "Response."

26. A. Rivellese et al., "Effect of Dietary Fibre on Glucose Control and Serum Lipoproteins in Diabetic Patients," *Lancet* 2:447–50 (1980); G. Riccardi et al., "Separate Influence of Dietary Carbohydrate and Fiber on the Metabolic Control in Diabetes," *Diabetologia* 26:116–21 (1984).

27. G. Riccardi and A. A. Rivellese, "Effects of Dietary Fiber and Carbohydrate on Glucose and Lipoprotein Metabolism in Diabetic Patients," *Diabetes Care* 14:1115–25 (1991).

28. J. M. Munoz, "Fiber and Diabetes," *Diabetes Care* 7:297–300 (1984); O. Pedersen et al., "Insulin Receptor Binding to Monocytes from Insulin-Dependent Diabetic Patients after a Low Fat, High-Starch, High-Fiber Diet," *Diabetes Care* 5:284–91 (1982).

29. M. J. Franz, "Nutrition Principles for the Management of Diabetes Related Complications," *Diabetes Care* 17:490–518 (1994).

30. V. A. Koivisto et al., "Insulin Binding to Monocytes in Trained Athletes," *J Clin Invest* 64:1011–15 (1979); B. Saltin et al., "Physical Training and Glucose Tolerance in Middle-Aged Men with Chemical Diabetes," *Diabetes* 28:S30–32 (1979); P. Bjorntorp et al., "The Effect of Physical Training on Insulin Production in Obesity," *Metabolism* 19:631–38 (1970); J. Le Blanc et al., "Effects of Physical Training and Adiposity on Glucose Metabolism and 25I-Insulin Binding," *J Appl Physiol* 46:235–39 (1979).

Chapter 17. Weight Control Vegetarian-Style

1. Steiger, chairman, Federal Trade Commission, Testimony of Janet D. before the Subcommittee on Regulation, Business Opportunities and Energy of the House Committee on Small Business, Mar. 26, 1990.

2. R. Sichieri, J. E. Everhart, and V. S. Hubbard, "Relative Weight Classifications in the Assessment of Underweight and Overweight in the United States," *Int J Obes* 16:303–12 (1992); National Center for Health Statistics, M. F. Najjar and M. Rowland, "Anthropometric Reference Data and Prevalence of Overweight," *Vital Health Statistics* 11, no. 238 (1987).

3. A. S. Levy and A. W. Heaton, "Weight Control Practices of US Adults Trying to Lose Weight," *Ann Intern Med* (in press); M. Serdula, "Weight Control Practices of US Adolescents and Adults," *Ann Intern Med* (in press).

4. NIH Technology Assessment Conference Panel, "Methods for Voluntary Weight Loss and Control," *Ann Intern Med* 116:942–49 (1992).

5. R. E. Beauchene et al., "Nutrient Intake and Physical Measurements of Aging Vegetarian and Nonvegetarian Women," *J Am Coll Nutr* 1:131 (1982); I. L. Rouse, B. K. Armstrong, and L. J. Beilin, "The Relationship of Blood Pressure to Diet and Lifestyle in Two Religious Populations," *J Hypertension* 1:65–71 (1983); N. Levin, J. Ratton, and T. Gilat, "Energy Intake and Body Weight in Ovo-Lacto Vegetarians," *J Clin Gastroenterol* 8:451–53 (1986); P. Millet et al., "Nutrient Intake and Vitamin Status of Healthy French Vegetarians and Nonvegetarians," *Am J Clin Nutr* 50:718–27 (1989).

6. J. S. Garrow, *Energy Balance and Obesity in Man* (New York: Elsevier, 1974); L. S. Braitman, E. Adlin, and J. L. Stanton, "Obesity and Caloric Intake: The National Health and Nutrition Examination Survey of 1971–75 (HANES I)," *J Chronic Dis* 38:727–32 (1985).

7. L. Lissner et al., "Dietary Fat and the Regulation of Energy Intake in Human Subjects," *Am J Clin Nutr* 46:886–92 (1987); A. Tremblay et al., "Impact of Dietary Fat Content and Fat Oxidation on Energy Intake in Human Subjects," *Am J Clin Nutr* 49:799–805 (1989); A. Tremblay et al., "Nutritional Determinants of the Increase in Energy Intake Associated with a High-Fat Diet," *Am J Clin Nutr* 53:1134–37 (1991); A. Kendall et al., "Weight Loss on a Low-Fat Diet: Consequence of the Imprecision of the Control of Food Intake in Humans," *Am J Clin Nutr* 53:1123–29 (1991).

8. L. Lissner et al., "Dietary Fat and the Regulation of Energy Intake in Human Subjects," *Am J Clin Nutr* 46:866–92 (1987).

9. Poehlman et al., "Resting Metabolic Rate."
10. Kendall et al., "Weight Loss."
11. Y. Schutz, J. P. Flatt, and E. Jequier, "Failure of Dietary Fat Intake to Promote Fat Oxidation: A Factor Favoring the Development of Obesity," *Am J Clin Nutr* 52:246–53 (1989); J. P. Flatt, "Energetics of Intermediary Metabolism," in *Substrate and Energy Metabolism in Man*, ed. J. S. Garrow and D. Halliday (London: John Libbey, 1985).
12. M. K. Hellerstein et al., "Measurement of de Nova Hepatic Lipogenesis in Humans Using Stable Isotopes," *J Clin Invest* 87:1844–52 (1991).
13. R. A. Mathieson et al., "The Effect of Varying Carbohydrate Content of a Very Low Caloric Diet on Resting Metabolic Rate and Thyroid Hormones," *Metabolism* 35:394–98 (1986).
14. M. J. Toth and E. T. Poehlman, "Sympathetic Nervous System Activity and Resting Metabolic Rate in Vegetarians," *Metabolism* 43:621–25 (1994); E. T. Poehlman et al., "Resting Metabolic Rate and Postprandial Thermogenesis in Vegetarians and Nonvegetarians," *Am J Clin Nutr* 48:290–13 (1988).
15. D. M. Dreon et al., "Dietary Fat: Carbohydrate Ratio and Obesity in Middle-Aged Men," *Am J Clin Nutr* 47:995–1000 (1988).
16. A. Tremblay et al., "Diet Composition and Postexercise Energy Balance," *Am J Clin Nutr* 59:975–79 (1994).
17. D. Rigaud et al., "Overweight Treated with Energy Restriction and a Dietary Fibre Supplement: A 6-Month Randomized, Double-Blind, Placebo-Controlled Trial," *Int J Obesity* 14:763–69 (1990); A. Astrup, E. Vrist, and F. Quaade, "Dietary Fibre Added to Very Low Calorie Diet Reduces Hunger and Alleviates Constipation," *Int J Obesity* 14:105–12 (1990).
18. K. H. Duncan, J. A. Bacon, and R. L. Weinser, "The Effects of High and Low Energy Density Diets on Satiety, Energy Intake, and Eating Time of Obese and Nonobese Subjects," *Am J Clin Nutr* 37:763–67 (1983).
19. V. M. Sardesai and T. H. Waldshan, "Natural and Synthetic Intense Sweeteners," *J Nutr Biochem* 2:236–43 (1991).
20. P. M. Suter, Y. Schutz, and E. Jequier, "The Effect of Ethanol on Fat Storage in Healthy Subjects," *New Engl J Med* 326:983–87 (1992).
21. N. D. Barnard, L. W. Scherwitz, and D. Ornish, "Adherence and Acceptability of a Low-Fat, Vegetarian Diet among Patients with Cardiac Disease," *J Cardiopulmonary Rehabil* 12:423–31 (1992); W. Insull et al., "Results of a Randomized Feasibility Study of a Low-Fat Diet," *Arch Int Med* 150:421–27 (1990).
22. R. D. Mattes, "Fat Preference and Adherence to a Reduced-Fat Diet," *Am J Clin Nutr* 57:373–81 (1993).
23. J. J. Duncan, N. F. Gordon, and C. B. Scott, "Women Walking for Health and Fitness: How Much Is Enough?" *J Am Med Assoc* 266:3295–99 (1991).

CHAPTER 18. THE VEGETARIAN ATHLETE

1. I. Fisher, "The Influence of Flesh Eating on Endurance," *Yale Med J* 13:205–21 (1907).
2. E. Berry, "The Effects of High and Low Protein Diet on Physical Efficiency," *Am Phys Ed Rev* 14:288–97 (1909).
3. J. C. Whorton, *Crusaders for Fitness* (Princeton, N.J.: Princeton University Press, 1982).
4. Berry, "Effects of High and Low Protein."
5. N. Pritikin, "The Brave Soldiers in the Ironman Army Travel on Their Stomachs," *Runner's World* (Feb. 1984), 127; L. Fishman, "They're Glitz, Glam and Veg," *Veg Times*, (Feb. 1994), 60–63.
6. N. Hanne, R. Dlin, and A. Rostein, "Physical Fitness, Anthropometric and Metabolic Parameters in Vegetarian Athletes," *J Sports Med* 26:180–85 (1986).
7. J. E. Cotes et al., "Possible Effect of a Vegan Diet upon Lung Function and the Cardiorespiratory Response to Submaximal Exercise in Healthy Women," *J Physiol* 209:30P–32P (1970).
8. M. S. Plomden and D. Bernardot, "Position of the American Dietetic Association and the Canadian Dietetic Association for Physical Fitness and Athletic Performance," *J Am Diet Assoc* 93:691–96 (1993).
9. S. H. Short and W. R. Short, "Four Year Study of University Athletes' Dietary Intake," *J Am Diet Assoc* 82:632–45 (1983); L. M. Burke and R. S. D. Read, "Diet Patterns of Elite Australian Male Triathletes," *Physician Sportmed* 15:140 (1987).
10. J. R. Brotherhood, "Nutrition and Sports Performance," *Sports Med* 1:350–89 (1984).
11. National Research Council, *Recommended Dietary Allowances*, 10th ed. (Washington, D.C.: National Academy Press, 1989), chapter 6.
12. Plomden and Bernardot, "Position of the American Dietetic Association."
13. I. Gontzea, P. Sutzescu, and S. Dumitrache, "The Influence of Muscular Activity on the Nitrogen

Balance and on the Need of Man for Proteins," *Nutr Rep Int* 10:35–43 (1974).

14. I. Celejowa and M. Homa, "Food Intake, Nitrogen and Energy Balance in Polish Weight Lifters during a Training Camp," *Nutr Metabol* 12:259–74 (1970).

15. V. R. Young, "Protein and Amino Acid Metabolism in Relation to Physical Exercise," in *Nutrition and Exercise* (New York: Wiley, 1986), 9–32.

16. M. Colgan, *Optimum Sports Nutrition* (Ronkonkoma, N.Y.: Advanced Research Press, 1993).

17. N. A. Breslau et al., "Relationship of Animal Protein-Rich Diet to Kidney Stone Formation and Calcium Metabolism," *J Clin Endocrinol Metabol* 66:140–46 (1988).

18. B. M. Brenner, T. W. Meyer, and T. H. Hostetter, "Dietary Protein Intake and the Progressive Nature of Kidney Disease: The Role of Hemodynamically Medicated Glomerular Injury in the Pathogenesis of Progressive Glomerular Sclerosis in Aging Renal Ablation, and Intrinsic Renal Disease," *N Engl J Med* 307:652–59 (1982).

19. P. Kontessis et al., "Renal, Metabolic and Hormonal Responses to Ingestion of Animal and Vegetable Proteins," *Kid Int* 38:136–44 (1990).

20. A. R. Sherman and B. Krammer, "Iron, Nutrition, and Exercise," in *Nutrition in Exercise and Sport*, ed. I. Wolinsky and J. F. Hickson (Boca Raton, Fla.: CRC Press, 1989), 291–300.

21. Ibid.

22. O. D. Vellar, "Studies on Sweat Loss of Nutrients," *Scand J Clin Lab Invest* 21:157–67 (1968).

23. R. Pate, "Sports Anemia: A Review of the Current Research Literature," *Phys Sports Med* 11:115–26 (1983); Expert Scientific Working Group, "Summary of a Report on Assessment of the Iron Nutritional Status of the United States Population," *Am J Clin Nutr* 42:1318–30 (1985).

24. M. R. Williamson, "Anemia in Runners and Other Athletes," *Phys Sports Med* 9:73–78 (1981).

25. E. Eichner, "'Sports Anemia': Poor Terminology of a Real Phenomenon: Gatorade," *Sports Sci Exch* 1, no. 6 (1988); E. Eichner, "The Anemia of Athletes," *Phys Sports Med* 11:122–25 (1986).

26. M. Colgan, S. Fielder, and L. A. Colgan, "Micronutrient Status of Endurance Athletes Affects Hematology and Performance," *J Appl Nutr* 43:17–30 (1991); D. Clement and R. Asmundson, "Nutritional Intake and Hematological Parameters in Endurance Runners," *Phys Sports Med* 10:37–43 (1982).

27. R. B. Moore et al., "Maintenance of Iron Status in Healthy Men during an Extended Period of Stress and Physical Activity," *Am J Clin Nutr* 58:923–27 (1993); D. Roberts and D. J. Smith, "Training at Moderate Altitude: Iron Status of Elite Male Swimmers," *J Lab Clin Med* 120:387–91 (1992).

28. J. L. Beard, "Are We at Risk for Heart Disease Because of Normal Iron Status?" *Nutr Rev* 51:112–15 (1993); E. D. Weinberg, "Roles of Iron in Neoplasia," *Biol Trace Element Res* 34:123–140 (1992).

29. W. M. Sherman and D. R. Lamb, "Nutrition and Prolonged Exercise," in *Perspectives in Exercise Science and Sports Medicine Prolonged Exercise*, ed. D. R. Lamb and R. Murray (Indianapolis, Ind.: Benchmark Press, 1988), 213–80; J. Ivy, "Muscle Glycogen Synthesis after Exercise: Effect of Time of Carbohydrate Ingestion," *A Appl Physiol* 64:1480–85 (1988); J. Zachwieja, "Influence of Muscle Glycogen Depletion of the Rate of Resynthesis," *Med Sci Sports Exer* 23:44–48 (1991).

30. J. R. Brotherhood, "Nutrition and Sports Performance," *Sports Med* 1:350–89 (1984).

31. D. L. Costill, "Carbohydrate Nutrition before, during and after Exercise," *Fed Proc* 44:364–68 (1985).

32. E. Horton, "Metabolic Fuels, Utilization, and Exercise," *Am J Clin Nutr* 49:931–32 (1989); J. Durnin, "The Energy Cost of Exercise," *Proc Nutr Soc* 44:273 (1985).

33. A. Z. Belko et al., "Effects of Exercise on Riboflavin Requirements: Biological Validation in Weight Reducing Women," *Am J Clin Nutr* 41:270–77 (1985); A. Z. Belko et al., "Effects of Exercise on Riboflavin Requirements of Young Women," *Am J Clin Nutr* 37:509–17 (1993); A. Z. Belko et al., "Effects of Aerobic Exercise and Weight Loss on Riboflavin Requirements of Moderately Obese, Marginally Deficient Young Women," *Am J Clin Nutr* 40:553–61 (1984).

34. J. Bergstrom et al., "Effect of Nicotinic Acid on Physical Working Capacity and on Metabolism of Muscle Glycogen in Man," *J Appl Physiol* 26:170–76 (1969); D. Hilsendager and P. Karpovich, "Ergogenic Effect of Glycine and Niacin Separately and in Combination," *Res Q* 35:S389–92 (1964); L. Carlson, R. Havel, and L. Ekelund, "Effect of Nicotinic Acid on the Turnover Rate and Oxidation of the Free Fatty Acids of Plasma in Man during Exercise," *Metabolism* 12:837–45 (1963).

35. Tin-May-Than et al., "The Effect of Vitamin B_{12} on Physical Performance Capacity," *Br J Nutr* 40:264–73 (1978); H. J. Montoye et al., "Effects of Vitamin B_{12} Supplementation on Physical Fitness and Growth of Young Boys," *J Appl Physiol* 589–92 (1955); H. Montoye, "Vitamin B_{12}: A Review," *Res Q* 56:308–13 (1955).

36. M. E. Visagie, J. P. DuPlessies, and N. F. Laubscher, "Effects of Vitamin C Supplementation on Black Mineworkers," *S Afr Med J* 49:889–92 (1975).

37. G. Keren, "The Effect of High Dosage Vitamin C Intake on Aerobic and Anaerobic Capacity," *J Sports Med Phys Fitness* 20:145–48 (1980); H. Howard and B. Segesser, "Ascorbic Acid and Athletic Performance," *Ann NY Acad Sci* 258:458–64 (1975).

38. D. K. Bowles et al., "Effects of Acute Submaximal Exercise on Skeletal Muscle Vitamin E," *Free Rad Res Comm* 14:139–43 (1991); Y. Kobayashi, "Effect of Vitamin E on Aerobic Work Performance in Men during Acute Exposure to Hypoxic Hypoxia" (thesis, University of New Mexico, 1974).

39. F. Couzy, P. Lafargue, and C. Y. Guezennec, "Zinc Metabolism in the Athlete: Influence of Training, Nutrition, and Other Factors," *Int J Sports Med* 4:263–66 (1990); H. W. Lane, "Some Trace Elements Related to Physical Activity: Zinc, Copper, Selenium, Chromium, and Iodine," in *Nutrition in Exercise and Sport*, ed. I. Wolinsky and J. F. Hickson (Boca Raton, Fla.: CRC Press, 1989), 301–307.

40. R. A. Anderson and H. N. Guttman, "Trace Minerals and Exercise," in *Exercise, Nutrition and Energy Metabolism*, ed. E. S. Horton (New York: Macmillan, 1988), 180–95.

41. K. P. Jones et al., "Comparison of Bone Density in Amenorrheic Women due to Athletics, Weight Loss, and Premature Menopause," *Obstet Gynecol* 66:5–8 (1985).

42. C. Christiannsen et al., "Prevention of Early Postmenopausal Bone Loss: Controlled 2-Year Study in 315 Normal Females," *Eur J Clin Invest* 10:273–79 (1980).

43. J. M. Lutter, "Mixed Message about Osteoporosis in Female Athletes," *Physician Sportsmed* 11:154–65 (1983).

44. C. E. M. Cann et al., "Decreased Spinal Mineral Content in Amenorrheic Women," *J Am Med Assoc* 251:626–29 (1984); B. L. Drinkwater et al., "Bone Mineral Content of Amenorrheic and Eumenorrheic Athletes," *N Engl J Med* 311:277–81 (1984); J. Lindberg et al., "Exercise Induced Amenorrhea and Bone Density," *Ann Int Med* 101:647–48 (1984).

45. T. Lloyd et al., "Collegiate Women Athletes with Irregular Menses during Adolescence Have Decreased Bone Density," *Obstet Gynecol* 72:639–42 (1988).

46. B. R. Goldin et al., "Estrogen Excretion Patterns and Plasma Levels in Vegetarian and Omnivorous Women," *New Engl J Med* 307:1542–47 (1982); J. C. Barbosa et al., "The Relationship Among Adiposity, Diet, and Hormone Concentrations in Vegetarian and Nonvegetarian Postmenopausal Women," *Am J Clin Nutr* 51:798–803 (1990); P. I. Musey et al., "Effect of Diet on Oxidation of 17B-Estradiol in Vivo," *J Clin Endocrinol Metab* 65:792–95 (1987); K. M. Pirke et al., "Dieting Influences the Menstrual Cycle: Vegetarian versus Nonvegetarian Diet," *Fertility Sterility* 46:1083–88 (1986).

47. D. P. Rose et al., "Effect of a Low-Fat Diet on Hormone Levels in Women with Cystic Breast Disease. I. Serum Steroids and Gonadotrophins," *J Natl Cancer Inst* 78:623–26 (1987); R. L. Prentice et al., "Dietary Fat Reduction and Plasma Estradiol Concentration in Healthy Postmenopausal Women," *J Natl Cancer Inst* 82:129–34 (1990); D. P. Rose et al., "High-Fiber Diet Reduces Serum Estrogen Concentrations in Premenopausal Women," *Am J Clin Nutr* 54:520–25 (1991); K. M. Pirke et al., "Dieting Influences the Menstrual Cycle."

48. A. B. Pedersen et al., "Menstrual Differences due to Vegetarian and Nonvegetarian Diets," *Am J Clin Nutr* 53:879–85 (1991).

49. S. M. Brooks et al., "Diet in Athletic Amenorrhoeas," *Lancet* 1:559–60 (1984).

50. J. Slavin, J. Lutter, and S. Cushman, "Amenorrhoea in Vegetarian Athletes," *Lancet* 1:1974–75 (1984).

51. B. Magnesson, L. Hallberg, L. Rossander, et al., "Iron Metabolism and 'Sports Anemia'," *Acta Med Scand* 216:157–64 (1984).

52. K. R. Price and G. R. Fenwick, "Naturally Occuring Oestrogens in Foods—a Review," *Food Addit Contam* 2:73–106 (1985); Y. Folman and G. S. Pope, "Effect of Norethisterone Acetate, Dimethylstilbesterol, Genistein and Coumestrol on Uptake of [^{3}H]oestradiol by Uterus, Vagina, and Skeletal Muscle of Immature Mice," *J Endocrinol* 44:213–18 (1969).

53. K. H. Myburgh, "Low Bone Density Is an Etiologic Factor for Stress Fracture in Athletes," *Ann Intern Med* 113:754–59 (1990).

54. Drinkwater et al., "Bone Mineral Content"; Lindberg et al., "Exercise Induced Amenorrhea."